Lecture Notes in Computer Science 4987

Commenced Publication in 1973
Founding and Former Series Editors:
Gerhard Goos, Juris Hartmanis, and Jan van Leeuwen

Lecture Notes in Computer Science 4987

Commenced Publication in 1973
Founding and Former Series Editors:
Gerhard Goos, Juris Hartmanis, and Jan van Leeuwen

Editorial Board

David Hutchison
Lancaster University, UK
Takeo Kanade
Carnegie Mellon University, Pittsburgh, PA, USA
Josef Kittler
University of Surrey, Guildford, UK
Jon M. Kleinberg
Cornell University, Ithaca, NY, USA
Alfred Kobsa
University of California, Irvine, CA, USA
Friedemann Mattern
ETH Zurich, Switzerland
John C. Mitchell
Stanford University, CA, USA
Moni Naor
Weizmann Institute of Science, Rehovot, Israel
Oscar Nierstrasz
University of Bern, Switzerland
C. Pandu Rangan
Indian Institute of Technology, Madras, India
Bernhard Steffen
University of Dortmund, Germany
Madhu Sudan
Massachusetts Institute of Technology, MA, USA
Demetri Terzopoulos
University of California, Los Angeles, CA, USA
Doug Tygar
University of California, Berkeley, CA, USA
Moshe Y. Vardi
Rice University, Houston, TX, USA
Gerhard Weikum
Max-Planck Institute of Computer Science, Saarbruecken, Germany

Xiaohong Gao   Henning Müller
Martin J. Loomes   Richard Comley
Shuqian Luo (Eds.)

Medical Imaging
and Informatics

2nd International Conference, MIMI 2007
Beijing, China, August 14-16, 2007
Revised Selected Papers

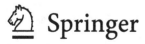 Springer

Volume Editors

Xiaohong Gao
Martin J. Loomes
Richard Comley
Middlesex University
School of Computing Science The Burroughs
NW4 4BT London, United Kingdom
E-mail: {x.gao; m.loomes; r.comley}@mdx.ac.uk

Henning Müller
University of Applies Sciences Sierre
TecnoArk 3
3960 Sierre, Switzerland
E-mail: henning.mueller@sim.hcuge.ch

Shuqian Luo
Capital Medical University
No. 10 Xitoutiao You An Men
100069 Beijing, China
E-mail: shuqian_liu@yahoo.com.cn

Library of Congress Control Number: 2008930311

CR Subject Classification (1998): I.4, I.5, I.2.10, J.3, I.3

LNCS Sublibrary: SL 6 – Image Processing, Computer Vision,
Pattern Recognition, and Graphics

ISSN   0302-9743
ISBN-10   3-540-79489-1 Springer Berlin Heidelberg New York
ISBN-13   978-3-540-79489-9 Springer Berlin Heidelberg New York

Springer is a part of Springer Science+Business Media

springer.com

© Springer-Verlag Berlin Heidelberg 2008
Printed in Germany

Typesetting: Camera-ready by author, data conversion by Scientific Publishing Services, Chennai, India
Printed on acid-free paper   SPIN: 12263424   06/3180   5 4 3 2 1 0

Preface

This series constitutes a collection of selected papers presented at the International Conference on Medical Imaging and Informatics (MIMI2007), held during August 14–16, in Beijing, China. The conference, the second of its kind, was funded by the European Commission (EC) under the Asia IT&C programme and was co-organized by Middlesex University, UK and Capital University of Medical Sciences, China.

The aim of the conference was to initiate links between Asia and Europe and to exchange research results and ideas in the field of medical imaging. A wide range of topics were covered during the conference that attracted an audience from 18 countries/regions (Canada, China, Finland, Greece, Hong Kong, Italy, Japan, Korea, Libya, Macao, Malaysia, Norway, Pakistan, Singapore, Switzerland, Taiwan, the United Kingdom, and the USA). From about 110 submitted papers, 50 papers were selected for oral presentations, and 20 for posters. Six key-note speeches were delivered during the conference presenting the state of the art of medical informatics. Two workshops were also organized covering the topics of "Legal, Ethical and Social Issues in Medical Imaging" and "Informatics" and "Computer-Aided Diagnosis (CAD)," respectively. This series presents the cutting-edge technology applied in the medical field, which can be epitomized by the second and sixth papers in the session of "Medical Image Segmentation and Registration," on the application of bio-mimicking techniques for the segmentation of MR brain images. Paper 4 in the session of "Key-Note Speeches" describes the pioneering work on frameless stereotactic operations for the removal of brain tumors, whereas the paper entitled "CAD on Brain, Fundus, and Breast" was presented in the session of "Computer-Aided Detection (CAD)."

A special tribute is paid to Paolo Inchingolo from the University of Trieste, Italy, one of the key-note speakers, who sadly passed away due to sudden illness. Professor Inchingolo specialized in health-care systems and tele-imaging. His paper appears as the second in the session of "Key-Note Speeches."

The editors would like to thank the EC for their financial support and also the China Medical Informatics Association (CMIA) for their support. Special thanks go to the reviewers who proof-read the final manuscripts of the papers collected in this book, in particular, Tony White, Ray Adams, Stephen Batty, Christian Huyck, and Peter Passmore.

January 2008

Xiaohong Gao
Henning Müller
Martin Loomes
Richard Comley
Shuqian Luo

Organization Committee

General Co-chairs	Debing Wang, China
	Martine Looms, UK
	Davide Caramella, Italy
Executive Chair	Yongqin Huang, China
Program Co-chairs	Shuqian Luo, China
	Edward M. Smith, USA
Publication Chair	Henning Müller, Switzerland
Organizing Committee Chair	Ying Liang, China
Organization Chair	Xiaohong Gao, UK

International Programme Committee

David Al-Dabass, Norttingham Trent University, UK
Yutaka Ando, National Institute of Radiological Sciences, Japan
Franclin Aigbithio, Wolfson Brain Imaging Centre, Cambridge, UK
Richard Bayford, Middlesex University, UK
Stephen Batty, Institute of Cognitive Neuroscience, UCL, UK
Roald Bergstrøm, President of the 24th EuroPACS Conference, Norway
Hans Blickman, Dept. of Radiology UMC, Netherlands
Jyh-Cheng Chen, National Yang-Ming University, Taiwan, China
Hune Cho, Kyungpook National University, Korea
John Clark, University of Cambridge, UK
Richard Comley, Middlesex University, UK
Andrzej Czyzewski, Gdansk University of Technology, Poland
Robert Ettinger, Middlesex University, UK
Mansoor Fatehi, Iranian Society of Radiology, Iran
Huanqing Feng, University of Science and Technology of China
Haihong Fu, Beijing Union Hospital, China
Hiroshi Fujita, Gifu University, Japan
W. Glinkowski, Medical University of Warsaw, Poland
Sean He, University of Technology, Sydney, Australia
H.K. Huang, University of California San Francisco, USA
Jacob Hygen, KITH, Norway
Paolo Inchingolo, Universita' di Trieste, Italy
Theodore Kalamboukis, Athens University of Economics and Business, Greece
Myeng-ki Kim, Seoul National University, Korea

Michio Kimura, Hamamatsu University, Japan
Inger Elisabeth Kvaase, Directorate for Health and Social Affairs, Norway
Thomas Lehmann, Aachen University, Germany
Hua Li, Institute of Computing Technology, China
Qiang Lin, Fuzhou University, China
Subin Liu, Peking University, China
Tianzi Jiang, National Laboratory of Pattern Recognition, China
Peter Passmore, Middlesex University, UK
Lubov Podladchikova, Rostov State University, Russia
Hanna Pohjonen, Consultancy of Healthcare Information Systems, Finland
Jan Størmer, UNN, Tromso, Norway
Egils Stumbris, Riga Municipal Telemedicine Centre, Latvia
Yankui Sun, Tsinghua University, China
Yin Leng Theng, Nanyang Technological University, Singapore
Simon Thom, St Mary's Hospital, UK
Zengmin Tian, Navy General Hospital, China
Federico Turkheimer, Hammersmith Hospital, UK
Baikun Wan, Tianjin University, China
Boliang Wang, Xiamen University, China
Jim Yang, KITH, Norway
Jiwu Zhang, Eastman Kodak Company, China
Guohong Zhou, Capital University of Medical Sciences, China

Sponsors

European Commission IT&C Programmes
China Medical Informatics Association, China
Middlesex University, UK
Capital University of Medical Sciences, China

Table of Contents

Medical Informatics

PET, fMRI, Ultrasound and Thermal Imaging

3D Reconstruction and Visualization

Workshops

Legal, Ethical and Social Issues in Medical Imaging and Informatics

Computer-Aided Diagnosis (CAD)

Complexity Aspects of Image Classification

Andreas A. Albrecht

University of Hertfordshire
Science and Technology Research Institute
Hatfield, Herts AL10 9AB, UK

Abstract. Feature selection and parameter settings for classifiers are both important issues in computer-assisted medical diagnosis. In the present paper, we highlight some of the complexity problems posed by both tasks. For the feature selection problem we propose a search-based procedure with a proven time bound for the convergence to optimum solutions. Interestingly, the time bound differs from fixed-parameter tractable algorithms by an instance-specific factor only. The stochastic search method has been utilized in the context of micro array data classification. For the classification of medical images we propose a generic upper bound for the size of classifiers that basically depends on the number of training samples only. The evaluation on a number of benchmark problems produced a close correspondence to the size of classifiers with best generalization results reported in the literature.

1 Introduction

The most common method in automated computerised image classification is feature selection and evaluation, accompanied by various methods - predominantly machine learning-based - of processing labels attached to features that are expressed as numerical values or textual information (for a comprehensive overview in the context of medical image analysis we refer the reader to the review article [5] by K. Doi). The number of features extracted from ROIs in medical images varies depending upon the classification task. Usually, the 10 Haralick feature values are calculated [11], but in some cases up to 49 features are taken into account [7]. Apart from this approach, there are attempts to represent sample data by classification circuits without prior feature analysis, see [2,8]. From a complexity point of view, the calculation of a feature value can be carried out in polynomial time $n^{O(1)}$ in terms of the image size n. Therefore, under the assumption that correct image classification is computationally demanding, the core complexity of the problems must be inherent in one or more tasks that have to be carried out in order to complete the image classification. Potential candidates for such tasks are minimum feature selection and the complexity of classifiers in machine learning-based methods. Both problems are addressed in the present paper, where on the one hand we utilize the theory of parameterized complexity for the feature selection problem, and on the other hand the theory of threshold circuit complexity for parameter settings of classifiers.

X. Gao et al. (Eds.): MIMI 2007, LNCS 4987, pp. 1–4, 2008.

2   The Complexity of Feature Selection

At an abstract level, the feature selection problem has been proven to be $\mathcal{NP}$-complete [10]. In its decision problem version, the feature set problem is defined as follows [4]: *Input:* A set $\mathsf{E} \subseteq \{0,1\}^m \times \mathrm{T}$ of examples and an integer $k > 0$, where T is a set of target features and the binary values are related to m non-target features; *Output:* Positive return, if there exists $S \subseteq \{1, 2, ..., m\}$ of size k such that no two elements of E that have identical values for all the features selected by S have different values for the target feature; otherwise negative return.

Within the sub-classification of the $\mathcal{NP}$ class by parameterized complexity classes $\mathrm{FPT} \subseteq W[1] \subseteq \cdots \subseteq W[d] \subseteq \cdots \subseteq \mathcal{NP}$ (see [6]), the feature selection problem has been proven to be $W[2]$-complete, which raises the question about the potential accuracy of feature selection methods, see [1] and the literature therein. In the parameterized complexity hierarchy, FPT denotes the class of *fixed-parameter tractable problems*. The definition of the specific class FPT is motivated by the attempt to separate time complexity bounds for problems P in terms of $n = size(I)$, $I \in P$ is a particular instance, and a parameter k: $P \in \mathrm{FPT}$, if P admits an algorithm whose running time on instances I with (n, k) is bounded by $f(k) \cdot n^{O(1)}$ for an arbitrary function f. Thus, for fixed k, problems from FPT are solvable in polynomial time; see [6] for $P \in \mathrm{FPT}$. The classes $W[d]$ are defined by mixed type Boolean circuits (bounded fan-in gates and unbounded fan-in gates) with maximum d unbounded fan-in gates on any input-output path, i.e. $P \in W[d]$, if P uniformly reduces to the decision problem of circuits defining $W[d]$. The reduction algorithm has to be from FPT.

Thus, roughly speaking, given a two-class 2D/3D image classification problem (e.g., tumour/non-tumour ROI) with a potentially increasing number m of features extracted from images (e.g., $m = 10, ..., 49, ...$), along with a total number $|\mathsf{E}|$ of samples from both classes, then the problem to decide if $k < m$ features are sufficient to classify any sample correctly is $W[2]$-complete (in practice, of course, m is limited). In this context we note that algorithms or heuristics that solve or approximate the feature set problem can be used to verify if a set of features can be reduced to a proper subset on a given sample set.

In [1] we proved an $(m/\delta)^{c_1 \cdot \kappa} \cdot n^{c_2}$ time bound for finding minimum solutions $S_{\min}$ of a given feature set problem, where n ($\sim |\mathsf{E}| \cdot m$) is the total size of the problem instance, κ is a parameter associated with the fitness landscape induced by the instance, c_1 and c_2 are relatively small constants, and $1 - \delta$ is the confidence that the solution found within this time bound is of minimum size. In terms of parameterized complexity of $\mathcal{NP}$-complete problems, our time bound differs from an FPT-type bound by the factor $m^{c_1 \cdot \kappa}$ for fixed δ. The parameter κ is the maximum value of the minimum escape height from local minima of the underlying fitness landscape, where $\kappa \leq |S_{\min}|$ due to the nature of the feature set problem. Based on results from circuit complexity (see also [3]), one can argue that $|S_{\min}| \leq \log |\mathsf{E}|$, which is an estimation for the size of $S_{\min}$, but the elements of the set are still not known (here, we assume $\log |\mathsf{E}| << m$). An exhaustive search over all selections of $\log |\mathsf{E}|$ features out of m features would results in a time bound similar to the one mentioned above, but κ is an instance-specific parameter and can usually be chosen much smaller than $\log |E|$.

3   The Complexity of Classification Circuits

When evaluating feature values by machine learning methods, a major task is to establish the appropriate size of the machine learning tool (in terms of "neuronal" units, nodes in decision trees, number of threshold gates in classification circuits), see, e.g., [5,7,11]. We investigated a priori settings for the size of machine learning tools by utilizing results from the theory of circuit complexity, see [3,9] and the literature therein. Let us consider a two-class classification problem P that is encoded as a Boolean function f_P on n input variables, and we try to approximate f_P by a learning (training) procedure that returns a classification circuit $C(f_P)$. The aim is to achieve high generalization results on unseen data. The learning procedure employs Boolean training data $L(f_P) = \{(\sigma_1, ..., \sigma_n; \eta)\}$ and Boolean test data $T(f_P)$, where in real-world applications we usually have $m_{f_P} = |L(f_P)| << 2^n$ and $m_L := |L(f_P)| = \alpha \cdot |T(f_P)|$ for $\alpha \approx 2$ or $\alpha \approx 3$. In practice, $L(f_P)$ represents only a tiny fraction of all possible 2^n tuples defining f_P. In [3,9] we propose the following approach for a priori estimations of the circuit complexity, where the gates are unbounded fan-in threshold functions $y = \text{sign}(\sum_{i=1}^{s} \omega_i \cdot x_i - \vartheta)$ and the complexity is defined by the number of threshold gates that have to be trained on $L(f_P)$: the circuit $C(f_P)$ is approximated by a composition of two circuits:

$$C(f_P) = C[n_P \rightarrow n_L] \oplus C[n_L], \tag{1}$$

where n_P is the original size of each binary sample, $n_L := \lceil \log_2 m_L \rceil$ is the length of the encoding of samples, and $C[n_P \rightarrow n_L]$ is an n_L-output circuit that calculates the encoding of elements from $L(f_P)$. The encoding then becomes the binary input to the core classification circuit $C[n_L]$. For the complexity $S(\cdots)$ of two types of threshold circuits one can show

$$S(C[n \rightarrow n_L]) < 6.8 \cdot \sqrt{2^{n_L}} + 3 \cdot n_L, \tag{2}$$

$$S(C[n_L]) \leq 28 \cdot \sqrt{\frac{2^{n_L}}{n_L}} + 11 \cdot (n_L - \log_2 n_L) + 2, \tag{3}$$

which implies for $n_L \leq 15$:

$$S(C(f_P)) < 34.8 \cdot \sqrt{2^{n_L}} + 14 \cdot n_L - 11 \cdot \log_2 n_L + 2. \tag{4}$$

We note that the upper bound depends on the number of training samples only due to $n_L = \lceil \log_2 m_L \rceil$. Since the bound certainly overestimates the number of gates, the bound has been evaluated by an a posteriori analysis of the classifier complexity for best classification results published in the literature for a number of benchmark problems. From the analysis we concluded that approximately

$$\lceil 2.5 \cdot \sqrt{2^{n_L}} \rceil \approx \lceil 2.5 \cdot \sqrt{m_L} \rceil \tag{5}$$

threshold gates are sufficient to provide a high generalization rate. The approach has been utilized to achieve a high classification accuracy on CT images related to the diagnosis of focal liver lesions [8].

References

1. Albrecht, A.A.: Stochastic Local Search for the FEATURE SET Problem with Applications to Microarray Data. Appl. Math. Comput. 183, 1148–1164 (2006)
2. Albrecht, A., Loomes, M.J., Steinhöfel, K., Taupitz, M.: Adaptive Simulated Annealing for CT Image Classification. Int. J. Pattern Recogn. 16, 573–588 (2002)
3. Albrecht, A.A., Chashkin, A.V., Iliopoulos, C.S., Kasim-Zade, O.M., Lappas, G., Steinhöfel, K.: A priori Estimation of Classification Circuit Complexity. In: Daykin, J.W., Steinhöfel, K., Mohamed, M. (eds.) Texts in Algorithmics, vol. 8, pp. 97–114, King's College, London (2007)
4. Cotta, C., Moscato, P.: The k-Feature Set Problem is W[2]-complete. J. Comput. System Sci. 67, 686–690 (2003)
5. Doi, K.: Current Status and Future Potential of Computer-aided Diagnosis in Medical Imaging. British J. Radiol. 78, S3–S19 (2005)
6. Downey, R., Fellows, M.: Parameterized Complexity. Springer, Heidelberg (1998)
7. Gletsos, M., Mougiakakou, S.G., Matsopoulos, G.K., Nikita, K.S., Nikita, A.S., Kelekis, D.: A Computer-aided Diagnostic System to Characterize CT Focal Liver Lesions: Design and Optimization of a Neural Network Classifier. IEEE T. Inform. Techn. Biomed. 7, 153–162 (2003)
8. Hein, E., Albrecht, A., Melzer, D., Steinhöfel, K., Rogalla, P., Hamm, B., Taupitz, M.: Computer-assisted Diagnosis of Focal Liver Lesions on CT Images. Acad. Radiol. 12, 1205–1210 (2005)
9. Lappas, G., Frank, R.J., Albrecht, A.A.: A Computational Study on Circuit Size vs. Circuit Depth. Int. J. Artif. Intell. Tools. 15, 143–162 (2006)
10. Davies, S., Russell, S.: NP-completeness of Searches for the Smallest Possible Feature Set. In: Greiner, R. (ed.) Proceedings of the AAAI Symposium on Relevance, pp. 41–43. AAAI Press, Menlo Park (1994)
11. Susomboon, R., Raicu, D.S., Furst, J.: Pixel-based Texture Classification of Tissues in Computed Tomography. In: Proceedings DePaul CTI Research Symposium (2006)

The Open Three Consortium: An Open-Source Initiative at the Service of Healthcare and Inclusion

Paolo Inchingolo

Open Three Consortium, Higher Education in Clinical Engineering, DEEI,
University of Trieste, Trieste, Italy

Abstract. The Higher Education in Clinical Engineering (HECE) of the University of Trieste constituted in 2005 the Open Three Consortium (O3), an innovative open-source project dealing with the multi-centric integration of hospitals, RHIOs (Regional health information organizations) and citizens (care at home and on the move, and ambient assisted living), based on about 60 HECE bilateral cooperation Agreements with Hospitals, Medical Research Centers, Healthcare Enterprises, Industrial Enterprises and Governmental Agencies and on the International Networks ABIC-BME (Adriatic Balcanic Ionian Cooperation on Biomedical Engineering) and ALADIN (Alpe Adria Initiative Universities' Network). The collaboration with multiple open-source solutions has been extended, starting an international cooperation with the open-source based company Sequence Managers Software, Raleigh, NC, United States. The O3 Consortium proposes e-inclusive citizen-centric solutions to cover the above reported three main aspects of the future of e-health in Europe with open-source strategies joined to full-service maintenance and management models. The Users' and Developers' O3 Consortium Communities are based mainly on the HECE agreements.

Keywords: open-source; distributed health care; citizen-centric health-care; ambient assisted living; international cooperation communities.

1 Introduction

After an early experience (Figure 1) with the project Open-PACS (1991-95), aiming to distribute PACS services and to pioneer a surgical PACS by opening the AT&T Commview PACS installed in 1988 in Trieste [1], the Group of Bioengineering and ICT and the Higher Education in Clinical Engineering (HECE) of the University of Trieste started the project DPACS (Data and Picture Archiving and Communication System) in 1995.

The goal of DPACS (Figure 2) was "the development of an open, scalable, cheap and universal system with accompanying tools, to store, exchange and retrieve all health information of each citizen at hospital, metropolitan, regional, national and European levels, thus offering an integrated virtual health card of the European Citizens" in a citizen-centric vision [2]. In a decade, the idea of DPACS was widely diffused, and its basic concept can be found today in the European Union Research Programs, in particular in European Union's 7th Framework Program (FP7).

X. Gao et al. (Eds.): MIMI 2007, LNCS 4987, pp. 5–11, 2008.
© Springer-Verlag Berlin Heidelberg 2008

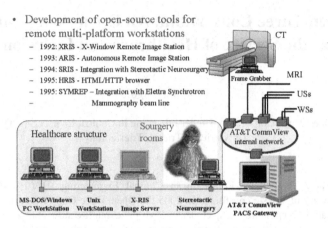

Fig. 1. The project Open-PACS (1991-1995)

A first version of DPACS was experimented in 1996-1997 at the Cattinara Hospital of Trieste. In 1998 the DPACS system was running routinely for managing all radiological images (CT, MRI, DR, US, etc.) as well as in the connection with the stereotactic neurosurgery. Some mono-dimensional signals such as ECGs were also integrated into the system.

Over the years, DPACS was enriched with the sections of anatomo-pathology, anesthesia and reanimation, clinical chemistry laboratory and others. Furthermore, at the beginning of 2000 its applications was progressively forwarded to the new emerging necessities of the future health care, health management and assistance to the world citizen, based on e-health (telemedicine) driven home-care, personal-care and ambient assisted living.

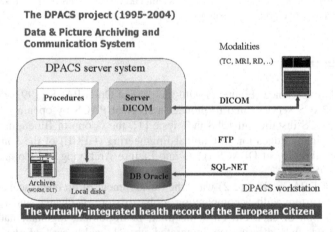

Fig. 2. The project DPACS (1995-2004) aiming to offer a virtually-integrated health record of the European Citizen

2 Materials and Methods

According to the considerations reported above several new needs have been pointed out and used to program new developments of the project such as as:

1) to have a multilingual approach to both client and server managing interfaces and for the presentation of medical contents);

2) to have a simple data & image display client interface, automatically updatable, highly portable from a PC or a MAC or a LINUX workstation to a palm or a cellular-based communicator;

3) to be able to connect with a wide variety of communication means, both fixed and mobile;

4) to offer a highly modular data & image manager/archiver, independent of the platform (UNIX/LINUX, WINDOWS, MAC) and of the selected database;

5) to improve the interoperability of both server and client system components among them and with all the other information systems components in the hospital and in the health enterprise;

6) to have an efficient and effective tool to "create" the integrated virtual clinical record in the hospital as well as at home or during the travel of a citizen.

The recognized importance of these strategies of DPACS for the future of Europe, presented as concluding lecture of the EuroPACS meeting in Oulu in 2002 [3], led the EuroPACS Society to entrust HECE with the organization of the 2004 EuroPACS meeting in Trieste, focusing on these themes. The successful "EuroPACS-MIR 2004 in the enlarged Europe" meeting held in Trieste in September 2004, with more than 400 participants from 47 Countries, witnessed the deep discussion on the organizational, standard-related and interoperability issues in all the contexts from the single department case up to the transnational integration [4].

Discussions in all the conference sessions, and especially the ones on interoperability in the workshop lasting one day on the world-wide IHE (Integrating the Healthcare Enterprise) project, gave strong results and guidelines for future work. First agenda on the round table was the question: "Is there a need for a transnational IHE committee in Central and Eastern Europe?" The IHE Workshop closed with the commitment to HECE of creating a transnational IHE committee for the Central and Eastern Europe, dealing with technical, harmonization and law-orienting activities in 22 Central and Eastern European Countries. Second, the same round table and most of the IHE workshop sessions underlined that the adoption of open standards and open source solutions is becoming a strictly mandatory path to facilitate a fast integration of health systems in Europe and worldwide, fostering this process in the transitional and developing Countries.

3 Results

3.1 Building Up the Open Three Consortium

HECE, together with BICT's laboratories HTL and OSL (Open Source Laboratory) at DEEI, started both these lines in 2005. In particular, in relation to the second one, the group of Trieste, who presented at Trieste's EuroPACS the new open-source version of their DPACS-2004 project [5], and the group of the Radiology Department of Padova, which presented the new open-source version of their Raynux /MARiS project [6], decided to fuse and integrate their projects and efforts. Hence, the "Open Three (O3) Consortium" Project was formally constituted by HECE (see www.o3consortium.eu). O3 deals [7] with open-source products for the three domains of the tomorrow's e-health, in the frame of the European e-health programs: hospital, territory and home-care / mobile-care /ambient assisted living (AAL) in a citizen-centric vision (Figure 3).

Open Hospital

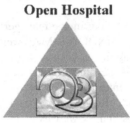

Open Territory   **Open Home & Mobile**
& RHIOs   **Care + Open AAL**

Fig. 3. The three domains of the Open Three (O3) Consortium

The main characteristics of the O3 open-source products are multi-language support, high scalability and modularity, use of Java and Web technologies at any level, support of any platform, high level of security and safety management, support of various types of data-bases and application contexts, treatment of any type of medical information, i.e. images, data and signals, and interoperability through full compliance to the "Integrating the Healthcare Enterprise" (IHE) world project, obtained by building up O3 as a collection of "bricks" representing the IHE "Actors", connecting each other through the implementation of a wide set of IHE Integration profiles [8].

3.2 First Set of Products of the Open Three Consortium

The first set of O3 products cover all the needs of image management in Radiology and in Nuclear Medicine at intra- and inter-Enterprise levels (Figure 4).

The most important are: O3-DPACS, the new version of DPACS [9] enriched with many new features such as, the XDS (Cross-Enterprise Clinical Document Sharing) and the XDS-I (Cross-Enterprise Document Sharing for Imaging) profiles, which allow images and data be exchanged very easily within any territorial environment; O3-RWS [10], a revolutionary radiological workstation, including managing of and access to MIRC (Medical Images Resource Center) data and structured report; O3-MARIS, a "super" RIS offering many new integration features and MIRC support; O3-XDS, one of the first XDS document repository and registry; O3-PDA, a first step toward the opening to the home-care and mobile-care world; O3-TEBAM allowing true reconstruction of the electrical brain in 3D in presence of pathologies.

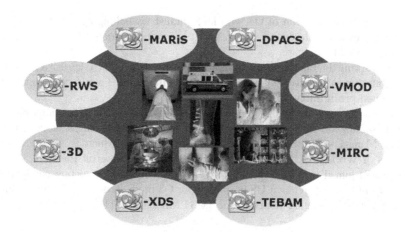

Fig. 4. The first set of O3 products

The O3 products have been tested successfully at the IHE 2005 Connectathon in Amsterdam and at the IHE 2006 Connectathon in Barcelona, gaining compliance to 19 IHE actors and 15 IHE profiles, having passed more than 300 tests with most of the European market brands.

3.3 Organization of the Open Three Consortium

From the organizational point of view, the O3 Community is made up of all the institutions having an agreement with HECE. In particular, those belonging to the international networks ABIC-BME (Adriatic Balcanic Ionian Cooperation in Biomedical Engineering) and ALADIN (Alpe Adria Initiative Universities Network), and the institutions - about 60 health-care and industrial enterprises and governmental agencies - have a bilateral agreement active with HECE. In the O3 Community, the O3 Users' Community and the O3 Developers' Community are identified. Every member of the O3 Community can in principle ask to participate in both communities.

The Developers community started under the responsibility and administration of HECE, with main contributions from the Universities of Trieste and Padova, and lately Maribor in Slovenia, and grew with many other European and US contributions, from universities and research centers and from industries. It provides the active members of the Users' Community with all the necessary project design, site analysis, implementation, logging, authoring, bugs' solving, and high-level 24/7 full-risk service. Additionally, training is highly cared by HECE, starting with preparing clinical engineering professionals at three different levels, offering both traditional and e-learning courses with particular skills in Clinical Informatics, Health Telematics, E-health integration standards and IHE-based interoperability, and also provision of specific courses and training on site.

Furthermore, selected radiologists of the Active Users' Community – where O3 is running (in Italy, from Trieste, Padova, Pisa and Siena, and in Slovenia from Maribor) constitute a Medical Advisor Committee, which gives very precious feedback to the O3 Developers' Community.

The growing cooperation of O3 with large industries belonging to the O3 Community is another very interesting aspect, and it is especially focused on the integration with territory and home-care.

O3 is working in many western countries (Italy, Slovenia, Cyprus, Switzerland, United States, etc.) and now is being adopted also in the third world countries (thanks to the O3 non-profit initiative called O3-AID).

Some months ago, the collaboration with multiple open-source solutions has been extended, starting an international co-operation with the open-source based company Sequence Managers Software, Raleigh, NC, United States, which is one of the core companies of WorldVista. Their main products are a very powerful Electronic Medical record (EMR) joined with a Hospital Information System (HIS), counting nearly 10,000 installations in military and civil US hospitals. Our O3 products are now being introduced in these hospitals, integrating them with the SMS EMR and HIS [11].

4 Discussion

Thanks to the practical experimentation with the solutions described above, the experience of a 16-year study on the integration of health systems using ICT technologies, from the hospital department to the single citizen in the e-health context of the future information-based society, has shown that some key methodological and organizational elements are extremely relevant to the success of the e-health integration process.

From the point of view of the organization of our cooperative work with other user and developer centers, the initiative of the Open Three Consortium has proven its real efficiency and efficacy. All the O3 sub-systems can be adjusted to any scale including the national and the international. Being O3 completely developed as Open Source and with Java and Web technologies, being independent of database, OS, HW and language and 100% compliant with the IHE world-wide interoperability initiative, its reuse and portability are facilitated, fostering wide distribution in the world.

The choice of Open Source as the leading solution of O3 for the future of e-health anticipates a common trend in the industrialized and political world, evidenced last year by:

(1)   the position assumed by the Department of Health & Human Services and the Department of Defense of Unites States at the Open Source Strategy for Multi-Centre Image Management Workshop, held in March 2006 at Las Vegas (USA);

(2)   the decision announced by the world's biggest industries at the OSDL Joint Initiatives Face to Face Meeting Review – Health Care Information Exchange, held in May 2006 at Sophia-Antipolis (France);

(3)   finally the European Union with the Riga Declaration signed during the Intergovernmental Meeting of the European Commission "ICT for an Inclusive Society", held in June 2006 at Riga (Latvia). Interestingly, O3 was invited to all these three events.

The adoption of the O3 concept in Europe, in Asia, and in Africa, and, in particular, in the United States with the international cooperation with SMS – WorldVista opens new scenarios of world-wide cooperation fostering open-source multi-centric and citizen-centric solutions.

5 Conclusions

In conclusion, the O3 Consortium seems to represent a significant contribution that will really support the increase of e-health integration, not only in the local region, but also across Europe and the world.

O3 links vital processes in the moving and integration of information thanks to an e-integration approach that started five years ago with our ALADIN network (Alpe Adria Initiative Universities' Network - www.aladin-net.eu), one of the first citizen-centric initiatives in Europe. Within the Alpe-Adria Region (central and eastern Europe), O3 is demonstrating relevant actions in cross-border eRegion development that improves the way people work together, live together and grow together, without frontiers. The strong cooperation recently started with the Faculty of Medicine of the University of Maribor is an important testimony of this process. From this region, O3 is fostering the widest international cooperation and integration, with China, Japan, USA, Brazil, etc., reinforcing the synergy with the European industry and the power of Europe to approach and gain the non-European markets increasingly, in particular in American and Far East Countries.

References

1. Diminich, M., Inchingolo, P., Magliacca, F., Martinolli, N.: Versatile and open tools for LAN, MAN and WAN communications with PACS. In: Held, B., Ciskowski, P. (eds.) Comput. Biomed., pp. 309–316. Comp. Mech. Pub, Southampton (1993)
2. Fioravanti, F., Inchingolo, P., Valenzin, G., Dalla Palma, L.: The DPACS Project at the University of Trieste. Med. Informat. 22(4), 301-314 (1997)
3. Inchingolo, P., et al.: New trends of the DPACS project. In: Niinimaki, Ilkko, Reponen (eds.) Proceedings o20th EuroPACS, pp. 205–208. Oulu University Press (2002)
4. Inchingolo, P., Pozzi Mucelli, R. (eds.): EuroPACS-MIR 2004 in the Enlarged Europe. EUT, Trieste (2004) ISBN: 88-8303-150-4
5. Inchingolo, P., et al.: DPACS-2004 becomes a java-based open-source modular system. Idem, pp. 271-276 (2004)
6. Saccavini, C.: The MARIS project: open-source approach to IHE radiological workflow software. Idem, pp. 285–287 (2004)
7. Inchingolo, P.: The Open Three (O3) Consortium Project. In: Open Source Strategy for Multi-Center Image Management (2006), https://www.mcim.georgetown.edu/MCIM
8. Inchingolo, P., et al.: O3-DPACS Open-Source Image-Data Manager/Archiver and HDW2 Image-Data Display: an IHE-compliant project pushing the e-health integration in the world. In: Comput. Med. Imag. Graph., vol. 30, pp. 391–406. Elsevier Science, Amsterdam (2006)
9. Beltrame, M., Bosazzi, P., Poli, A., Inchingolo, P.: O3-DPACS: a Java-based, IHE compliant open-source data and image manager and archiver. In: IFMBE Proceed. Medicon 2007 (2007)
10. Faustini, G., Inchingolo, P.: O3-RWS: a Java-based, IHE-compliant open-source radiology workstation. In: IFMBE Proceed. Medicon 2007 (2007)
11. Inchingolo, P., Lord, B.: International medical data collaboration with multiple open-source solutions. In: Open Source Strategy for Multi-Center Image Management, St. Louis Missouri, USA (2007), http://www.mcim.georgetown.edu/MCIM2007

Extending the Radiological Workplace Across the Borders

Hanna Pohjonen[1,2], Peeter Ross[2,3], and Johan (Hans) Blickman[4]

[1] Rosalieco Oy, Espoo, Finland
[2] Inst. of Clin. Med., Tallinn Univ. of Technology, Estonia
[3] East-Tallinn Central Hospital, Tallinn, Estonia
[4] Dept. of Radiology, UMC St. Radboud, Nijmegen, The Netherlands
hanna.pohjonen@rosalieco.fi

Abstract. Emerging technologies are transforming the workflows in healthcare enterprises. Today, several vendors offer holistic web-based solutions for radiologists, radiographers and clinicians - a single platform for all users. Besides traditional web, streaming technology is also emerging to the radiological practice in order for improving security and enabling the use of low network bandwidths.

The technology does not set limitations any more: today, the digital workplace knows no boundaries; remote reporting, off-hour coverage, virtual radiologists are all ways to offer imaging services in a non-traditional way. The challenge, however, is to provide trust over distance – across organizational or even national boundaries. In the following three different aspects important in building trust in remote reporting are discussed: 1) organizational change issues, 2) continuous feedback and 3) legal implications.

Keywords: web, streaming, remote reporting, cross-border.

1 Introduction

Thus far dedicated stand-alone PACS workstations have dominated the way how radiologists work and web-based tools have been used for delivering images to clinicians mainly. The main reasons for not using web for diagnostic work have been the lack of diagnostic and sophisticated analysis tools - like 3D reconstruction - in web solutions.

This is changing: today several vendors offer holistic web-based solutions for radiologists, radiographers and clinicians - a single platform for all users. These solutions provide the radiologists with diagnostic tools, advanced image processing methods as well as meeting folders all in web.

The technology does not set limitations any more: today, the digital workplace knows no boundaries; remote reporting, off-hour coverage, virtual radiologists are all ways to offer imaging services in a non-traditional way. The challenge, however, is to provide trust over distance – across organizational or even national boundaries.

X. Gao et al. (Eds.): MIMI 2007, LNCS 4987, pp. 12–17, 2008.

2 Material and Methods

2.1 Traditional Web

The web-based solution provides healthcare professionals with enterprise-wide access to all patient data and analysis functions. Such anytime, anywhere pervasive coverage matches the highly nomadic workflows of many healthcare practitioners, and has the potential to significantly impact clinical workflows.

Consultations between clinicians and radiologists become easier and more efficient when the same platform is used and the professionals can log in using any end-terminal regardless of their profile. Consultations can occur via a web conference as well – the same screen can be shared by the clinician and the consulting radiologist – or by a resident and a senior radiologist.

Web-based diagnostics integrated with web RIS enables a virtual radiological environment to be built, where radiologists can remotely use viewing tools and RIS via VPN across organizational or national borders. Pervasive access to image data and analysis tools at home while on-call can eliminate many late-night trips into the radiology department to diagnose studies involving trauma and emergency cases.

The new generation web-architecture enables built-in redundancy and easy software/hardware updates. The platform is adjustable for different end-terminals and network bandwidths and overall training times can be significantly reduced. By introducing systems that minimize support and maintenance the overall burden on IT departments can be greatly reduced.

Web client applications can be thin and thus require minimal configuration and setup activities on the client side. This is important for today's large or ASP-based configurations in which many users must be quickly and easily hooked up to the system.

2.2 Streaming Technology

Besides traditional web, streaming technology is also emerging to the radiological practice. Streaming is a broad term that refers to sending portions of data from a source to a client for processing or viewing, rather than sending all the data first before processing or viewing. In the imaging field streaming technology is used to overcome various limitations such as limited bandwidth connections, clients that are not powerful enough for the computation tasks required, and the handling of large data sets.

There are two types of streaming relevant in the imaging field. Intelligent downloading is a form of streaming whereby only the data required for immediate viewing or processing are downloaded to a client. In general, processing of the data occurs locally on the client. Additional downloading may occur in the background in anticipation of other viewing or processing requests.

In adaptive streaming of functionality data are not downloaded to clients, only frame-buffer views of the data or results of data analyses are streamed. The power of the server is used to render final screen images which are then compressed and transmitted to client devices.

In other cases, streaming of functionality transmits data to clients in accordance with various parameters and preferences regarding performance goals, bandwidth consumption, and available client resources. The data are then processed locally on the client.

In other words, the goal of the technology for adaptive streaming of functionality is to provide remote access to full system functionality, using the best combinations of local and remote processing of medical data.

3 Results

The main advantages of streaming technology include

1) Effective use of bandwidth: streaming technology can use bandwidth in a manner that can be well estimated, and in many cases such bandwidth usage is more efficient than with traditional web-based solutions (involving data downloading).
2) Increased security and data consistency: because data can be prevented from being downloaded to local clients, and only streamed for interactive viewing, an additional level of data security can be provided. Streams can also be required to be encrypted. Additionally, streaming requires only a single copy of data to be stored, which is accessed as needed, rather than maintaining multiple copies in order to meet distribution demands.
3) Access to full clinical functionality: by offering access to exactly the same system features and interfaces on all access devices and at all locations, users become more comfortable, efficient and standardized regarding daily workflows. Handheld mobile/wireless devices can provide clinicians with enterprise-wide access to all patient data and analysis tools on a pervasive basis.
4) Predictable scalability: streaming systems scale linearly with the number of users, the number of sites, and the amount of data handled.

4 Discussion

The workflow of clinicians is patient-centric and also highly nomadic – rarely are they able to accomplish all necessary tasks by remaining at a single location for an extended period of time (an office, for example). However, clinicians have difficulty in moving outside their own environments because of the need to have access to those IT systems that support their work. Similarly, contacts with patients at the bedside can be challenging because disparate sources of patient data need to be assembled for effective communication. There is also a clear need to extend the workplace outside the organizational or even national borders – for both clinicians and radiologists.

Therefore pervasive and mobile access to patient data and analysis tools can open up new avenues of communication, both amongst professionals and with patients, as well as new avenues of mobility to support nomadic workflows.

When extending the workplace across organizational and national borders, the technology is not the limiting factor. With traditional web and especially combined with streaming technology we can build a secure and trusted workplace which knows no boundaries. The issue, however, is to build trust over distance – between the service providers and the customers for the reporting service. In the following three aspects important in building trust are discussed: organizational change issues, feedback and legal issues.

4.1 Organizational Change Issues

When outsourcing reporting service the factors in the current organizational environment that will enhance or hinder the development or implementation of the service should be considered:

- What groups will support the development of the remote reporting service? Why?
- What groups will block the development of the remote reporting service? Why?
- How will you convey the message to gain support or buy-in for the development of the remote reporting service in your organization?
- What problems or pitfalls can you anticipate that will affect the success of the remote reporting service?

Only when the organization is ready and prepared for integrating remote reporting as part of the radiological operation of a hospital, there is a chance in succeeding to build trust in the service.

The remote reporting service provider should be tightly involved side in the organizational change management of the customer. The customer should get familiar with the 'face' of the service provider in order to build trust. The backgrounds of the project champion and the core project team, their skills and abilities to execute the business case strategy should be described. The personnel needs, the roles of the key project team members, and the role of an outside council if any should be identified. Staffing requirements and organizational structure in terms of responsibilities and reporting relationships should be clarified. At least the following questions should be answered:

- What are the roles and responsibilities of the project champion and the project team?
- Who are the key leaders, what is their experience with similar projects?
- Does the project team have training or learning needs to support the success of the proposed project?
- Describe the function of outside supporting professional services, if any.
- What are the reporting relationships between the key project team members?

4.2 Continuous Feedback

When buying a remote reporting service the customer wants proof of quality, known and accepted processes and protocols, transparency, possibilities for peer review and double blind readings from time to time. On the other hand, the service provider expects access to the relevant data, feedback on discrepancies and learning from other specialists.

Feedback – both from radiologists but also from clinicians - is essential in building and maintaining trust in a remote reporting situation where the service provider is not in the same building or not even in the same country; ensuring transparency in performance and quality indicators is a prerequisite for a self-sustainable remote radiology business case. The users (i.e. the customers for the remote reporting) should be able to give digital feedback easily and in a user-friendly way.

At the same time learning is enabled by systematic automation of feedback on different levels between participants in the healthcare process. Constructive feedback creates a safe environment for individual self-improvement. The feedback software should be easy to use and preferably desktop-integrated with the local RIS/PACS.

4.3 Legal Implications

In building remote reporting business case you should consider the main issues that may arise from the need to manage personal information in a manner that takes into consideration both individual sensitivities and the need to provide healthcare practitioners (and, potentially, patients, administrators and others) with access to health records. In particular, you need to demonstrate that you have understood the trust and security implications arising from the legal and clinical environment in which the remote reporting service is to operate.

The following issues should be discussed and agreed on between the service provider and the customer:

- How will patient information be stored, transmitted and used so that it is kept confidential and only shared with those individuals who have a legitimate need to see it? Will encryption and electronic signatures be needed? How will patient consent be recorded and, if necessary, used to govern access to information?
- How all actions performed will be associated with the identifiable individual who performed those actions? What manual and automated facilities will be required to maintain and subsequently process any audit trail / security log etc.?
- What processes will be used to address disaster recovery and business continuity?
- Who will provide the service and who, ultimately, will be responsible for the care of the patient – will clinical responsibility be shared, in fact, between several clinicians?
- How much will the patient be told about how their information is used and how will their informed, voluntary consent be obtained? Who, under what circumstances, may act on behalf of the patient to grant or withhold consent?
- What legislation governs the capture, storage, dissemination and destruction of information? Are there different legal considerations in different relevant countries? What are the legal implications if the information management process fails to achieve the required or expected Quality of Service as might be described in terms of confidentiality, integrity (e.g. completeness and correctness), and availability (e.g. timeliness) of information?

- Will the service be offered locally, nationally or internationally? If so will the radiologists involved need to be qualified and insured to practice in another country? Will it be necessary for them to revalidate their qualifications or take new ones?
- If the service is to be provided online, how will contracts be created and entered into and how will payments be collected?

In conclusion, building trust in remote reporting is a complex and challenging task that should be carefully considered from several points of view in order to assure a self-sustainable remote reporting service.

From Frame to Framless Stereotactic Operation—Clinical Application of 2011 Cases

Zeng-min Tian, Wang-sheng Lu, Quan-jun Zhao, Xin Yu, Shu-bin Qi, and Rui Wang

Department of Neurosurgery, Navy General Hospital of PLA, Beijing 100037, China
tianzengmin@vip.sina.com

Abstract. Stereotactic operations were performed with the frameless stereotactic instrument (named as CAS-R-2) manufactured by ourselves rather than traditional stereotactic frame. The aim of this study was to assess the clinical usefulness, accuracy and safety of the frameless stereotactic instrument. We retrospectively reviewed 2011 patients aged between 0.2 to 89 years (with mean of 30.7 years) with CT/MRI image-guided frameless stereotactic surgery between January 1997 to April 2007. The accuracy of position and improvement of symptom was observed. The surgical procedures were successful. All targets were pointed accurately in just one go during the operation. Follow-up being performed 3 to 48 months (averaged 24 months) after the operation, the total effective rate was 93.3% without serious surgery-related complications. Compared with the traditional frame stereotactic operations, this method has some advantages, such as releasing the patients pain, convenient to the doctors, extending the range of indications and increasing the safety and effectiveness of the operations.

Keywords: Surgical operation, Robotics, CT/MRI image, Frameless stereotaxy.

1 Introduction

Recent developments in neuro-navigation, stereotactic frames and computer aided technique have contributed to minimal invasive procedure in neurosurgery field. Stereotactic operation has been clinically employed over the last half century with traditional frames in place, which has several limitations, including bulky, interference in the surgical exposure, correlative pain and without feedback to the surgeon about anatomical structures encountered in the procedure[1,2]. Consequently, frameless stereotactic technique became an important research direction of neurosurgery. Based on the experience of more than 3000 framed stereotactic operations, we designed and manufactured a new frameless stereotactic equipment with navigating function, named CAS-R-2 (Computer Assistant Surgery-Robot, type 2) in 1997. During January 1997 ~ April 2007, we performed 2011 cases of frameless stereotactic operations successfully using CAS-R-2 robot system and obtained good results. The study protocol was approved by the local ethical committee, and formal consent was obtained from all patients or their closest relatives before inception of the study.

X. Gao et al. (Eds.): MIMI 2007, LNCS 4987, pp. 18–24, 2008.

2 Materials and Methods

2.1 Patient Population

We prospectively reviewed 2011 patients (1203 males and 808 females with age range of 0.2~89 years; i.e., mean=30.7 years) who had undergone frameless CT/MRI image-guided stereotactic operations with CAS-R-2 robot system. Among these 2011 cases, 844 cases had brain tumors of various forms (360 with astrocytoma range from low-grade astrocytoma to multiple glioblastoma, 342 with cystic and cyst-solid craniopharyngioma, 51 with brain metastases, 30 with cystic acoustic neuroma, 22 with germinomas, 17 with pituitary adenomas, 10 with meningioma, 6 with ependymoma, and 6 with gelatin cyst); 569 were with functional neurosurgical diseases (210 with epilepsy, 182 with Parkinsons diseases, 57 with mental diseases,120 with other diseases); 279 patients underwent neural stem cell transplatation; 157 underwent biopsy for brain lesions; and 76 and 13 were intracerebral hemorrhage and brain abscess respectively, 42 cases were hydrocephalus and arachnoids cyst (combined with endoscope surgery), 17 and 14 cases were with metal foreign body and intracerebral small sources respectively.

2.2 Stereotactic Equipment, CAS-R-2

The CAS-R-2 robot system used in this study, was collaboratively developed from traditional stereotactic frame and CAS-R-1 system over the period of ten years by the Navy General Hospital and Beijing University of Aeronautics and Astronautics. The CAS-R-2 robot system mainly consists of five components. They are computer-assisted planning system, intraoperative navigation system, intellective mechanical arm with five-degree freedom, locking controller of mechanical arm and recognizing part of marker. The robotic construction fulfils the functions of reconstructing and displaying three-dimensional(3D) model based on the patients radiological data, calculating a 3D reference coordinate corresponding to the target and planning the track of puncture, providing a real-time navigation through a mapping between the operation space of four markers and pattern space, serving as a operation platform for the surgeons (Fig. 1).

2.3 Operative Method

Anesthesia: 1582 patients were performed stereotactic operation under local anesthesia; 429 under local anesthesia combined with intravenous anesthesia, most of them being infant and elderly who could not tolerate local anesthesia.

The operation had following steps: 1).The four markers were placed on the patients scalp. The markers were usually like electrocardio-electrode piece obviously visiable on computerized tomography (CT) or small lipid beads on magnetic resonance imaging (MRI). 2). After patient had undergone a CT or MRI scan, the CT/MRI image information were transmitted to CAS-R-2 main computer through PACS local network system. Surgeons had formulated a feasible surgical plan including lesion border, target point and puncturing track by

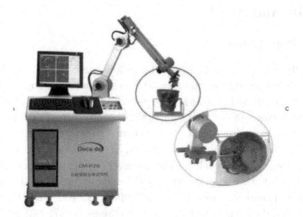

Fig. 1. The CAS-R-2 robot system. The instrument roughly consists of computer, software and mechanical arm with five-degree freedom.

three-dimensional reconstruction of the image data. 3). After the anesthesia, a patient's head was immobilized with a shaping pillow to keep it in a stable position. The system had been registered at the beginning of the operation by touching the probe tip to markers on the patients scalp. 4). Navigating puncture: Operators performed navigating puncture using intelligent mechanical arm, simulating the track of needle on the screen in real-time. When mechanical arm arrived at the precise position, the operators locked the direction and position of arm immediately. 5). After the mechanical arm guided puncture needle arrived at the target, the operators began corresponding surgical manipulation, such as evacuating fluid and injecting drugs (Figs. 2, 3).

3   Results

No case needed to be aborted because of the registration failure. The surgical operations were successful in all cases. Overall, 553 operations were performed based on the guidance of CT , whilst 1458 operations based on MRI. The whole procedure starting from transmitting the CT/MRI image into computer to mechanical arm arriving at the accurate direction and position took about 20-30 minutes. All targets were pointed accurately in just one go during the operations of 2011 cases. Follow-up took place in 3 to 48 months (with average of 24 months) after the operation. The early effective rate was 93.3% without serious surgical complication. 844 were with intracavitary and intratumoral irradiation for brain tumors (cystic brain tumors were injected isotope ^{32}P after evacuation for cyst, solid tumor were transplanted isotope ^{125}I or after being loaded ^{192}Ir and mixed solid and cystic tumors were treated by intracavitary irradiation and gamma knife surgery). 569 were the deep-lesion damaging of functional neurosurgical disease (epilepsy treated by depth electroencephalogram EEG electrode producing amygdale and hippocampus lesions with radiofrequency techniques; Mental disease and

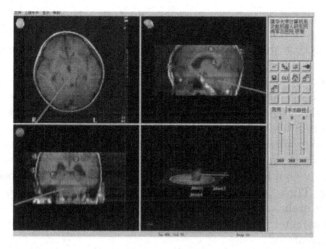

Fig. 2. Surgical plan for brain lesions. The plan includes lesion border, target point and puncturing track formulated by three-dimensional reconstruction of the image data.

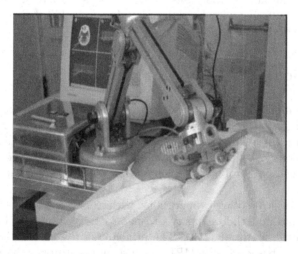

Fig. 3. The biopsy procedure for brain stem lesions. When mechanical arm arrives at the accuracy position according the surgical plan, it guides puncture needle to arrive at target followed by biopsy on the operation platform.

Parkinson's disease treated by producing special lesions with radiofrequency techniques). 157 were biopsy. Most cases had positive results except four cases with inconclusive tissue diagnosis, including inflammation. 76 were evacuation for hemorrhage including 29 putamen hemorrhages, 25 thalamic, 17 subcortical and 5 in other locations, 16~23 ml being aspirated (accounting for 40%~80% of the total volume of hematoma, 40~60 ml) and the drainage tube was left in target place for 1~3 days followed by an injection of urokinase. 13 were evacuation for brain deep abscess, and aspirate 5∼20 ml abscess fluid, then located a drainage tube followed by injecting antibiotic. Before beginning the fistulation of hydrocephalus and arachnoids cyst, we first established a best plan on entry point and puncture track using CAS-R-2 and then began to endoscope-assisted fistulation in 42 cases. Metal foreign body and small sources were removed in 31 cases.

All frameless operations were successfully carried out without side effects attributable to the usage of the system. The error of the locating precision by the robot system in practice was less than 1.0mm, which was tested through an ex vivo study. Most patients were fit to have liquid food 2∼ 4 hour after the operation and resumed their daily activities on the following day. During the early postoperative period, five (0.3%) patients with brain tumors developed surgical complications. Three cases presented intracranial hematoma due to biopsy. One showed severe brain edema and one had additional neurological deficit (oculomotor paralysis) after intratumoral irradiation. All patients have recovered after conservation treatment.

All cases were followed up in 3∼48 months (average 24 months) after operation. The total efficiency of operation in 2011 cases was 93.3%, including being cured clinically in 1034 cases (51.4%), remarkably recovered in 843 cases (41.9%), and inefficacy in 106 cases (5.3%). Disease progression happened in 23 cases (1.1%) suffering with hemiplegia, and coma, whilfist five patients died (0.3%) because of disease progression.

4   Discussions

The frameless stereotactic neurosurgery is a directional study in the international neurosurgery field. The study involved the knowledge of multi-discipline, including robotics, microelectrode, image processing, virtual reality and minimal invasive surgery [1-4]. We have developed the frameless stereotactic instruments, a practical CAS robot system based on plentiful stereotactic operation experience.

The frameless strereotactic operations with robot assistance enhance the safety of patients and the dexterity of operators, avoiding the limitations of traditional framed operations [5-6]. The principle of the method is to establish a reference frame based on CT/MRI image scanning, to plan the procedure of the brain operation and carry out virtual operation, finally to accomplish the assisted location of intelligent mechanical arm with multi-sensor. The clinical practice shows that it can decrease the patients pain and psychological burden without the need of mounting a frame on the head of the patient. The computer assisted surgical planning system can improve the accuracy of locating lesion and the visualization of procedure, which makes the surgical operating more convenient and decreases the subsequent damage. The error of locating precision by the robot system in practice is less than 1.0mm. It not only applies to traditional strereotactic operation field (the biopsy of brain deep diseases, the lesion of nuclear cluster in deep brain of Parkinsonism, intratumor irradition), but also applies to those patients who are not adapted to fix the frame or present with multiple brain lesion. In a way, the operative process is similar to the traditional one. Neurosurgeons can easily control it. It is suitable to common indications of stereotactic operation.

Compared with the similar robotic systems developed in the other countries in the field, our system can be characterised as [6-9]: 1). Collecting the importing medical images: based on numerous existing CT/MRI machines, whilst the locating software can acquire several data of CT/MRI images in various formats, leading to the wider range of applications; 2). Locating software system: 3-D images can demonstrate the volume of the lesion, definite the target on the screen of computer, automatically execute coordinates transformations and map to the angle coordinates of mechanical arms; 3).Simulating the operating pathway: it shows the puncturing track chosen by surgeons using CAS-R-2 machine in real time, providing navigations of puncturing target; 4). Capable robot system: the tail end of five joint mechanical arms can both show the target position, carry puncture needle, endoscope and other surgical instruments, and can fix the instrument in order to make it under a stable pose directing to the target.

The modern stereotactic neurosurgery aiming at minimal invasive is developed towards accuracy, programmable, and intelligent direction. The successfully application of brain frameless stereotactic operation also reflects this trend. In terms of safety, accuracy and convenience of the CAS-R-2 robot system, the system is reliable and will become a new neurosurgical tool providing a platform for neurosurgeons.

5 Conclusions

Robot-assisted neurosurgery is feasible. This new technology may enhance surgical safety and convenience. We believe continued improvement in computer assisted technology will promise much wider use of robot-assisted system in stereotactic surgery.

Acknowledgements

This work was supported by the National Science Foundation of China, the Ministry of Science and Technology of China, and the Chinese Scientific Association.

References

1. Apuzzo, M.L.: New dimensions of Neurosurgery in the Realm of High Technology: Possibilities, Practicalities, Realities. Neurosurgery 38, 625–639 (1996)
2. Friets, E.M., Strohbehn, J.W., Roberts, D.W.: Curvature-based nonfiducial registration for the Frameless Stereotactic Operating Microscope. IEEE Trans Biomed Eng. 42, 867–878 (1995)
3. Kikinis, R., Gleason, P.L., Moriarty, T.M., Moore, M.R., Alexander, E., Stieg, P.E.: Computer-assisted Interactive Three-dimensional Planning for Neurosurgical Procedures. Neurosurgery 38, 640–651 (1996)

4. Spivak, C.J., Pirouzmand, F.: Comparison of the reliability of brain lesion localization when using traditional and stereotactic image-guided techniques: a prospective study. J. Neurosurg 103, 424–427 (2005)
5. Woodworth, G.F., McGirt, M.J., Samdani, A., Garonzik, I., Olivi, A., Weingart, J.D., et al.: Frameless Image-guided Stereotactic Brain Biopsy Procedure: Diagnostic Yield, Surgical Morbidity, and Comparison with the Frame-based Technique. J. Neurosurgery 104, 233–237 (2006)
6. Holloway, K.L., Gaede, S.E., Starr, P.A., Rosenow, J.M., Ramakrishnan, V., Henderson, J.M., et al.: Frameless Stereotaxy Using Bone Fiducial Markers for Deep Brain Stimulation. J. Neurosurgery 103, 404–413 (2005)
7. Treuer, H., Klein, D., Maarouf, M., Lehrke, R., Voges, J., Sturm, V., et al.: Accuracy and Conformity of Stereotactically Guided Interstitial Brain Tumour Therapy Using I-125 Seeds. Radiotherapy Oncology 77, 202–209 (2005)
8. Tian, Z., Wang, T., Liu, Z., Zhao, Q., Du, J., Liu, D.: Robot Assisted System in Stereotactic Neurosurgery. Aca J. PLA Postgraduate Med School 1, 4–5 (1998)
9. Tian, Z., Zhao, Q., Wang, T., Du, J., Liu, D., Lu, H.: Use of robot in frameless stereotactic neurosurgery. Chinese J. Minimally Invasive Neurosurgery 5, 129–130 (2000) (in Chinese)

Medical Image Segmentation Based on the Bayesian Level Set Method

Yao-Tien Chen[1] and Din-Chang Tseng[2]

[1] Department of Computer Science and Information Engineering,
Yuanpei University, HsinChu, 30015, Taiwan
ytchen@mail.ypu.edu.tw
[2] Department of Computer Science and Information Engineering,
National Central University, Chungli, 32001, Taiwan
tsengdc@ip.csie.ncu.edu.tw

Abstract. A level set method based on the Bayesian risk is proposed for medical image segmentation. At first, the image segmentation is formulated as a classification of pixels. Then the Bayesian risk is formed by false-positive and false-negative fractions in a hypothesis test. Through minimizing the average risk of decision in favor of the hypotheses, the level set evolution functional is deduced for finding the boundaries of targets. To prevent the propagating curves from generating excessively irregular shapes and lots of small regions, curvature and gradient of edges in the image are integrated into the functional. Finally, the Euler-Lagrange formula is used to find the iterative level set equation from the derived functional. Comparing with other level-set methods, the proposed approach relies on the optimum decision of pixel classification; thus the approach has more reliability in theory and practice. Experiments show that the proposed approach can accurately extract the complicated shape of targets and is robust for various types of images including high-noisy and low-contrast images, *CT*, *MRI*, and ultrasound images; moreover, the algorithm is extendable for multiphase segmentation.

Keywords: image segmentation, level set method, Bayesian risk, hypothesis test.

1 Introduction

Nowadays a large number of various medical images [1, 2] are generated from hospitals or medical centers with sophisticated image acquisition devices, such as computed tomography (*CT*), magnetic resonance (*MRI*), ultrasound image (*US*), X-ray diffraction, electrocardiogram (*ECG*), and positron emission tomography (*PET*). Medical image segmentation is a technique assisting doctors to process and analyze the medical images, so that doctors can make better diagnosis, accurately examine disease symptoms, and support their decisions in a variety of clinical works. For medical imagery, a main goal of image segmentation is to accurately extract the shape of targets from various types of medical images. Over these decades, many approaches have been developed to achieve the goal; active contour is one of the most powerful methods.

X. Gao et al. (Eds.): MIMI 2007, LNCS 4987, pp. 25–34, 2008.
© Springer-Verlag Berlin Heidelberg 2008

The level set method was started by Osher and Sethian [3] in 1988. Since then, a great variety of geometric deformable models have been developed in response to the ever-increasing demands on image segmentation. Chan and Vese [4] proposed an active contour model working with no reliance on the gradient to stop the propagation process. With the stopping force based on Mumford-Shah segmentation formulas [5], the model becomes an energy-minimizing segmentation and given as

$$\frac{\partial \phi}{\partial t} = \delta_0(\phi) \left[\mu \, div \left(\frac{\nabla \phi}{|\nabla \phi|} \right) - v - \lambda_1 (g - c_1)^2 + \lambda_2 (g - c_2)^2 \right], \tag{1}$$

where g denotes the image gray levels, $\delta_0(\phi)$ is the Dirac measure (the derivative of the Heaviside function), c_1 is the average of g inside the propagating curve, and c_2 is the average of g outside the propagating curve; $\mu \geq 0$, $v \geq 0$, and λ_1, $\lambda_2 > 0$ are fixed parameters. Chan et $al.$ also proposed active contours without edge for vector-valued images [6] and multiphase segmentation [7].

Lee and Seo [8] proposed a level set-based partial differential equation (*PDE*) based on the modified fitting term of the Chan-Vese model for the bimodal segmentation. The energy functional is designed to obtain a stationary global minimum; thus the energy functional has a unique convergence state, the evolution algorithm is invariant to the initialization, and level set function can set an appropriate termination criterion. Martin et $al.$ [9] proposed a level-set active segmentation based on the maximum likelihood estimation to improve the segmented results for several different noise models and showed that the regularity term could be efficiently determined by using the minimum description length (*MDL*) principle. They assume that noise can be described by members of the exponential family, such as *Gaussian*, *Gamma*, *Poisson*, or *Bernoulli* distribution. The active contour model is given as

$$\frac{\partial \phi}{\partial t} = \varepsilon \big(F_j(x, y) - \lambda \, k(x, y) \big) |\nabla \phi(x, y)|, \tag{2}$$

where $F_j(x, y) = \dfrac{1}{2} \left[\log(\hat{\sigma}_f^{\,2}) - \log(\hat{\sigma}_b^{\,2}) + \dfrac{(g(x, y) - \hat{m}_f)^2}{\hat{\sigma}_f^{\,2}} - \dfrac{(g(x, y) - \hat{m}_b)^2}{\hat{\sigma}_b^{\,2}} \right]$;

$g(x, y)$ is gray level of pixel (x, y); $\hat{m}_f$ and $\hat{m}_b$ are the maximum likelihood estimates of gray-level mean in foreground and background, respectively; $\hat{\sigma}_f^{\,2}$ and $\hat{\sigma}_b^{\,2}$ are the maximum likelihood estimates of gray-level variance in foreground and background, respectively; ε is a constant; λ obtained from *MDL* principle is a weighting coefficient for the regularity term; and $k(x, y)$ is the curvature of the level set function ϕ at (x, y).

The segmentation algorithm for medical images needs to face more challenges, such as the complicated structure of organs and tissues, the noise influences caused by the imaging devices, the anatomical variation in patients, and high-noisy/low-contrast contents. For applications on organ extraction and brain cortical region segmentation, more accurate and effective techniques are pursued. Suri et $al.$ [10] gave a review of the state-of-the-art 2-D and 3-D cerebral cortex segmentation techniques on three different classes: region-based, boundary-based, and fusion of region- and boundary-based techniques. Goldenberg et $al.$ [11] proposed an approach for 3-D brain cortex segmentation. The method is based on the coupled surface model that is derived as a minimization of the variational geometric framework. The surface evolution is performed using the fast geodesic active contour approach; numerical scheme combining semi-implicit additive operator splitting (*AOS*) [12] propagation scheme, level set representation, narrow band approach, and the fast marching method. Chenoune *et al.* [13] proposed a segmentation of cardiac cine-*MR* images and myocardial deformation assessment using level set methods. First, the level set method proposed by Osher and Fedkiw [14] is modified by introducing an additional region-based constraint. Then, it is applied on a 2D+*t* (*i.e.*, 3-D pseudo-volume by stacking the 2-D images) dataset to detect endocardial contours.

In this paper, we propose a level set method based on the Bayesian risk to segment various medical images. At first, by minimizing the risk of misclassification, the level set evolution functional is deduced. To prevent the propagating curves from generating excessively irregular shapes and lots of small regions, curvature and gradient of edges in the image are integrated into the functional. Finally, the Euler-Lagrange formula is used to find the iterative level set equation from the derived functional so that the propagating curves can move towards and stop at the boundaries of targets.

2   The Bayesian Risk

In this section, the basic concept of Bayesian risk [15, 16] is introduced and which will be used to classify pixels into several groups based on the similar characteristics. Then, based on the risk we derive the level set evolution functional.

Suppose an image comprise foreground and background pixels to be classified. Classification of the image can be represented by two hypotheses: a null hypothesis H_1 where the foreground is absent, and an alternative hypothesis H_2 in which the foreground is present. The classifier is used to determine which hypothesis is correct; that is, the classifier must choose one of two decisions, Θ_1: the classifier declares that the foreground is absent, or Θ_2: the foreground is present. In the hypothesis test, there are four conditional probabilities used for the combinations of hypothesis and decision. (*i*) $P(\Theta_1|H_1)$ is the probability that the classifier declares the foreground absent when it is actually absent. (*ii*) $P(\Theta_2|H_1)$ is the probability that the classifier declares the foreground present when it is actually absent. (*iii*) $P(\Theta_1|H_2)$ is the probability that the classifier declares the foreground absent when it is actually present. (*iv*) $P(\Theta_2|H_2)$ is the probability that the classifier declares the foreground present when it is actually present.

$P(\Theta_2|H_1)$, called type I risk, is the probability of rejecting the null hypothesis H_1 when it is true; while $P(\Theta_1|H_2)$, called type II risk, is the probability of accepting H_1 when H_1 is false. For each combination of hypothesis and decision, there exists an associated loss. The losses of $P(\Theta_1|H_1)$, $P(\Theta_2|H_1)$, $P(\Theta_1|H_2)$, and $P(\Theta_2|H_2)$ are denoted as $l(1,1)$, $l(2,1)$, $l(1,2)$, and $l(2,2)$, respectively. $l(1,1)$ and $l(2,2)$ are the losses of correct decision while $l(2,1)$ and $l(1,2)$ are the losses of incorrect decision. $l(1,1)$ and $l(2,2)$ are expected to be low or zero; $l(2,1)$ and $l(1,1)$ (also $l(1,2)$ and $l(2,2)$) are mutually inverse; thus $l(2,1)$ and $l(1,2)$ are expected to be high. For images, the Bayesian risk for classifying a pixel into foreground or background is given by [15, 16]

$$r = l(1,1)P(H_1)P(\Theta_1|H_1) + l(2,1)P(H_1)P(\Theta_2|H_1)$$

$$+ l(1,2)P(H_2)P(\Theta_1|H_2) + l(2,2)P(H_2)P(\Theta_2|H_2). \tag{3}$$

As the general rule, we set the losses $l(1,1) = l(2,2) = 0$ and $l(1,2) = l(2,1) = 1$, if the classifier makes the right decisions; thus the Bayesian risk can be rewritten as

$$r = P(H_1)P(\Theta_2|H_1) + P(H_2)P(\Theta_1|H_2). \tag{4}$$

Let R be the region consisting of two disjoint phases (zones) ω_1 and ω_2. The phase ω_1 contains all pixels that lead the classifier to choose decision Θ_1, whereas ω_2 contain all pixels that result in decision Θ_2. The two hypotheses, H_1 and H_2, are associated with probability density functions (*pdfs*) $P(g|H_1)$ and $P(g|H_2)$ respectively, where g denotes a pixel. The risk $P(\Theta_2|H_1)$ is the integral of $P(g|H_1)$ over the phase ω_2 and $P(\Theta_1|H_2)$ is the integral of $P(g|H_2)$ over the phase ω_1. Thus the total risk for the two-zone case is

$$r = \int_{\omega_1} P(H_2)P(g|H_2)dxdy + \int_{\omega_2} P(H_1)P(g|H_1)dxdy. \tag{5}$$

3 The Level Set Models

The Bayesian risk will be used to deduce the level set evolution functional for segmentation. An image is taken as a function $g(x, y) : \Omega \to R$, where (x, y)'s denote spatial coordinates and Ω is an open subset of R^2. The image is formed by two phases (zones) which may consist of several disconnected parts. We denote these phases as ω_i, $i = 1, 2$, and the boundary of ω_i is $\partial\Omega$. Assuming that phase ω_i is represented by a Lipschitz function $\phi(x, y)$, called level set function, such that

$$\begin{cases} \phi(x, y) < 0, & \text{if } (x, y) \in \omega_1, \\ \phi(x, y) > 0, & \text{if } (x, y) \in \omega_2, \\ \phi(x, y) = 0, & \text{if } (x, y) \in \partial\Omega. \end{cases} \tag{6}$$

We denote the evolving curve as C and it is completely determined by level set function ϕ. To describe a region in which ϕ is greater than zero or not, a unit step function called Heaviside function is used. The Heaviside function H and its Dirac measure δ_0 are defined as

$$H(\phi) = \begin{cases} 1, & \text{if } \phi \geq 0, \\ 0, & \text{if } \phi < 0, \end{cases} \tag{7}$$

and

$$\delta_0(\phi) = \frac{d}{d\phi} H(\phi). \tag{8}$$

In the two-phase segmentation, the proposed approach is based on minimizing the functional containing *Bayesian* and *regularity* terms, and is described as

$$F(C, \phi) = F_B(C, \phi) + F_R(C, \phi), \tag{9}$$

where $F_B(C, \phi)$ is the *Bayesian* term and $F_R(C, \phi)$ is the *regularity* term; curve C is represented by zero level set (*i.e.*, $\phi(x, y) = 0$). The statistical decision theories are generally used for decision making. Here we apply minimizing the Bayesian risk to find the boundaries of targets in an image and the Bayesian term is defined as

$$F_B(C, \phi) = \int_{\omega_2} P(\omega_1) P(g|\omega_1) dxdy + \int_{\omega_1} P(\omega_2) P(g|\omega_2) dxdy. \tag{10}$$

To prevent the curve from generating excessively irregular shape and lots of small regions, we set the *regularity* term [4] as

$$F_R(C, \phi) = v \int_{\Omega} \delta_0(\phi(x, y)) |\nabla \phi(x, y)| dxdy, \tag{11}$$

where $v \geq 0$ is the constant for weighting the *regularity* term.

Assuming that the gray levels of image pixels are *Gaussian* distribution and mutually independent (*i.e.*, approximately independent and identically distributed). The *pdf* of image pixels is expressed by

$$P(g|\omega_i) = \frac{1}{\sqrt{2\pi}\sigma_i} \exp\left[\frac{-(g - \mu_i)^2}{2\sigma_i^2}\right], i = 1, 2, \tag{12}$$

where g denotes the random variable of pixel gray levels; μ_i and σ_i are the mean and variance of phase ω_i. To eliminate the exponential form of the *Gaussian* function, we take logarithm to make the functional of *Bayesian* term as

$$F_B(C, \phi) = \int_{\omega_2} \ln P(\omega_1) - \frac{1}{2}\left(\ln(2\pi\sigma_1^2) + \frac{(g - \mu_1)^2}{\sigma_1^2}\right) dxdy$$
$$+ \int_{\omega_1} \ln P(\omega_2) - \frac{1}{2}\left(\ln(2\pi\sigma_2^2) + \frac{(g - \mu_2)^2}{\sigma_2^2}\right) dxdy. \tag{13}$$

Based on finding the minimum extremal of the functional $F(C, \phi)$, the evolving curve C will approach the target boundary. The functional $F(C, \phi)$ is minimized by solving the associated Euler-Lagrange equation. Consequently, the level set equation for evolution process is given as

$$\frac{\partial \phi}{\partial t} = \delta_0(\phi)\left\{v \, div\left(\frac{\nabla \phi}{|\nabla \phi|}\right) - \left[\ln P(\omega_1) - \frac{1}{2}\left(\ln\left(2\pi\sigma_1^2\right) + \frac{(g - \mu_1)^2}{\sigma_1^2}\right)\right]\right.$$
$$\left. + \left[\ln P(\omega_2) - \frac{1}{2}\left(\ln\left(2\pi\sigma_2^2\right) + \frac{(g - \mu_2)^2}{\sigma_2^2}\right)\right]\right\}, \tag{14}$$

with initial condition $\phi(x, y, t = 0) = \phi_0(x, y)$ in Ω and boundary condition

$$\frac{\delta_0(\phi)}{|\nabla \phi|} \frac{\partial \phi}{\partial \vec{n}} = 0 \text{ on } \partial\Omega, \tag{15}$$

where $\vec{n}$ is the unit normal at the boundary $\partial\Omega$ and $\dfrac{\partial\phi}{\partial\vec{n}}$ is the normal derivative of ϕ at the boundary. In Eq.(14), we use a conservative statistical procedure [17] to estimate two priori probabilities $P(\omega_1)$ and $P(\omega_2)$. During the processing, if the pixel number in phase ω_1 is increasing (decreasing), the probability $P(\omega_1)$ must be increased (decreased). Thus, $P(\omega_1)$ and $P(\omega_2)$ are initially set 1/2; then, if ω_1 phase is increased (i.e., pixel number at $(i+1)th$ iteration is greater than that at ith iteration in ω_1), we accordingly modify the priori probability.

4 Experiments

Three kinds of experiments were executed to evaluate the performance of boundary extraction (edge detection). They are high-noisy and low-contrast image segmentation, multi-phase image segmentation, and medical image segmentation.

Level set function is represented by discrete grids, and zero level set is identified by linear interpolation. For spatial derivative approximation of level set equations, first order upwind approximations [14] were used to keep the numerical solution stable when computing derivatives.

At first, to understand the ability of level set methods for edge detection, a high-noisy synthetic image of a blurred-boundary circle target was used to examine the three mentioned level set methods: Chan-Vese level set method [4], Martin's level set method [9], and the proposed Bayesian level set method as shown in Fig. 1. From the results, we can see that all three methods can detect the target boundary, but the proposed method produces the smoothest and most matched contour.

Medical images are a special category of images in their characteristics and purposes. Segmentation on *CT* images is useful for checking aneurysms, calcifications, brain tumors, or other abnormalities. Two *CT* abdominal images shown in Fig. 2 (a) and (b) were segmented as results shown in Fig. 2 (c) and (d). In Fig. 2 (c), the boundary of a spurious tumor has been extracted at the top left of the liver for further processes. Although a few blood vessels and normal parts have also been extracted, these regions are certainly ignored for diagnosis applications. There are no interested regions found in Fig. 2 (d).

Brain image segmentation in *MRI* delineates the neuroanatomical structures to provide quantification of cortical atrophy and assistance in diagnosis. The brain structures, cerebrospinal fluid (*CSF*), gray matter (*GM*), and white matter (*WM*), are used to quantify the evolution of many lesions like brain atrophy, hydrocephalus, and brain tumors. The purpose of brain cortical segmentation is to accurately extract the *CSF*, *GM*, and *WM* boundaries. In *MRI* images, brightness contrast of tissues is dependent on the proton spin density (*PD*), spin-lattice relaxation time (*T*1), and spin-spin relaxation time (*T*2) of the tissues being imaged. We used the proposed multiple-phase method to extract the boundaries of *CSF*, *GM*, and *WM*. *T*1- and *T*2-weighted *MRI* images shown in Fig. 3 (a) and (b) were segmented as results shown in Fig. 3 (c) and (d). As indicated by the segmented results, we can find that these boundaries are correctly extracted. The segmented regions for *T*1-weighted *MRI* image are respectively shown in Fig. 3 (e) to (h), where black regions stand for the segmented results.

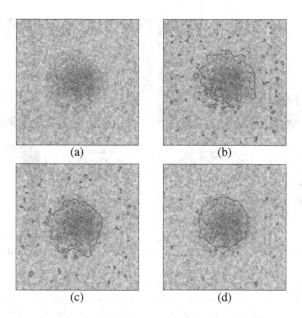

Fig. 1. A low-contrast and high-noisy image of a blurred-boundary target. (a) The original image. (b) The segmented result of Chan-Vese model. (c) Result of Martin's model. (d) Result of the proposed approach.

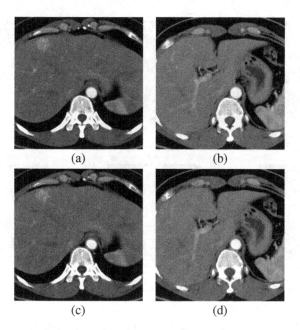

Fig. 2. Boundary extraction of *CT* abdominal images. (a) and (b) The original images. (c) and (d) The segmented results.

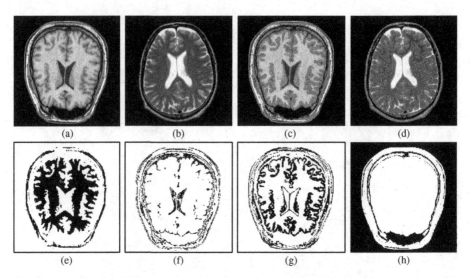

Fig. 3. *WM*, *GM*, and *CSF* boundary extraction from human-brain $T1$- and $T2$- weighted *MRI* image using the proposed multiple-phase level set model. (a) and (b) The original images. (c) and (d) The extracted results. (e) The region of $\phi_1 < 0$ and $\phi_2 < 0$ for $T1$-weighted *MRI* image. (f) The region of $\phi_1 < 0$ and $\phi_2 > 0$. (g) The region of $\phi_1 > 0$ and $\phi_2 < 0$. (h) The region of $\phi_1 > 0$ and $\phi_2 > 0$.

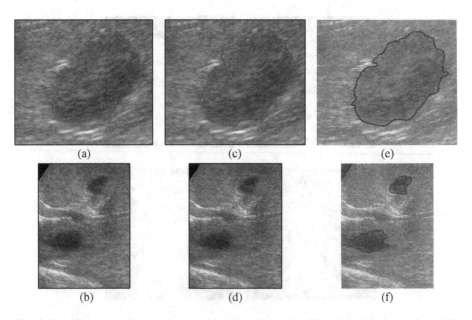

Fig. 4. Boundary extraction of ultrasound images. (a) and (b) The original images. (c) and (d) The extracted boundaries. (e) and (f) The manual-traced boundaries.

Ultrasound images are obtained by emitting and receiving reflects of high-frequency sound waves. The reflected sound wave echoes are recorded and displayed as an image. Segmentation on ultrasound images is useful for examining body's internal organs, heart, liver, spleen, pancreas, and kidneys. Two ultrasound images shown in Fig. 4 (a) and (b) were segmented. The boundary of a tumor was accurately extracted as shown in Fig. 4 (c), and the boundaries of two spurious tumors were extracted as shown in Fig. 4 (d). The manual-traced boundaries are shown in Fig. 4 (e) and (f) for comparison. Due to the influence of imaging devices, such as speckles and random noises, the quality of images are heavily degraded; however, the proposed approach is still able to extract satisfactory boundaries of interested targets.

5 Conclusions

In this paper, level set methods were proposed for image segmentation in which the Bayesian risk was used to develop the segmentation algorithms. At first, the image segmentation was formulated as a classification of pixels. Then the Bayesian risk is formed by false-positive and false-negative fractions in a hypothesis test. Through minimizing the risk of misclassification, the level set evolution functional was deduced for finding the boundaries of targets. To prevent the propagating curves from generating excessively irregular shape and lots of small regions, curvature and gradient of images were integrated in the functional. Finally, we used Euler-Lagrange formula to minimize the functional to derive the level set evolution equations. The generated level set equations were useful for segmenting various kinds of medical images; moreover, the developed equations and algorithms are easily extended for multiphase segmentation.

The proposed approach has the following advantages: (*i*) The statistical decision theories are integrated into the derivation of level set method; hence the boundaries of targets can be more accurately extracted. (*ii*) The proposed approach takes the pixel distribution into the segmentation, so that the local noises have less influence to the propagating process. (*iii*) Many complicated shapes, such as corners, cavities, convexity, and concavities can be extracted at one time; the proposed approach is highly compatible with the medical image segmentation. (*iv*) The proposed method can be easily extended to facilitate the multiphase and 3-D surface segmentation.

References

1. Armstrong, P., Wastie, M.L.: Diagnostic Imaging. Blackwell Scientific Publications, London (1989)
2. Bryan, G.J.: Diagnostic Radiography: A Concise Practical Manual. Churchill Livingstone Inc., New York (1987)
3. Osher, S., Sethian, J.A.: Fronts propagating with curvature-dependent speed: algorithms based on Hamilton-Jacobi formulations. Journal of Computational Physics 79, 12–49 (1998)
4. Chan, T.F., Vese, L.A.: Active contours without edges. IEEE Trans. Image Processing 10, 266–277 (2001)

5. Mumford, D., Shah, J.: Optimal approximation by piecewise smooth functions and associated variational problems. Commun. Pure Appl. Math. 42, 577–685 (1989)
6. Chan, T.F., Sandberg, B.Y., Vese, L.A.: Active contours without edges for vector-valued images. Journal of Visual Communication and Image Representation 11, 130–141 (2000)
7. Chan, T.F., Vese, L.A.: A level set algorithm for minimizing the Mumford-Shah functional in image processing. In: Proc. IEEE Workshop on Variational and Level Set Methods in Computer Vision, Vancouver, BC, Canada, pp. 161–168 (2001)
8. Lee, S.-H., Seo, J.K.: Level set-based bimodal segmentation with stationary global minimum. IEEE Trans. Image Processing 15, 2843–2852 (2006)
9. Martin, P., Refregier, P., Goudail, F., Guerault, F.: Influence of the noise model on level set active contour segmentation. IEEE Trans. Pattern Anal. Mach. Intell. 26, 799–803 (2004)
10. Suri, J.S., Liu, K., Singh, S., Laxminarayan, S.N., Zeng, X., Reden, L.: Shape recovery algorithms using level sets in 2-D/3-D medical imagery: A state-of-the-art review. IEEE Trans. Information Technology in Biomedicine 6, 8–28 (2002)
11. Goldenberg, R., Kimmel, R., Rivlin, E., Rudzsky, M.: Cortex segmentation: A fast variational geometric approach. IEEE Trans. Medical Imaging 21, 1544–1551 (2002)
12. Weickert, J., ter Haar Romeny, B.M., Viergever, M.A.: Efficient and reliable scheme for nonlinear diffusion filtering. IEEE Trans. Image Processing 7, 398–410 (1998)
13. Chenoune, Y., Delechelle, E., Petit, E., Goissen, T., Garot, J., Rahmouni, A.: Segmentation of cardiac cine-MR images and myocardial deformation assessment using level set methods. Computerized Medical Imaging and Graphics 29, 607–616 (2005)
14. Osher, S., Fedkiw, R.: Level Set Methods and Dynamic Implicit Surfaces. Springer, New York (2003)
15. Casella, G., Berger, R.L.: Statistical Inference, Calif Wadsworth & Brooks/Cole, CA (1990)
16. Strickland, R.N.: Image-Processing Techniques Tumor Detection. Marcel Dekker Inc., New York (2002)
17. Mendenhall, W., Sincich, T.: Statistics for Engineering and The Sciences. Prentice-Hall, New Jersey (1994)

A Worm Model Based on Artificial Life for Automatic Segmentation of Medical Images

Jian Feng, Xueyan Wang, and Shuqian Luo

College of Biomedical Engineering, Capital Medical University,
Beijing 100069, China
sqluo@ieee.org

Abstract. An intelligent deformable model called worm model is constructed. The worm has a central nervous system, vision, perception and motor systems. It is able to memorize, recognize objects and control the motion of its body. The new model overcomes the defects of existing methods since it is able to process the segmentation of the image intelligently using more information available rather than using pixels and gradients only. The experimental results of segmentation of the corpus callosum from MRI brain images show that the proposed worm model is able to segment medical images automatically and accurately. For those images that are more complex or with fragmentary boundaries, the predominance of the worm model is especially clear.

1 Introduction

The correct classification of human organs in medical image can provide computer -assisted diagnosis for clinicians, and is the groundwork of some image processing, such as the 3D reconstruction and the visualization of medical images. Several segmentation algorithms exist, but they are far from perfect. The available methods to segment medical image include threshold value segmentation algorithm, edge detection algorithm using differential operators, region growing method and clustering segmentation algorithm. Traditional segmentation algorithms for medical image are based on the information of the pixel intensity and/or the gradient of intensity [1]. Artificial life based segmentation of medical image is fairly new. Recent researches show that the method using deformable model based on artificial life is effective to segment image because it can take full advantage of local and global information [2-5]. Abbreviated to Alife, Artificial Life was officially put forward in an artificial life seminar in the U.S. on September 21st, 1987. According to its founder, Alife is a manmade system that has natural life characteristic [6, 7].

In this paper, an intelligent deformable model called worm model is constructed. The worm has a central nervous system, vision system, perception system and locomotion system. It can memorize, recognize objects and control the motion of its body. It overcomes the defects of the current existing methods since it is able to process the segmentation of the image intelligently using more available information, rather than only using pixels and gradients. Its ability to segment the corpus callosum (CC) from MRI brain images shows that the worm model could segment images automatically and accurately. For those images that are more complex or with fragmentary boundary, the predominance of the worm model is especially clear.

X. Gao et al. (Eds.): MIMI 2007, LNCS 4987, pp. 35–43, 2008.

2 Method

2.1 The Construction of the Worm Model

The worm model, no larger than several pixels, is made up of many nodes, and it possesses 'head', 'neck' and 'body'. The 'head' is the function section, which has a nerve center system, vision system, perception system, and it also can memorize information and give off orders. The 'neck' and the 'body' are locomotion parts.

The worm's eyes are located in the head, they are able to emit lines of sight to produce the sense of vision. It has fan-shaped eyeshot, each line of sight is less than 7 pixels by considering the actual size of targets. In order to make a rational vision scope for the worm model, we define that the angle between each line is 15 degrees, and the angle between the first line of sight and the body is 15 degrees, too. Then the angle between the seventh line of sight and the body will be up to 105 degrees, so it can provide a rational vision scope for the worm to search for targets.

The perception organ, located in the head, has two functions. Firstly, the perception organ is a useful supplement for the vision organ. Because the field of eyeshot is just in front of the neck, it cannot see the fields out of its eyeshot. Then it has to use its perception organ to perceive those fields. Secondly, the perceptual organ can be used as a sensor and a trigger. When the worm is in very dangerous surroundings, for instance, its head is too close to the edge, the perceptual organ will trigger the worm to take urgent measures to avoid collision. If the perceptual organ has detected the finishing information, it would trigger the worm to stop searching or moving immediately.

The function of the worm's neck is to harmonize locomotion. By changing the values of the orientation profile and/or the length profile in the neck, it will look up or look down to change its eyeshot, thus it can adjust itself during moving.

The worm's body is the locomotion center. The worm will go forward or backward by changing the slope values of the orientation profile and/or the length profile in the body.

2.2 The Worm's Cognition System

The worm's life system includes nerve center system, perception system, vision system and motor system (Figure 1).

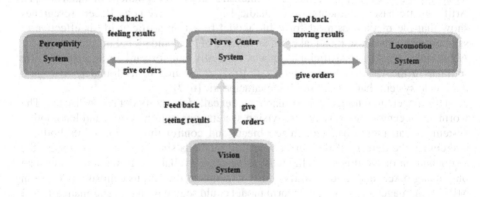

Fig. 1. The worm's life system

The nerve center system is composed of cognition system, memory system and feedback processing system. The Back Propagation Nerve Net is used in the cognition system. Because there are 7 lines of vision in the eyeshot and each line is less than 7 pixels, the vision information will be transformed into 7×7 matrix before it is sent to the brain. Thus the number of the input layer nodes is 49. Based on the actual requirements, it is determined that the number of the output layer nodes be 3. Experimental results indicate better results are obtained when the number of the concealed layer nodes is about half the number of the input layer nodes. For this reason, the number of the concealed layer nodes is 25.

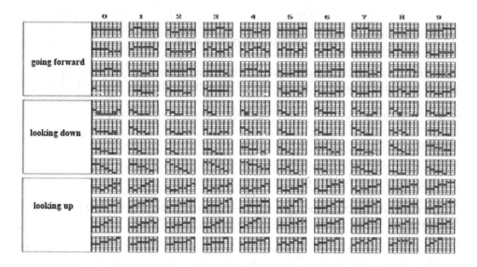

Fig. 2. Training samples for the worm

The output codes represent the worm's locomotion directions, which include going forward, looking up and looking down respectively. Training samples are changed to concur with the actual instance in MR images, while at the same time to ensure that the recognition ratio of the training samples is higher than 98% (Figure 2).

2.3 The Worm's Cognition Process

There are four steps in the process of the worm's cognition.

Step 1. The nerve center commands the vision organ to emit lines of vision within its eyeshot to detect the edge of the image.

Step 2. The vision system will rectify the vision information, and then send it to the nerve center system.

Because the worm has a fan-shaped eyeshot, and the length of the vision lines is used to form the vision matrix, the vision information has to be twisted. For example, a beeline is translated into a folded line when it is captured by the vision system (Figure 3a, b). Thus, the vision information is rectified before it is sent to the nerve center system.

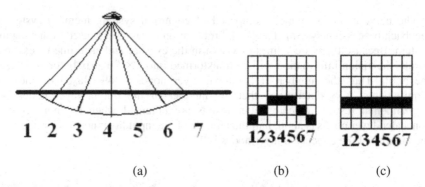

Fig. 3. The rectification of the vision codes

The vision information is rectified with geometry knowledge. The fourth line of vision is made as the benchmark line. The angle between the third line or the fifth line and the benchmark line is $\dfrac{\pi}{12}$, thus, the third and the fifth line can be described as following:

$$L(i) = L(i) \cdot \cos \frac{\pi}{12} \qquad i = 3, 5; \tag{1}$$

The second and the sixth, the first and the seventh line can be described respectively as following:

$$L(i) = L(i) \cdot \cos \frac{\pi}{6} \qquad i = 2, 6; \tag{2}$$

$$L(i) = L(i) \cdot \cos \frac{\pi}{4} \qquad i = 1, 7; \tag{3}$$

After being rectified, the vision codes are able to incarnate the true instance of the detected edge (Fig. 3c).

Step 3. The nerve center system identifies and processes the vision matrix, then gives off a locomotion order as well as memorizes the current moving direction and track.

Step 4. During the locomotion, the worm has sense of touch. When the worm is in very dangerous surroundings, such as its head is too close to the edge, the perception organ will trigger the worm to take urgent measures to avoid it. If the perception organ has detected the finishing information, it would trigger the worm to stop immediately.

3   Results and Analysis

3.1   The Segmentation Results Using the Worm Model

Firstly, convert a MR image into a binary image, and then place a worm model on the top of this image. Based on prior experience, the worm can automatically find the

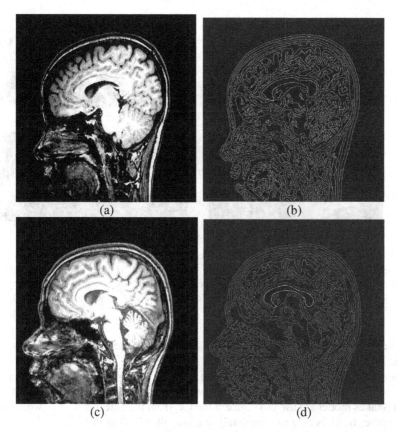

Fig. 4. The segmentation results using the worm model

corpus callosum. It will then go down to the CC's center where it will divide into four little worms in order to detect edges in different directions. These worms are commanded to detect image edges in four different directions: up-left, up-right, bottom-left, and bottom-right. Lastly, the detecting tracks are memorized when the image edges are detected completely. Figure 4b and 4d show the segmentation results using the worm model.

3.2 Comparison with Other Methods

Comparison with Other Methods. We process the image shown in Figure 5 using other methods, such as Canny operator, Sobel template and region growing method. After several experiments, the optimal parameters for each method are obtained. The threshold gray gradient value is 128 in Canny operator, while it is 80 in Sobel template, and the growing threshold value is 12 in region growing method. The image processed by these methods shows that there are discontinuities in the vault of the CC (Figure5a, b, c). However, there is no discontinuity in the vault when the worm model is used (Figure 5d).

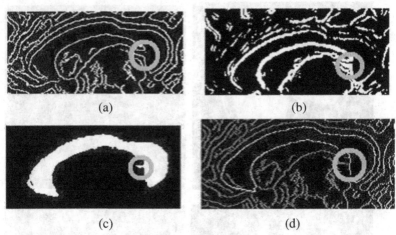

(a)   (b)

(c)   (d)

Fig. 5. Comparison with Canny operator, Sobel template and region growing method: (*a*) Segmented by Canny operator, the edge in the vault of the CC is discontinuous; (*b*) Segmented by Sobel template, the edge in the vault of the CC is discontinuous; (*c*) Segmented by region growing method, the edge of the CC is wrong; (*d*) Segmented by the worm model, the edge in the vault of the CC is continuous.

Comparison with the Snakes Model. Segmenting the CC using Snakes model required locating the CC and drafting the edge by hand. The worm model, however, segments the CC automatically only using a few prior experiences, thus getting rid of the dependence on manual work. Figure 6a shows errors are incurred at the vault edge when Snakes model are used to segment the CC from the MR image. The worm model, on the other hand, is able to completely segment the CC (Figure 6b).

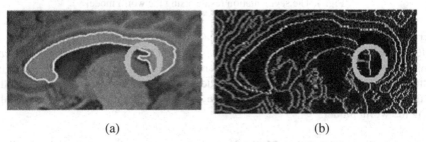

(a)   (b)

Fig. 6. Comparison with Snakes model: (*a*) Segmented by Snakes model, the edge in the vault of the CC is not correct; (*b*) Segmented by the worm model, the edge in the vault of the CC is continuous.

3.3 Quantitative Comparison with Other Methods

Quantifying the segmentation result of a medical image, there is no golden standard for the evaluation [1]. In order to quantitatively compare with other algorithms, an experimental model is constructed as shown in Figure 7a. The target edge is an ellipse (Figure 7b), which is interrupted by four small shapes. These shapes, two being round and two being rectangular, represent pliable and sharp interruption to the target edge, and their gray values are chosen respectively as 32 and 64, which are close to the gray value of the target edge.

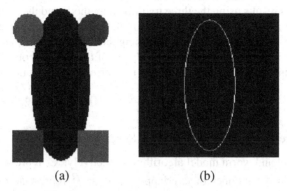

(a)   (b)

Fig. 7. The experimental image

The experimental model is processed using each of the different methods, namely, Canny operator, Sobel template, region growing method, Snakes model and worm model. The same parameter from each method is used as the one stated before. The segmenting results are shown in Figure 8. For easy comparison and calculation, the result from the region growing method is processed to only distill the edge (Figure 8d).

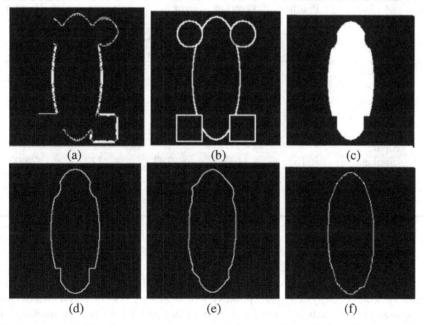

(a)   (b)   (c)

(d)   (e)   (f)

Fig. 8. The segmenting results of different methods: (a) Segmenting result using Canny operator; (b) Segmenting result using Sobel template; (c) Segmenting result using region growing method; (d) The edge of the region growing result; (e) Segmenting result using Snakes model; (f) Segmenting result using worm model.

After subtracting target image (Figure 7b) from the segmenting images (Figure 8a, b, d, e, f), five sorts of data are obtained. The first sort of data is the number of the pixels in the standard segmentation result. The second sort is the number of the pixels in the segmentation results using the three traditional methods and the worm model. The third sort is the number of overlapping pixels in the corresponding place. The fourth sort is the number of error pixels within the 8-neighbors of the corresponding correct pixels. The last sort is the number of error pixels out of the 8-neighbors of the corresponding correct pixels. We define the measure of the correct ratio as following:

$$C_i = \frac{\alpha_i + \beta_i}{\gamma_i} \times 100 \quad i = 1, 2, 3, 4, 5 \tag{4}$$

Where, i represents Canny operator, Sober template, region growing algorithm, Snakes model and worm model algorithm respectively; C represents the correct ratio; α represents the number of overlapping pixels; β represents the number of error pixels within the 8-neighbors; γ represents the number of the CC pixels segmented by the five algorithms.

The target image in Table 1 has a continuous edge and 392 pixels. It shows that the worm model method has remarkable advantage.

Table 1. Quantitative comparison of different methods

	Pixels	Overlap-ping pixels	error pixels within 8-neighbors	error pixels out of 8-neighbors	Correct ratio (%)
Canny operator	1301	233	425	643	50.58
Sobel template	1970	322	522	1126	42.84
region growing	520	112	277	131	74.81
Snakes model	516	105	287	124	75.97
worm model	452	139	248	65	85.62

4 Conclusions

An artificial life model is introduced to segment medical images. This model has nerve center system, vision system, perception system and motor system, and it also has some life characteristic, such as memorizing, cognizing and locomotion controlling. The model is able to take full advantage of local information because it has alterable eyeshot and flexible deformation. As a result, it can automatically segment the target using more information than just pixels and gradients, and it can also overcome the inadequacies of the traditional algorithms. Furthermore, it has a high intelligence and only need a few prior experiences.

In this study, we simply segment the CC based on binary images, and only give the worm some elementary life characteristics. Future investigations will involve directly segmenting the grayscale image to enhance the life characteristics of the worm model, and apply this model to 3D reconstruction of medical images.

Acknowledgement

This work was supported by grant from the National Natural Science Foundation of China (No. 60472020).

References

1. Luo, S., Zhou, G.: Medical image processing and analysis, pp. 65–138. Science Press, Beijing (2003)
2. Montagnat, J., Delingette, H., Ayache, N.: A review of deformable surfaces: topology, geometry and deformation. Image and Vision Computing 19, 1023–1040 (2001)
3. Pizer, S., Fletcher, P., Fridman, Y., Fritsch, D., Gash, A., Glotzer, J., Joshi, S., Thall, A., Tracton, G., Yushkevich, P., Chaney, E.: Deformable m-reps for 3D medical image segmentation. International Journal of Computer Vision 55, 85–106 (2003)
4. Shen, D., Davatzikos, C.: An adaptive-focus deformable model using statistical and geometric information. IEEE Transactions on Pattern Analysis and Machine Intelligence 22, 906–913 (2000)
5. Sebastian, T.B., Tek, H., Crisco, J.J., Kimia, B.B.: Segmentation of carpal bones from CT images using skeletally coupled deformable models. Medical Image Analysis 7, 21–45 (2003)
6. Huang, W., Pan, Z.: Applications of Artificial Life in Computer Graphics. Journal of Computer-Aided Design & Computer Graphics 17, 1383–1388 (2005)
7. McInerney, T., Hamarneh, G., Sheton, M., Terzopoulos, D.: Deformable organisms for automatic medical image analysis. Medical Image Analysis 6, 251–266 (2002)

An Iterative Reconstruction for Poly-energetic X-ray Computed Tomography

Ho-Shiang Chueh[1], Wen-Kai Tsai[1], Chih-Chieh Chang[1], Shu-Ming Chang[1], Kuan-Hao Su[1], and Jyh-Cheng Chen[1,2,*]

[1] Department of Biomedical Imaging and Radiological Sciences, National Yang-Ming University, Taipei, Taiwan

[2] Department of Education and Research, Taipei City Hospital, Taipei, Taiwan, R.O.C.
*jcchen@ym.edu.tw

Abstract. A beam-hardening effect is a common problem affecting the quantitative ability of X-ray computed tomography. We develop a statistical reconstruction for a poly-energetic model, which can effectively reduce beam-hardening effects. A phantom test is used to evaluate our approach in comparison with traditional correction methods. Unlike previous methods, our algorithm utilizes multiple energy-corresponding blank scans to estimate attenuation map for a particular energy spectrum. Therefore, our algorithm has an energy-selective reconstruction. In addition to the benefits of other iterative reconstructions, our algorithm has the advantage in no requirement for prior knowledge about object material, energy spectrum of source and energy sensitivity of the detector. The results showed an improvement in the coefficient of variation, uniformity and signal-to-noise ratio demonstrating better beam hardening correction in our approach.

Keywords: beam-hardening, poly-energetic, iterative reconstruction.

1 Introduction

X-ray computed tomography had provided anatomic information for more than 3 decades. The modern X-ray computed tomography can provide more quantitative information about geometry and density. A beam-hardening effect is a major reason affecting accuracy of quantitative results[1]. Several correction methods for beam-hardening have been reprinted, such as linearization and dual energy methods[2-5]. In these post-processing beam hardening correction methods, energy-independent projections can be calculated from energy-dependent raw projections and then be applied with mono-energetic reconstruction. It is easy to reduce the beam-hardening effect. However, the main disadvantage is the material dependence. A statistical reconstruction for poly-energetic model has been presented in 2001 by Elbakri and Fessler[6,7]. They have also showed several benefits in the statistical method. They assume the object is comprised of several known non-overlapping tissue types and the attenuation coefficient is modeled as the product of the energy-dependent mass attenuation coefficient and the energy- independent density of the tissue. They also assume the mass attenuation coefficients of the several tissue types are known. This method can reduce beam hardening because it estimates the energy-independent

X. Gao et al. (Eds.): MIMI 2007, LNCS 4987, pp. 44–50, 2008.

density. For our algorithm, it is also an iterative reconstruction for the poly-energetic model. However, the difference is that we assume the energy spectrum is comprised of several sub-energy spectrums. The expected photon flux for each sub-spectrum can be respectively calculated by an energy-corresponding blank scan and attenuation map. The energy-corresponding blank scan can be obtained by different filters. We also assume there is a relationship between attenuations for a particular sub-energy spectrum to another. Then, we can formulate a maximum-likelihood function for the poly-energetic model and develop an iterative algorithm to estimate a discrete attenuation map for the particular energy spectrum. Because the sub-energy spectrum is relatively narrow compared to the original energy spectrum, the beam hardening can be reduced. In addition to the benefits of statistical reconstruction, our algorithm has the advantage in being knowledge-free to tissue type and mass attenuation coefficients.

The first section describes a background and discusses a difference between our algorithm and other published method. The next section explains our statistical reconstruction for poly-energetic X-ray computed tomography. Then, several results generalized by different methods for comparison are showed in section 3. Finally, we discuss and summarize the results in section 4 and 5, respectively.

2   Iterative Reconstruction Algorithm

For a ray of infinitesimal width, the expected photon flux detected along a particular projection line L_j is given by:

$$\bar{y}_j(\varepsilon) = I_j(\varepsilon) \exp\left[-\int_{L_j} \mu(\bar{x}, \varepsilon) dl\right] \tag{1}$$

where y_j represents the photon flux measured at the jth in N detectors and $\bar{y}_j$ is its expectation. The $I_j(\varepsilon)$ is the initial photon flux detected by the jth detector. It incorporates the energy dependence of the incident ray and detector sensitivity. The integral in the exponent is taken over the line L_j and μ is X-ray attenuation coefficient, which is dependent on spatial coordinates and beam energy. The goal of any CT algorithm is to reconstruct the attenuation map μ from the measured data $[y_1,...,y_N]$.

In our statistical reconstruction algorithm, we assume the energy spectrum ε is comprised of K sub-energy spectrums. For the kth sub-energy spectrum, the expected photon flux is given by:

$$\bar{y}_j(\varepsilon_k) = I_j(\varepsilon_k) \exp\left[-\int_{L_j} \mu(\bar{x}, \varepsilon_k) dl\right] \tag{2}$$

and $I_j(\varepsilon) = \sum_{k=1}^{K} I_j(\varepsilon_k)$, $\bar{y}_j(\varepsilon) = \sum_{k=1}^{K} \bar{y}_j(\varepsilon_k)$. We also assume a ratio of attenuation for kth sub-energy spectrum to the particular sub-energy spectrum is known.

$$r_k = \mu(\varepsilon_k)/\mu(\varepsilon_1) \tag{3}$$

where $r_1=1$ and the ε_1 is the particular sub-energy spectrum.

Therefore, the expected photon flux for the whole energy spectrum is expressed by:

$$\bar{y}_j(\varepsilon) = \sum_{k=1}^{K} I_j(\varepsilon_k) \exp\left[-r_k \int_{L_j} \mu(\bar{x},\varepsilon_1) dl\right] \tag{3}$$

For image reconstruction, we parameterize the three-dimensional object space using isotropic voxels. Let $\mu = [\mu_1, \cdots, \mu_p]^T$ be the vector of unknown attenuation coefficient, where T stands for transpose. The expected count number of detected photon can be calculated by

$$\bar{d}_j = \sum_{k=1}^{K}\left[b_{jk}\exp\left(-r_k[A\mu]_j\right)\right], \quad j=1,\cdots,N \tag{4}$$

where the d_j and $\bar{d}_j$ are measured and expected count number at jth detector, respectively. The b_{jk} is the count number measured at jth detector for kth energy spectrum. The notation $[A\mu]_j$ denotes the inner product $\sum_{i=1}^{p} a_{ij}\mu_i$. This inner product can be interpreted as the line integral of the discrete attenuation along jth ray. The $A=\{a_{ij}\}$ is a system matrix, which is an intersection length for jth ray at ith voxel.

Each count of measurement can be looked upon as a random variable associated with an approximate Poisson process. The log-likelihood function can be expressed as

$$L(\mu) = \sum_{j=1}^{N}\left\{d_j \ln\left[\sum_{k=1}^{K}\left(b_{jk} e^{-r_k[A\mu]_j}\right)\right] - \sum_{k=1}^{K}\left(b_{jk} e^{-r_k[A\mu]_j}\right)\right\} \tag{5}$$

The first differential of log-likelihood function can be expressed as

$$\frac{\partial L(\mu)}{\partial \mu_i} = \sum_{j=1}^{N}\left\{\frac{d_j \sum_{k=1}^{K}\left(-r_k a_{ij} b_{jk} e^{-r_k[A\mu]_j}\right)}{\sum_{k=1}^{K}\left(b_{jk} e^{-r_k[A\mu]_j}\right)} + \sum_{k=1}^{K}\left(r_k a_{ij} b_{jk} e^{-r_k[A\mu]_j}\right)\right\} \tag{6}$$

$$\frac{\partial L(\mu)}{\partial \mu_i} = \sum_{j=1}^{N} a_{ij}\left\{\frac{-d_j \sum_{k=1}^{K} r_k \bar{d}_{jk}}{\sum_{k=1}^{K} \bar{d}_{jk}} + \sum_{k=1}^{K} r_k \bar{d}_{jk}\right\} \tag{7}$$

A gradient algorithm[8;9] updates the attenuation coefficient vector by

$$\mu_i^{n+1} = \mu_i^n + \frac{\mu_i^n}{\sum_{j=1}^{N} d_j a_{ij}} \frac{\partial L(\mu)}{\partial \mu_i} \tag{8}$$

The n is iteration number. For accelerating reconstruction, an order-subset technique is utilized[10-12].

$$\mu_i^{n,s+1} = \mu_i^{n,s} + \frac{\mu_i^{n,s}}{\sum_{j \in S(s)} d_j a_{ij}} \sum_{j \in S(s)} a_{ij} \left\{ \frac{-d_j \sum_{k=1}^{K} r_k \overline{d}_{jk}}{\sum_{k=1}^{K} \overline{d}_{jk}} + \sum_{k=1}^{K} r_k \overline{d}_{jk} \right\} \qquad (9)$$

The order-subset algorithm updates all estimates of attenuation in the iteration. The s is subset number. The $S(s)$ contains the rays in subset s.

3 Results

The projection data is scanned by our home-made microCT. The isotropic voxel size is 30 μm with 8 folds binning. The fan and cone angles are 6.7 and 5.0 degrees, respectively. Uniform water in a cylindrical plastic tube was scanned by 360 projections in 180 degree. The diameter of tube is 16.5mm. The peak voltage is 50kVp.

We compared three procedures, (a) using a mono-energetic reconstruction to data without filter, (b) using a mono-energetic reconstruction to data with 0.5 mm aluminum filter, and (c) using our poly-energetic reconstruction to data without filter. For the poly-energetic, we use two blank scans acquired with and without 0.5mm aluminum filter. However, the measured projections are only acquired without the filter and the same as procedure (a). The mono-energetic and poly-energetic reconstructions are both order-subset gradient algorithm with 10 subsets. All the images are obtained after 3 iterations (seen in Fig. 1). Theoretically, to apply a 0.5mm aluminum filter can effectively reduce the beam hardening because it can attenuate soft X-ray. The higher gray value at edge is observed on Image obtained from procedure (a). It is a typical beam hardening artifact. For assessment of image quality, a coefficient of variation (CV), uniformity and signal-to-noise ratio (SNR) in the same region-of-interest (ROI) that fully covers the water region are showed in Table 1. According to the results on Table 1, the image obtained by our algorithm has the best improvement in CV, uniformity and SNR. An uniformity improvement can be easy observed in profiles of tomography obtained from procedure (b) and (c) (seen in Fig. 2). The results fully demonstrate our algorithm can effectively reduce beam-hardening effect better than others.

Table 1. The comparison of CV, uniformity and SNR for the three conditions

Parameter	Condition (a)	Condition (b)	Condition (c)
CV	5.1%	3.7%	2.7%
Uniformity	13.3%	9.4%	6.8%
SNR	25.83 dB	28.6 dB	31.44 dB

※ The CV is defined as $CV = \sigma/\overline{X}$. C contains the voxels in the ROI. The σ and $\overline{X}$ are standard deviation and mean of gray values in the ROI, respectively. The uniformity is defined as Uniformity $= \left(\overline{X}_H - \overline{X}_L \right)/\overline{X}$. The $\overline{X}_H$ is mean of voxels for upper 25% gray value in the ROI and $\overline{X}_L$ is for lower 25%. The SNR is defined as $SNR = 20\log(\overline{X}/\sigma)$ [3].

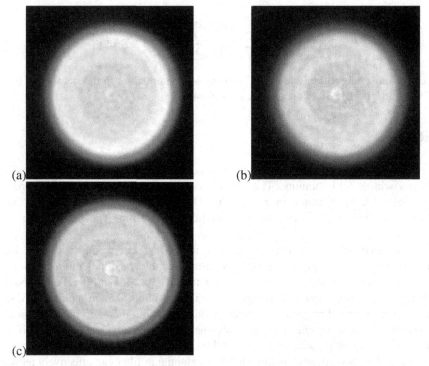

Fig. 1. The images obtained from the three conditions. All images have been linearly normalized from maximum to minimum. Image (a) is a tomograph reconstructed by mono-energetic reconstruction from the data without filter. Image (b) is a tomograph reconstructed by mono-energetic reconstruction from the data with 0.5mm aluminum filter. Image (c) is a tomograph reconstructed by poly-energetic reconstruction from the data without filter.

4   Discussion

In this study, we compared three different procedures. All the results were obtained in the same acquisition parameters, included voltages of tube, current of tube and exposure time. Because no any correction was applied in the procedure A, the results showed more serious beam hardening effect compared to the other procedures. The gray value in central area is lower than edge. The contrast can be shown in Figure 1 (a) and Figure 2. The difference between procedure A and B is the filter. In the procedure B, the 0.5 mm Aluminum filter was applied to stop the soft X-ray and reduced the beam hardening effect. Therefore, the results of procedure B were more uniform (seen in Figure 1 and 2) compared to the results of procedure A. This method is a hardware way to reduce beam hardening effect. It is widely applied in computed tomography. In the procedure C, we used the same data set as procedure A, but different in blank scan. The two blank scans were used in procedure C for the expectation of two sub-energy. Because only one scan is needed by our statistical reconstruction as well as the procedure A, the radiological dose and scan time in our method are the same as the procedure A.

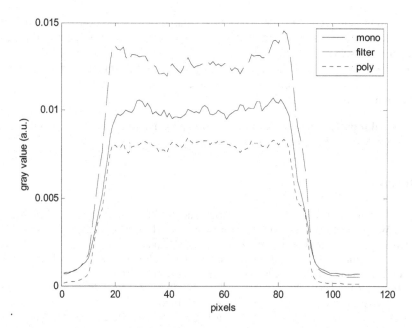

Fig. 2. The dashed line on top is a profile through Image (a) in Fig. 1. The solid line in the middle is a profile through image (b) in Fig. 1. The dotted line on bottom is a profile through image (c) in Fig. 1.

Using our poly-energetic reconstruction, the beam hardening effect can be reduced without the filter. It is specially advantage in soft X-ray computed tomography. In low voltage X-ray condition, most radiological signal will be stopped by the filter. In the post-processing beam hardening correction methods, few parameters are probably adjusted with object characteristics. However, our method is completed object-independent. The ratio r (seen in equation (3)) is possibly changed with different X-ray source, filter, voltage and detector, but no parameter is needed change with object. Comparing to Elbakri's poly-energetic reconstruction [6,7], our method is knowledge-free to material. It is no necessary to know the mass attenuation coefficient of material and segmentation. For single slice reconstruction of 30 iterations, the elapsed time of poly-energetic reconstruction is 43.5 sec and almost the same as mono-energetic reconstruction. There are three major benefits compared to present method of beam hardening correction: (1) no need filter in acquisition, (2) object-independence, (3) material knowledge-free and (4) the reconstruction speed as well as mono-energetic reconstruction.

5   Conclusions

The statistical reconstruction for poly-energetic X-ray computed tomography developed by us has been demonstrated to effectively reduce beam hardening effect, and improve the CV, uniformity and SNR. Our poly-energetic reconstruction is a high feasibility approach, because radiological dose, reconstruction time and scan time as well as mono-energetic method. The beam hardening correction can be achieved without requirement of prior knowledge of object material, energy spectrum of source and energy sensitivity of detector.

The study in this paper is only tested by the uniform object. In future, we will apply our algorithm to more complex object and find its potential in preclinical application.

Acknowledgments. This work was supported by National Science Council under grant NSC95-2622-B-010-004-CC3.

References

1. Li, W., Gill, R., Corbly, A., Jones, B., Belagaje, R., Zhang, Y., Tang, S., Chen, Y., Zhai, Y., Wang, G.M., Wa, A., Hui, K., Westmore, M., Hanson, J., Chen, Y.F., Simons, M., Singh, J.P.: High-Resolution Quantitative Computed Tomography Demonstrating Selective Enhancement of Medium-Size Collaterals by Placental Growth Factor-1 in the Mouse Ischemic Hindlimb. Circulation 113, 2445–2453 (2006)
2. Alvarez, R.E., Macovski, A.: Energy-Selective Reconstructions in X-ray Computerized Tomography. Phys. Med. Biol. 21(5), 733–744 (1976)
3. Van de, C.E., Van, D.D., Sijbers, J., Raman, E.: An Energy-Based Beam Hardening Model in Tomography. Phys. Med. Biol. 47(23), 4181–4190 (2002)
4. Brooks, R.A., Di, C.G.: Beam Hardening in X-ray Reconstructive Tomography. Phys. Med. Biol. 21(3), 390–398 (1976)
5. Macovski, A., Alvarez, R.E., Chan, J.L., Stonestrom, J.P., Zatz, L.M.: Energy Dependent Reconstruction in X-Ray Computerized Tomography. Comput. Biol. Med. 6(4), 325–336 (1976)
6. Elbakri, I.A., Fessler, J.A.: Statistical image Reconstruction For Polyenergetic X-ray Computed Tomography. IEEE Trans Med Imaging 21(2), 89–99 (2002)
7. Idris, A.E., Fessler, J.A.: Segmentation-free Statistical Image Reconstruction for Polyenergetic X-ray computed Tomography with Experimental Validation. Phys. Med. Biol. 48(15), 2453–2477 (2003)
8. Lange, L., Fessler, J.A.: Globally Convergent Algorithms for Maximum a Posteriori Transmission Tomography. IEEE Trans Med Imaging 4(10), 1430–1438 (1995)
9. Erdogan, H., Fessler, J.A.: Monotonic Algorithms for Transmission Tomography. IEEE Trans. Med. Imaging 18(9), 801–814 (1999)
10. Beekman, F.J., Kamphuis, C.: Ordered Subset Reconstruction for X-ray CT. Phys. Med. Biol. 46(7), 1835–1844 (2001)
11. Erdogan, H., Fessler, J.A.: Ordered Subsets Algorithms for Transmission Tomography. Phys. Med. Biol. 44(11), 2835–2851 (1999)
12. Kamphuis, C., Beekman, F.J.: Accelerated Iterative Transmission CT Reconstruction Using an Ordered Subsets Convex Algorithm. IEEE Trans Med Imaging 17(6), 1101–1105 (1998)

Application of Tikhonov Regularization to Super-Resolution Reconstruction of Brain MRI Images

Xin Zhang, Edmund Y. Lam, Ed X. Wu, and Kenneth K.Y. Wong

Department of Electrical and Electronic Engineering,
University of Hong Kong,
Pokfulam Road, Hong Kong
{xinzhang,elam,ewu,kywong}@eee.hku.hk

Abstract. This paper presents an image super-resolution method that enhances spatial resolution of MRI images in the slice-select direction. The algorithm employs Tikhonov regularization, using a standard model of imaging process and reformulating the reconstruction as a regularized minimization task. Our experimental result shows improvements in both signal-to-noise ratio and visual quality.

Keywords: Super-resolution Reconstruction, MRI, Tikhonov Regularization.

1 Introduction

Magnetic Resonance Imaging (MRI) is a non-invasive diagnostic technique to produce computerized images of internal body tissues. Its major goal is to maximize the image spatial resolution so as to provide accurate information for investigators. In this sense, only the improvement of in-plane resolution is not enough. To obtain high-resolution (HR) data in 3-D, the spatial resolution of the standard MRI protocol does not suffice [1], such as diffusion-weighted imaging (DWI) and echo-planar imaging (EPI). That is because acquiring HR images, especially in slice-select direction, would result in the reduction in signal-to-noise ratio (SNR). SNR is proportional to the main magnetic field strength. The decrease in SNR might be obviated by the usage of higher magnetic field scanners, but the corresponding changes in both T_1 and T_2 would further reduce the gain in SNR at the ultrahigh-field-strength MRI [2]. Moreover, higher magnetic strength would both increase inhomogeneity and introduce distortion artifacts into images. Therefore, super-resolution technique, as a post-processing method, has been introduced to enhance the resolution of MRI images.

Image super-resolution reconstruction is to restore a HR image from several low-resolution (LR) images taken from the same scene, but from slightly different view points [3]. Although these images may be translated, blurred, rotated, or corrupted with noise, they can be useful to provide different information for a HR image. Recently the method has been used for the improvement of MRI image

X. Gao et al. (Eds.): MIMI 2007, LNCS 4987, pp. 51–56, 2008.

quality. This application attracted a number of super-resolution reconstruction algorithms to be used in it. Irani and Peleg [4] introduced the Iterative Back Projection (IBP) into the reconstruction. Peled and Yeshurun [5] first presented an implementation of IBP into MRI data, which aimed to reconstruct images of human white matter fiber tract from Diffusion Tensor Imaging (DTI). IBP, because of its simplicity and easy implementation, was frequently utilized in the early development of super-resolution. But the algorithm was also known for its low rate of convergence and sensitivity to noise. Then Hsu *et al.* [6] proposed the application of wavelet-based Projection onto Convex Sets (POCS) super-resolution into cardiovascular MRI images. It extracted information from the non-stationary effect of heart and blood vessels in the successive images to reconstruct a HR image. As for stationary objects, such as the brain, it is not effective to perform a good reconstruction. But requirements of high quality brain MRI images are increasing now in both the neurology and the medicine. Therefore, we take Tikhonov regularization into this application to obtain a brain MRI image super-resolution reconstruction.

Tikhonov regularization is the most commonly used method in the regularization to ill-conditioned problems. In these problems, even small changes in input can result in wild oscillations in the approximation of a solution. In general, image restoration is ill-conditioned and difficult to find out a unique solution directly. Such is the case in MRI image super-resolution reconstruction. To achieve a reasonable solution, we use Tikhonov regularization to reformulate the problem as a regularized unconstrained minimization problem. Then it has a unique minimizer, i.e., the reasonable solution for the reconstruction problem.

In this work we take use of Tikhonov regularization into brain MRI image super-resolution reconstruction. This technique is utilized on a simulation and real brain MRI images to demonstrate the applicability and performance of the super-resolution reconstruction in MRI.

2   Methods

2.1   Observation Model

To perform a super-resolution reconstruction, the first step is to formulate an observation model that relates the original HR image to the acquired LR images. We consider the following problem:

$$Y = Hf + n, \tag{1}$$

where Y and f are vectors of length m representing the acquired LR images and the original HR image respectively, and H is an $m \times m$ linear operator that characterizes the degrading process. n is the vector of length m that represents the additive Gaussian white noise contaminating the measurement. So the problem is to determine the HR image given acquired LR images with the degradation matrix and the additive noise.

2.2   Tikhonov Regularization

Generally, the super-resolution reconstruction is an ill-posed problem because of an insufficient number of LR images and ill-conditioned degrading operator. It is necessary to rely on a regularization to stabilize the inversion of ill-posed problem. Here we take use of Tikhonov regularization for the reconstruction. Through the regularization, the problem (1) is replaced by the problem of seeking an estimate x to minimize the Lagrangian:

$$\min_f \left[\|Y - Hf\|_2^2 + \alpha \|Cf\|_2^2 \right] , \tag{2}$$

where the operator C is generally a high-pass filter, and $\| \cdot \|$ represents L_2 norm. The first term measures the fidelity of the solution to the data while the second term manages the smoothness of the solution. α denotes the Lagrange multiplier, commonly referred to as the regularization factor, that controls the tradeoff between the two terms. C is often chosen as the Laplacian operator to smooth the solution. So the minimizer of (2) expressed as normal equations is:

$$H^T Y = (H^T H - \alpha C^T C)f . \tag{3}$$

where H and C are block Toeplitz matrices. Equation (3) can be solved by Conjugate Gradient (CG), because it is more advantageous than others to solve large, sparse and symmetric positive definite linear system.

2.3   Signal-to-Noise Ratio (SNR)

When it comes to a method for digital image restoration, one should ensure that SNR is not compromised. Because super-resolution reconstruction belongs to the category, it is necessary to take SNR into account. In general, SNR is defined as the ratio of the mean pixel values to the standard deviation of the pixel values outside an interest. For the purpose of demonstrating the improvement of the method, this definition is still satisfactory.

3   Results

3.1   Simulation

A high-SNR, HR (64×64, 1 mm in-plane) image is shifted and contracted so as to create 4 images (32×32). The first two images are acquired with 0- and 1-mm shift in the phase-encode direction, and copies of the two images are shifted by 1 mm in the frequency-encode direction to get the other two images. Then Gaussian white noise is added to the four LR images to give them a SNR of 25dB. A part of one of the LR shifted images with additive noise is shown in Fig. 1A.

The reconstructed image after Tikhonov regularization is shown in Fig. 1B. The original HR image is shown for comparison in Fig. 1C. During the simulation, SNR in LR images has been chosen from 5dB to 25dB. All reconstructed

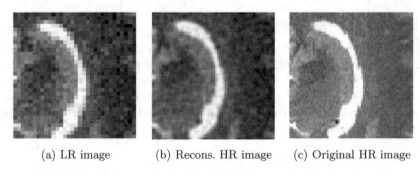

(a) LR image   (b) Recons. HR image   (c) Original HR image

Fig. 1. Images in a simulated reconstruction(regularization factor = 1.1)

images show the corpus callosum clearer than LR images and at the same time, decrease the impact of noise effectively.

3.2   Brain Imaging

We perform super-resolution reconstruction on human brain data. Owing to an inherent characteristic of MRI modality, the super-resolution postprocessing method could only be employed in the slice-select direction [10]. So in this case we set the slice thickness in LR images wide enough to acquire HR data with the same slice width as the reconstructed image. It is intended to analyze the improvement of the super-resolution reconstruction method. Our goal is to achieve a result whose image quality is as close as that of HR data, based on acquired LR images. The resolution in LR slices is set to be 1 mm, and the slice thickness is 4 mm. The first set of LR slices will include 28 slices. The second set of LR slices is slightly shifted up in the slice-select direction by 1 mm. The third and fourth set is shifted in the direction by 2 mm and 3 mm, respectively. Then in the first set, we extract one column of every slice in the same index to obtain the first LR image. Taking use of the same procedure, we achieve the other three LR images. They make up of the four LR images for a reconstruction.

One of LR images is shown in Fig. 2A. Figure 2B is the reconstructed HR image and Figure 2C is a HR image for a comparison. As the comparison shows, the reconstructed image contains clearer information thanks to the high resolution. So the improvement in the result is obvious. SNR is 11.53dB and 8.01dB in reconstructed HR image and original HR image, respectively.

4   Discussion and Conclusion

In this work, we investigate the possibility of using Tikhonov regularization to perform super-resolution reconstruction in human brain MRI images. Simulation result shows Tikhonov regularization is effective to be used in the super-resolution reconstruction. It is amenable to noise, to a large extent. The range of original SNR in LR images is from 5dB to 25dB in the simulation. The reconstructed image is always able to provide more readable information than noisy

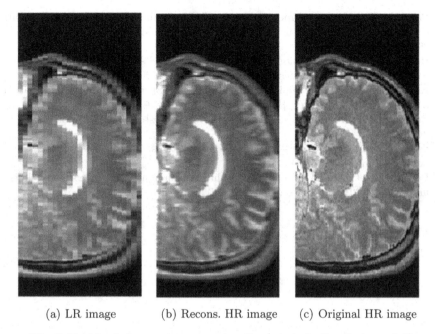

(a) LR image   (b) Recons. HR image   (c) Original HR image

Fig. 2. Real brain images in a reconstruction(regularization factor = 1.2)

LR images. In the real data experiment, these LR images are extracted from the four sets of LR slices. The reconstructed image in the slice-select direction presents clearer details than LR image because of the higher resolution, and gives acceptable SNR values.

To conclude, Tikhonov regularization is applicable to super-resolution reconstruction of brain MRI images. It works well to improve the resolution in the slice-select direction of MRI data without the loss of SNR.

Acknowledgment

This work was supported in part by the University Research Committee of the University of Hong Kong under Grant Number URC-10207440.

References

1. Greenspan, H., Oz, G., Kiryati, N., Peled, S.: MRI inter-slice reconstruction using super resolution. Magn. Reson. Imaging. 20, 437–446 (2002)
2. Eyal, C., Siuyan, L., Noga, A., Amos, F., Daniel, F.: Resolution enhancement in MRI. Magn. Reson. Imaging 24, 133–154 (2006)
3. Lam, E.: Noise in superresolution reconstruction. Optics Letters 28, 2234–2236 (2003)
4. Irani, M., Peleg, S.: Motion analysis for image enhancement: resolution, occlusion, and transparency. J. Vis. Comm. Image. Rep. 4, 324–335 (1993)

5. Peled, S., Yeshurun, Y.: Superresolution in MRI: Application to human white matter fiber tract visualization by diffusion tensor imaging. Magn. Reson. Med. 45, 29–35 (2001)
6. Hsu, J.T., et al.: Application of wavelet-based POCS super-resolution for cardiovascular MRI image enhancement. In: Proc. of ICIG 2004, pp. 524–575 (2004)
7. Katsaggelos, A.K. (ed.): Digital Image Restoration Sprintger Series in Information Sciences, vol. 23. Springer, Heidelberg (2003)
8. Banham, M.R., Katsaggelos, A.K.: Digital Image Restoration Sig. Proc. Mag. 14, 24–41 (1997)
9. Saad, Y.: Iterative methods for sparse linear systems, 1st edn. PWS Publ., Company, Boston, Mass (1996)
10. Peeters, R., et al.: The use of super-resolution techniques to reduce slice thickness in functional MRI. Int. J. of. Imag. Sys. Tech. 14, 131–138 (2004)

A Simple Enhancement Algorithm for MR Head Images[*]

Xiaolin Tian[1], Jun Yin[1], Yankui Sun[2], and Zesheng Tang[1,2]

[1] Faculty of Information Technology, Macau University of Science and Technology, Macao
[2] Department of Computer Science and Technology, Tsinghua University, Beijing, China
xltian@must.edu.mo, handsonyin2005@yahoo.com.cn,
syk@tsinghua.edu.cn, ztang@must.edu.mo

Abstract. In this paper, a simple enhancement algorithm for MR head images has been presented. The algorithm is based on histogram equalization but new adaptive reassigning rules have been involved, which approaches a non-linear gray level mapping. Comparing with other existing enhancement algorithms based on equalization, the new algorithm needs not calculate local histograms window by window but dynamically assigning new gray levels according to statistical info in related histogram, which makes the new algorithm natively faster. Testing results on different MR Head images have been reported and compared with several existing algorithms, which have shown that the new algorithm is not only faster but also reached better enhancement results.

Keywords: Medical image enhancement, MR head image, Histogram equalization, Non-linear mapping.

1 Introduction

The digital format of Magnetic Resonance Image(MRI) lends itself to a wealth of image enhancement techniques, which could provide details of internal organs to support activities such as disease diagnosis and monitoring, and surgical planning. Over the years different techniques have been studied to enhance MRI[1][2]. These methods can be classified as:

   i). Statistical or time/spatial domain methods.
   ii). Localized or adaptive algorithms.
   iii). Frequency domain techniques.

Histogram equalization techniques are statistical methods in time/spatial domain. Conventional histogram equalization algorithm [3] is simple and effective but may not get satisfied results from MRI. Some MRI enhancement results by conventional histogram equalization algorithm have been shown in the second row of figure 1 below. To improve enhancement results, many localized (or adaptive) histogram equalization algorithms have been proposed [4][5], which consider a local window for each individual pixel and computes the new intensity value based on the local histogram equalization. These localized algorithms usually improve results but they

---

[*] Supported by the National Natural Science Foundation of China (No. 30470487).

X. Gao et al. (Eds.): MIMI 2007, LNCS 4987, pp. 57–62, 2008.

are very time consuming even though there are some fast implementations for updating the local histograms [6].

In this paper, a new approach to improve conventional histogram equalization algorithm has been proposed, which is not based on localizing histogram in smaller spatial areas (local windows), but equalizing the histogram according to statistical characters of histogram of the whole image. In the other word, the new algorithm only calculates histogram once during the enhancement, so it is much faster than algorithms, which need calculate local histograms one by one.

The new algorithm is working as a non-linear mapping function between original MRI and enhanced MRI. It keeps some gray levels unchanged but reassigns new values to some selected gray levels. Usually to design a non-linear mapping should figure out a non-linear function first, or if an analytical formula is harder to design, a curve of mapping rule should be given out. Both of them are not easy to be obtained [7]. The new algorithm avoids figuring out any non-linear functions or curves, but just simply enhances MRI by the info offered by histogram. It is much simple but result is satisfied.

2 Method

The major steps of the new algorithm have been listed below based on the conventional histogram equalization algorithm[3]. The new added parts have been marked and highlighted in bold:

```
Notation:
    H is the histogram array of an image.
    Zmax is the maximum gray level in the image.
    Hint is an integer of the histogram.
    Z denotes the old levels.
    R denotes the new levels.
    Each Z will be mapped onto an interval [left(Z),
    right(Z)].


Approach:
Step1:  Read an image, evaluate its histogram and store
    it in the array H. Let Havg be its average value.
```

Step1.1(new added):
```
    Let N is the total pixel number in the image (size
    of input image),
    For Z = 0 to Zmax do:
      Begin
        If (H(Z)  >  k*N ) H(Z)=0
      End
Step2:  Set R = 0, Hint = 0
Step3:  For Z = 0 to Zmax do:
  Begin
      Set left(Z) = R, and Hint = Hint + H(Z)
      While Hint > Havg, do:
```

```
        Begin
          Hint = Hint - Havg,  R = R + 1.
        End
      Set right(Z) = R and define the value of new(Z)
      according to the average of left(Z) and right(Z),
      that means new(Z) = R( [left(Z) + right(Z)]/2 )
      where R(x) is a function of x to round x to the
      nearest integer.
    End
Step4:  For all pixels P of the image do:
    Begin
      If  left(f(P)) equals to right(f(P))
      then set the new value of the pixel P to the
          left(f(P))
      Else set the new value of the pixel P to the
          new(f(P)).
    End
End of algorithm.
```

The new algorithm has introduced a new parameter 'k' in the step 1.1, which is a key parameter to decide if the gray level should be ignored in further processing steps.

3 Results

The proposed algorithm has been tested on different MR head images, which are obtained from a hospital in TianJin, China. Two other exiting algorithms have been tested either to compare enhancement effects. They are classical enhancement algorithms; one is conventional histogram equalization algorithm [3], which is working in spatial domain and another is wavelet based enhancement algorithm [8], which is working in transform domain. All testing results haves shown that the enhanced effects of the new algorithm are better than both of the results from the conventional histogram equalization algorithm [3], and the wavelet transform algorithm [8].

There is a parameter k in the new algorithm. Different k had been tested in a training image set and k=0.2 has been selected for MR head images. So k=0.2 has been used for all testing. We believe k could be dynamically decided, which will be one of our further works in the future.

Several typical testing result images have been shown in the figure 1 below. For comparison purpose, results of the conventional histogram equalization algorithm [3] and results of the wavelet based enhancement algorithm [8] have been shown in figure 1 either. The figure 1 is organized as three original MR images have been shown in the first row; their corresponding enhanced images by conventional histogram equalization algorithm have been shown in the second row. Corresponding result images enhanced by wavelet based algorithm have been shown in the third row and results from the new algorithm proposed in the paper have been shown in the fourth row.

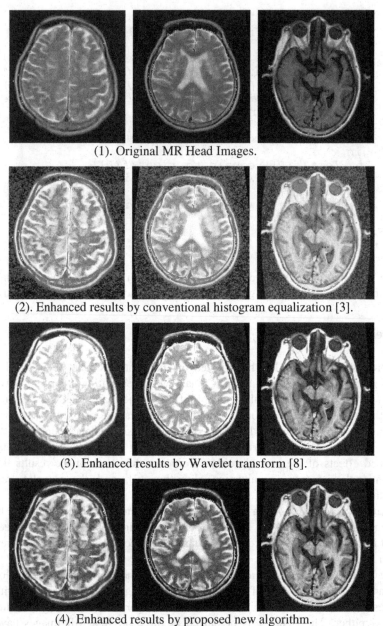

(1). Original MR Head Images.

(2). Enhanced results by conventional histogram equalization [3].

(3). Enhanced results by Wavelet transform [8].

(4). Enhanced results by proposed new algorithm.

Fig. 1. MRI with their enhanced images by different algorithms

4 Discussion and Conclusion

Testing results have shown that the new algorithm could get better enhancement results on all tested MR head images. From the figure 1 above, we could see that beside the new algorithm has the similar but still better result comparing with wavelet based algorithm in the third column, all other results from the new algorithm in the figure 1 had shown much better enhancement results compare with others.

Often, the quantitative measures of image processing results do not agree well with the preferences of the human eyes[9]. And the human eye is always the ultimate judge of whether the image processing results is acceptable or annoying. But we could use shapes of histogram to measure the enhancement results by different algorithms mentioned in the paper. Figure 2 below shows histogram of an original MRI in the figure 1, with histograms of its corresponding enhanced images by different algorithms shown in the figure 1.

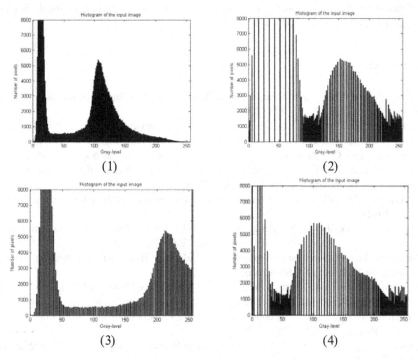

Fig. 2. Histograms of a MRI and its corresponding enhanced images in the first column of the figure 1

The histogram in (1) of figure 2 above shows the histogram of the first original MRI in the figure 1; (2) shows the histogram of corresponding enhanced image by conventional histogram equalization [3], which is the fist image of the second row in the figure 1; (3) shows the histogram of corresponding enhanced image by Wavelet transform [8], which is the fist image of the third row in the figure 1; (4) shows the histogram of corresponding enhanced image by the new algorithm proposed, which is the fist image of the fourth row in the figure 1. Form equalization's point of view, the new algorithm has the best enhancement result for it has more 'equal' histogram. This confirms our conclusion again that the new algorithm does have better enhancement result on MR head images.

Beside the better enhancement results, the new algorithm has also obvious predominance in its simple implement and faster processing speed. These advantages are native existed in its algorithm structure. First, the new algorithm is working in time/spatial domain so it does not need transferring and inverse transferring processing as wavelet based algorithms. Second, the new algorithm is still using a global histogram from the whole image to do the equalization, which is defiantly faster than those enhancement algorithms based on the localization. So the proposed algorithm has unassailable advantage on less complexity of algorithm, especially in less time cost comparing with these local window based equalization algorithms or algorithms based on Frequency/Transform domain techniques.

Acknowledgments. The work was supported by the National Natural Science Foundation of China (No. 30470487).

References

1. Carmi, E., Liu, S., Alon, N., Fiat, A., Fiat, D.: Resolution enhancement in MRI. Magnetic Resonance Imaging 24, 133–154 (2006)
2. Larrabide, A.A., Novotny, R.A.: A Medical Image Enhancement Algorithm Based on Topological Derivative and Anisotropic Diffusion. In: Proceedings of the XXVI I berian Latin-American Congress on Computational Methods in Engineering CILAMCE 2005, Brazilian Assoc. for Comp. Mechanics & Latin American Assoc. of Comp. Methods in Engineering, Guarapari, Esp´ırito Santo, Brazil (2005)
3. Pavlidis, T.: Algorithms for Graphics and Image Processing, pp. 50–54. Computer Science Press (1982)
4. Ju-lang, J., You-sheng, Z., Feng, X., Min, H.: Local Histogram Equalization with Brightness Preservation, Acta Electronica Sinica (2006)
5. Xian-min, W.: Research and Application of Adaptive Histogram Equalization Method. Information Technology & Informatization 4 (2005)
6. Eramian, M., Mould, D.: Histogram Equalization using Neighborhood Metrics. In: The 2nd Canadian Conference on Computer and Robot Vision (CRV 2005), pp. 397–404 (2005)
7. Rafael, C., Gonzalez, R.E.: Woods, Digital Image Processing, 2nd edn. Addison-Wesley Pub Co., Reading (2003)
8. Unser, M., Aldroubi, A.: A review of wavelets in biomedical applications. Proceedings of the IEEE 84(4), 626–638 (1996)
9. Castleman, K.R.: Digital Image Processing, ch. 17, p. 438. Prentice Hall, Inc., Englewood Cliffs (1996)

A Novel Image Segmentation Algorithm Based on Artificial Ant Colonies

Huizhi Cao, Peng Huang, and Shuqian Luo

College of Biomedical Engineering, Capital Medical University,
Beijing 100069, China
sqluo@ieee.org

Abstract. Segmentation is one of the most difficult tasks in digital image processing. This paper presents a novel segmentation algorithm, which uses a biologically inspired paradigm known as artificial ant colonies. Considering the features of artificial ant colonies, we present an extended model applied in image segmentation. Each ant in our model is endowed with the ability of memorizing a reference object, which will be refreshed when a new target is found. A fuzzy connectedness measure is adopted to evaluate the similarity between the target and the reference object. The behavior of one ant is affected by the neighboring ants and the cooperation between ants is performed by exchanging information through pheromone updating. The simulated results show the efficiency of the new algorithm, which is able to preserve the detail of the object and is insensitive to noise.

1 Introduction

The success of image analysis depends heavily upon accurate image segmentation algorithms. Image segmentation algorithms subdivide images into their constituent regions, with the level of subdivision depending on the problem being solved. Robust, automatic image segmentation requires the incorporation and intelligent utilization of global contextual knowledge. But the variability of the background, versatile properties of the target partitions that characterize themselves and the presence of noise make it difficult to accomplish the task. Considering the complexity, we often apply different methods in segmentation process according to the nature of the images. Region-based active contour models [1, 2] are widely used in image segmentation. In general, these region-based models have a number of advantages over gradient-based techniques for segmentation, including greater robustness to noise. However, the initial contour placement will affect the result of segmentation. Unsupervised fuzzy clustering, especially fuzzy c-means algorithm (FCM) [3-5], is widely employed in image segmentation. Based on minimum square error criterion, FCM algorithm can perform classification without the need to estimate the density distribution of the image. But when used in image segmentation, FCM algorithm has a serious limitation: it does not incorporate any spatial information. As a result, it is sensitive to noise and imaging artifacts. In this paper, we explore a novel approach to image segmentation with Artificial Ant Colonies.

X. Gao et al. (Eds.): MIMI 2007, LNCS 4987, pp. 63–71, 2008.

2   Related Work

Ramos [6] has explored the idea of using a digital image as an environment for artificial ant colonies. He observed that artificial ant colonies could react and adapt appropriately to any type of digital habitat. Ramos [7] has also investigated ant colonies based data clustering and developed an ant colony clustering algorithm referred to as ACLUSTER which he applied to a digital image retrieval problem. In doing so, Ramos [7] was able to perform retrieval and classification successfully on images of marble samples. Liu and Tang [8] have conducted similar work and have presented an algorithm for grey scale image segmentation using behavior-based agents that self reproduce in areas of interest. He and Chen [9] have provided an artificial cell model. In their models, each life is one individual unit, termed as a cell, which adheres to one pixel in the image. All of the cells bear similar structures but mutations may occur during the process of reproduction due to the influence of the environment. Hamarnehl [10] has shown how an intelligent corpus callosum agent, which takes the form of a worm, can deal with noise, incomplete edges, enormous anatomical variation, and occlusion in order to segment and label the corpus callosum in 2D mid-sagittal MR image slices of the brain.

3   Previous Model of Artificial Ant Colonies

As described by Chialvo and Millonas in [11], the state of an individual ant can be expressed by its position r, and orientation θ. Since the response at a given time is assumed to be independent of the previous history of the individual, it is sufficient to specify a transition probability from one place and orientation (r, θ) to the next $(r*, \theta*)$ an instant later. In previous works [6, 12, 13] transition rules were derived and generalized from noisy response functions, which in turn were found to reproduce a number of experimental results with real ants. The response function can effectively be translated into a two-parameter transition rule between the pixels by use of a pheromone weighting function:

$$W(\sigma) = (1 + \frac{\sigma}{1 + \delta\sigma})^{\beta} \tag{1}$$

This equation measures the relative probabilities of moving to a pixel r with pheromone density $\sigma(r)$. The parameter β is associated with the pheromone density, it controls the degree of randomness with which each ant follows the gradient of pheromone. As discussed in [6], for low values of β the pheromone concentration does not greatly affect its choice, while high values cause it to follow pheromone gradient with more certainty. $\frac{1}{\delta}$ is the sensory capacity, which describes the fact that each ant's ability to sense pheromone decreases somewhat at high concentrations. Considering that the ants have higher possibility to walk along the previous direction, Chialvo and Millonas[11] add an additional weighting factor $w(\Delta\theta)$, which ensures that very sharp turns are much less likely than turns through smaller angles, thus each ant in the colony have a probabilistic bias in the forward direction. Influenced by the concentration of pheromone in all the eight neighboring pixels, each individual in the ant colony can step in one of these pixels at each time step. Simultaneously, each individual leaves a constant amount η of pheromone at the pixel in which it is located at every time step t. This pheromone decays at each time step at a rate V. The normalized transition probabilities on the lattice to go from pixel k to pixel i at time t are given by [11]:

$$P_{ik} = \frac{W(\sigma_i)w(\Delta_i)}{\sum_{j/k} W(\sigma_j)w(\Delta_j)} \qquad (2)$$

The notation j/k indicates the sum over all the pixels j in the local neighborhood of k. Δ_i measures the magnitude of the difference in orientation from the previous direction at time t-1. A large number of ants can be placed on the image at random positions at time $t=0$. Then the movement of each ant is determined by the probability P_{ik}. Different from the pheromone deposition methods utilized in [11], Ramos added a new term which is not constant and related with a proposed correlation measures around local neighborhoods. The pheromone deposition T is defined as [6]:

$$T = \eta + p\Delta h \qquad (3)$$

Where η is a constant amount of pheromone; p is a constant; Δh is used to measure degrees of similarity between two different lattice windows, including three terms. The first term, computed through differences in simple averages, is responsible for finding differences on overall grey level intensity values, while the second measures differences on windows grey level homogeneity values through variance computations. The last term is computed through differences in two grey level histograms representative of two local neighborhoods. Δh is depicted as:

$$\Delta h = \left[a\frac{|m_1 - m_2|}{Max|m_1 - m_2|} + b\frac{|\sigma_1^2 - \sigma_2^2|}{Max|\sigma_1^2 - \sigma_2^2|} + c\frac{S}{S\max} \right] (a+b+c)^{-1} \qquad (4)$$

Where $(a+b+c) = 1$, m_1 means the grey level average intensities in one lattice window, while σ_1^2 represents the variance for the same window. S equals to the difference for all grey level intensities between two grey level histograms representative of two windows. Figure 1 shows part of our experimental results using the introduced model [6].

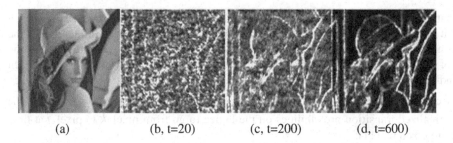

(a)   (b, t=20)   (c, t=200)   (d, t=600)

Fig. 1. Pheromonal fields for several iterations: (a) original image; (b) ~ (d) pheromonal fields after 20 iterations, 200 iterations and 600 iterations respectively.

4 Modeling Artificial Ant Colonies for Image Segmentation

When utilizing artificial ant colonies in image segmentation, we assume the ants in the system should have the ability to know what the "food" in their memory is. Thus they can find the pixels which are similar to the "food" in the image. Then the ants deposit pheromone on the pixels which will affect the motion of the ants. At each iteration step, the ants will change their position in the image according to certain rules. In the end, we can get the segmentation result through analyzing the pheromone distribution in the image. Implementation details will be described in the following.

4.1 What Is Food

The food in our algorithm can be described as a reference object which is memorized by the ants during image segmentation process. For simplicity, we select a r-radius neighborhood $N_r(o)$ of a pixel o in the image manually. Then the food in the ith ant's memory at time $t = 0$ can be initialized as:

$$F_{i,t\,=\,0} = N_r(o) \tag{5}$$

$$N_r(o) = \{e \in I \mid \|e - o\| < r\} \tag{6}$$

Where I represents the pixels in the image for segmentation . When an ant finds new food source, the food in ants' memory will be refreshed according to certain rules which will be introduced later on.

4.2 Finding Food Source

When the food is defined, the ants in the system have the tasks of finding pixels of similar property. In order to find these similarly pixels, ants are given the ability to compare pixels to the specific reference food for which they are looking for. If an ant is at the pixel c, $N_r(c)$ represents a r-radius neighborhood of the pixel c, then the comparison is controlled by the formula:

$$\mu_k(o,c) = \sqrt{\mu_\varphi(o,c)\mu_\psi(o,c)} \tag{7}$$

$$\mu_\varphi(o,c) = \frac{\min(m_o, m_c)}{\max(m_o, m_c)} \tag{8}$$

$\mu_\psi(o,c)$ is the homogeneity-based component which is often used in fuzzy connectedness algorithms [14]. m_o and m_c represent the grey level average intensities of $N_r(o)$ and $N_r(c)$ respectively. If $\mu_k(o,c)$ exceeds a threshold, the pixel c is defined as interesting to the ants searching for food source. When an ant i considers c as new food source, the food in the ant's memory at time $t = \tau$ will be refreshed as:

$$F_{i,t=\tau} = aN_r(c) + bF_{i,t=\tau-1} \tag{9}$$

Where a and b are constants.

4.3 Transition Rules

At each time step, the ants in the system will go from pixel k to pixel j. Different from [4], we assume the transition probability of an ant is also affected by other ants around it. The influence of other ants is confined in a given window W, the center of which is k. Then the normalized transition probability on the lattice to go from pixel k to pixel i at time t is defined as:

$$P_{ik} = \frac{W(\sigma_i)(w(\Delta_i) + E(\theta_i))}{\sum_{j/k} W(\sigma_j)(w(\Delta_j) + E(\theta_j))} \tag{10}$$

$$E(\theta) = \frac{N_{(w,\theta)}}{N_w} \tag{11}$$

Where N_w is the amount of ants in W, $N_{(w,\theta)}$ is the number of ants in W whose previous direction was θ. With the definition, the motion of ants is more like mass action, which can enhance the ants' ability of finding food source.

4.4 Pheromone Update

As discussed in section 4.2, an ant will consider the target as a food source when the value of $\mu_k(o,c)$ exceeds a threshold. During the process of finding food source, each ant has its own threshold λ. In our paper, the value of λ is between 0.6 and 0.9. Then the pheromone deposition T at pixel c can be defined as:

$$T_{(c)} = \begin{cases} \eta & if \mu_k(o,c) < \lambda \\ \eta + p\lambda & if \mu_k(o,c) \geq \lambda \end{cases} \tag{12}$$

Where η is a constant amount of pheromone; p is a constant.

5 Experiments and Results

To evaluate the feasibility of the proposed segmentation algorithm of artificial ant colonies, two sets of experiments are presented. The coefficients used for running these experiments are $\eta = 0.07, V = 0.015, \beta = 3.5, \delta = 0.2, p = 1.2$. The results of these experiments are described below.

The first example is based on a Printed Circuit Board (PCB) image with Gaussian noise [Fig.2 (a)]. The mean value of Gaussian white noise is 0 and the variance is 0.03.

Fig.2 (b) and Fig.2 (c) (from [9]) are segmentation results using median filter and Wiener adaptive filter respectively. From Fig.3 (a) to Fig.3 (c), we can find that more iterations have been done, more ants are close to the target. As shown in Fig.3 (c), our approach outperforms the two filter-based methods.

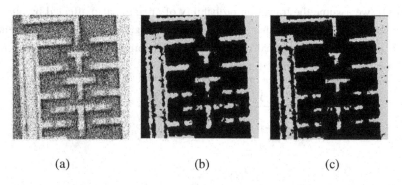

(a)   (b)   (c)

Fig. 2. Segmentation Results: (a) PCB image with Gaussian noise $(\mu = 0, \delta = 0.03)$; (b) thresholded image after 5×5 median filter; (c) thresholded image after 5×5 2D Wiener adaptive filter.

We use parts of phantom data provided by Brain Imaging Centre at Montreal Neurological Institute of McGill University to evaluate algorithm, 20% and 40%

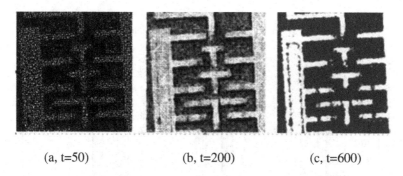

(a, t=50)   (b, t=200)   (c, t=600)

Fig. 3. Segmentation Results: (a) ~ (c) the segmentation results using artificial ant colonies for different iterations

bias-field, 0%, 3%and 5% noise. 15 images are chosen under every condition. We run the segmentation by the FCM and artificial ant colonies (AC) algorithm respectively, and then choose Jaccard Similarity Index (SI) to evaluate the segmentation results and similar level of manikin data. The SI can be defined as:

$$J(S_1, S_2) = \frac{|S_1 \cap S_2|}{|S_1 \cup S_2|} \qquad (13)$$

Where S1 and S2 are two pixel sets after segmentation.

Moreover, in the algorithm, we need to scrutinize if non-target pixels are recognized as target pixels or target pixels are recognized as non-target pixels mistakenly. Therefore, false negative ratio and false positive ratio of algorithm should be calculated at the meantime.

Table 1. Statistics of white matter segmentation result

noise	bias-field	false position	false negative	SI
0%	40%	7.07	0.84	0.92
	20%	5.32	1.05	0.93
	0%	4.03	1.46	0.95
3%	40%	7.23	0.63	0.88
	20%	6.44	0.83	0.91
	0%	5.12	1.28	0.91
5%	40%	7.81	1.02	0.86
	20%	6.53	1.09	0.87
	0%	3.09	2.45	0.90
average		5.84	1.18	0.90

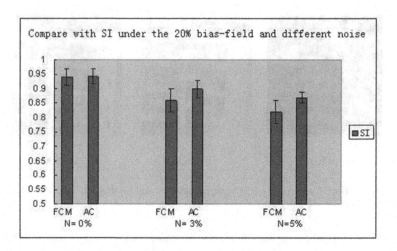

Fig. 4. Comparison with Jaccard Similarity Index (SI) of result using FCM, AC algorithm respectively under the 20% bias-field and different intensity of noise

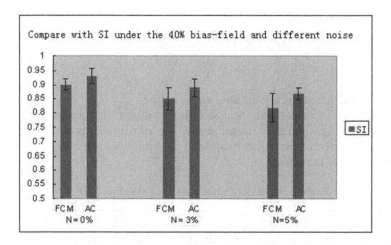

Fig. 5. Comparison with Jaccard Similarity Index (SI) of result using FCM, AC algorithm respectively under the 40% bias-field and different intensity of noise

When the value of SI is more close to 1, it means that the segmentation result is better. According to Fig.4 and Fig.5, AC algorithm presented in the paper can obtain more accurate result than FCM do when both noise and bias-field exist in images.

6 Discussion and Conclusion

In this paper, we have described a novel approach to image segmentation based on artificial ant colonies. This approach is a distributed algorithm based on a population of ants. Each ant constructs a candidate partition using the pheromone information accumulated by the others ants. Our experiments clearly indicate the robustness of the proposed approach to noise and its ability to retain the details of the partitions at the same time. A number of interesting aspects of our approach are currently being considered for further exploration. These include extending our model to 3D and creating realistic and more complex criteria during the process of finding food source.

Acknowledgements

The work is supported by National Natural Science Foundation of China, Grant number: 60472020.

References

1. Chan, T., Vese, L.: Active contours without edges. IEEE Trans. Image Processing 10, 266–277 (2001)
2. Paragios, N., Deriche, R.: Geodesic Active Regions for Texture Segmentation, Inria, Sophia Antipolis, France, Res. Rep.3440 (1998)
3. Pham, D.L.: Spatial Models for Fuzzy Clustering. Computer Vision and Image Understanding 84, 285–297 (2001)
4. Ahmed, M.N., Yamany, S.M., Mohamed, N., Farag, A., Moriarity, T.: A Modified Fuzzy C-Means Algorithm for Bias Field Estimation and Segmentation of MRI Dara. IEEE Trans. On Medical Imaging 21, 193–199 (2002)
5. Li, S.Z.: Markov Random Field Modeling in image Analysis, pp. 4–431. Springer, Heidelberg (2001)
6. Ramos, V., Almeida, F.: Artificial Ant Colonies in Digital Image Habitats - A Mass Behaviour Effect Study on Pattern Recognition. In: Dorigo, M., Middendorf, M., Stüzle, T. (eds.) Proceedings of ANTS 2000 - 2nd International Workshop on Ant Algorithms (From Ant Colonies to Artificial Ants), Brussels, Belgium, pp. 113–116 (2000)
7. Ramos, V., Muge, F., Pina, P.: Self-Organized Data and Image Retrieval as a Consequence of Inter-Dynamic Synergistic Relationships in Artificial Ant Colonies. In: Ruiz-del-Solar, J., Abraham, A., Köppen, M. (eds.) Frontiers in Artificial Intelligence and Applications, Soft Computing Systems - Design, Management and Applications, 2nd Int. Conf. on Hybrid Intelligent Systems, Santiago, Chile, vol. 87, pp. 500–509. IOS Press, Amsterdam (2002)
8. Liu, J., Tang, Y.Y.: Adaptive Image Segmentation With Distributed Behavior-Based Agents. IEEE Trans. Pattern Analysis and Machine Intelligence 21(6), 544–551 (1999)
9. He, H., Chen, Y.: Artificial Life for Image Segmentation. International Journal of Pattern Recognition and Artificial Intelligence 15(6), 989–1003 (2001)
10. Hamarneh1, G., McInerney, T., Terzopoulos, D.: Deformable Organisms for Automatic Medical Image Analysis. In: Niessen, W.J., Viergever, M.A. (eds.) MICCAI 2001. LNCS, vol. 2208, pp. 66–75. Springer, Heidelberg (2001)
11. Chialvo, D.R., Millonas, M.M.: How Swarms Build Cognitive Maps. In: Steels, L. (ed.) The Biology and Technology of Intelligent Autonomous Agents. NATO ASI Series, pp. 439–450 (1995)
12. Millonas, M.M.: A Connectionist-Type Model of Self-Organized Foraging and Emergent Behavior in Ant Swarms. Journal Theor. Biology 159, 529 (1992)
13. Millonas, M.M.: Swarms, Phase transitions, and Collective Intelligence. In: Langton, C.G. (ed.) Artificial Life III, Santa Fe Institute Studies in the Sciences of the Complexity, vol. 17, pp. 417–445. Addison-Wesley, Reading (1994)
14. Saha, P.K., Udupa, J.K., Odhner, D.: Scale-Based Fuzzy Connected Image Segmentation: Theory, Algorithms, and Validation. Computer Vision and Image Understanding 77, 145–174 (2000)

Characteristics Preserving of Ultrasound Medical Images Based on Kernel Principal Component Analysis

Tongsen Hu and Ting Gui

College of Information Engineering, Zhejiang University of Technology,
HangZhou, China
hts@zjut.edu.cn, guiting@zjc.zjut.edu.cn

Abstract. Kernel Principal Component Analysis (KPCA) is one of the methods available for analyzing ultrasound medical images of liver cancer. First the original ultrasound images need airspace filtering, frequency filtering and morphologic operation to form the characteristic images and these characteristic images are fused into a new characteristic matrix. Then analyzing the matrix by using KPCA and the principle components (in general, they are not unique) are found in order to that the most general characteristics of the original image can be preserved accurately. Finally the eigenvector projection matrix of the original image which is composed of the principle components can reflect the most essential characteristics of the original images. The simulation experiments were made and effective results were acquired. Compared with the experiments of wavelets, the experiment of KPCA showed that KPCA is more effective than wavelets especially in the application of ultrasound medical images.

Keywords: Ultrasound medical images, Kernel principal component analysis, Image processing, Characteristics extracting, Kernel function.

1 Introduction

One main problem of digital image processing is image analysis. The work of image analysis is to get the objective information and create the description of image through checking and measuring of the interested targets of the image. One important work of image analysis is to extract or measure the characteristic of the object. The characteristic of image can be divided into two aspects: one is statistical characteristic which is artificial definition and transformation such as histogram, quadrangle moment and frequency charts, the other is visual characteristic which is the natural characteristic of the area of image such as brightness, texture and contour etc.

There are two kinds of the description of an image area including the foundational technology of image processing such as the lines, the curves, the areas and the geometry characteristics and the further description of the relation and the structure among the areas. Normally characteristic of image area can include gray degree (including density, color), airspace, frequency, texture and geometry characteristic etc [1-3]. Normally image analysis tools include fractal, Gaussian-mixture-based,

X. Gao et al. (Eds.): MIMI 2007, LNCS 4987, pp. 72–79, 2008.

morphologic and wavelets etc [4-6]. Recently wavelets are widely used in the fields of digital image processing. For example, Risto, et al. used evolved wavelets transform to compress images [6], Yongqing Sun and Shinji Ozaw used wavelets to retrieve images [7]. In the same way, wavelets have also been tried in the field of medical image analysis and have got some development [8,9].

Though wavelets have made great progress in image analysis, it is only applied by one or two characteristics of the image such as low and high pass frequency. Kernel Principal Component Analysis (KPCA) is a new way from a new angle to analyze the ultrasound medical images: First the original ultrasound images need airspace filtering, frequency filtering and morphologic operation to form the characteristic images and these characteristic images are fused into a new characteristic matrix. Then analyzing the matrix by using KPCA and the principle components (in general, they are not unique) are found in order to that the most general characteristics of the original image can be preserved accurately. Last the eigenvector projection matrix of the original image which is composed of the principle components can reflect the most essential characteristics of the original images. The simulation experiments were made and effective results were acquired. The B-SCAN ultrasound images of liver cancer have been analyzed by KPCA in this paper. The result indicates that the method mentioned in this paper is better than 2- dimensional wavelets transform.

2 Theory

2.1 KPCA

Principle Component Analysis (PCA) is a method to find the most general characteristics from an object by analyzing all the characteristics of the object. There is a mathematical description of this method: given an original data matrix: $X=(x_{ij})_{m\times n}$, where $i=1,2,\ldots,m$, $j=1,2,\ldots,n$; it can be rewritten to the vector form: $X=(X_1,X_2,\ldots X_n)$; The purpose of using PCA is to find the most general index values which can reflect and preserve the original information of the object. Sothe n-dimensional linear combination of the original vector: $lX=l_1X_1+l_2X_2+\ldots+l_nX_n$, demands the variety of $Z=lX$ to be as far as possible large and the vector l be a standard vector. The l (not unique) which we sought is the general index value to satisfied the conditions [10].

Until Vapnik introduced the concept of kernel function to the high-dimensional linear space and created the concept of Support Vector Machine (SVM) in 1995 and Schölkopf, et al. led kernel space into PCA in 1998[11,12], the theory of KPCA had been formed. After Cristianini and Sha we-Taylor developed KPCA in extending the linear space to nonlinear space in 2000, the concept of KPCA is eventually perfected [13-15]. The theory of the KPCA is to map the problem of the nonlinear space into a high-dimensional linear space through choosing the kernel function, and then uses PCA to find the general index values which preserve the most general information of the original data. But there is no efficient way to determine a suitable kernel function. Now most of the people choose the kernel functions just according to the results of the experiments [10,15,16].

2.2 Application

Today KPCA is widely used in the fields of the image analysis. Ryoheis, et al. used KPCA to enhance the images of spacecraft anomaly in the fields of remote image detection [17]. Kwangs and Guohui He also applied KPCA to extract and analyze the characteristics in the fields of face recognition. They mapped the tested face sample images into the high-dimensional linear feature space through KPCA and they have made some progress [18,19]. KPCA is also used in medical image processing. For example, K S Kim at al. created the distinguishing system of blood cell image used KPCA to analyze the blood cells' characteristics and extract their general characteristics [20]. In the same way, there are other studies using KPCA to enhance and analyze the medical images [21, 22].

3 Method

In this paper the B-SCAN ultrasound medical images of liver cancer are mapped into the high-dimension linear feature space through KPCA using the similar method that mentioned in literature [18, 19]. In this paper the polynomial kernel function was chosen to be the kernel function.

The formula of polynomial kernel function:

$$K(x, y) = (x \bullet y + c)^d \text{ . } c \geq 0, \text{ d is Integer} \tag{1}$$

The following are the steps of the application of KPCA in this paper:

There is the pretreatment before the process: a) transfer the original B-SCAN ultrasound image of liver cancer to a vector matrix: $B = (b_{ij})$, where, $i = 1, \cdots, m, j = 1, \cdots n$; b) Eq. (1) is chosen to be the kernel function in this paper and the parameters are defined as follows: c=1, d=4; c) rewrite the x and y in the Eq. (1) to x_i and x_j, where x_i and x_j represent the elements of the vector matrix B which are contiguous to each other. So the Eq. (1) was transformed into Eq. (2):

$$f(x_i, x_j) = (x_i \bullet x_j + 1)^4 \text{ . } c \geq 0, \text{ d is Integer} \tag{2}$$

1. Filter the original images with airspace filter, frequency filter and dispose the original images with morphological arithmetic operator to fuse to a new feature matrix $V = (v_{ij}), i = 1, \cdots, m; j = 1, \cdots, n$.

2. Map the Formula (2) into the fused feature matrix V, build a new kernel matrix: X=f(V), where, f() is the Formula (2).
3. Calculate the mean value and standard deviation of the kernel matrix with Formula (3), Formula (4).

$$\bar{X} = \frac{1}{n}\sum_{i=1}^{n} x_{ij} \tag{3}$$

$$S_j = \sqrt{\frac{1}{n-1}\sum_{i=1}^{n}(x_{ij} - \bar{X})^2} \tag{4}$$

4. Standardize the matrix $X_{ij} = (x_{ij})$ with Formula (5), calculate the correlative matrix $R = (r_{ij})$ with Formula (6), (R is symmetrical matrix) .

$$Y_{ij} = (Y_{ij})_{m\times n} = \frac{X_{ij} - \bar{X}_j}{S_j} \tag{5}$$

$$Y_{ij} = (Y_{ij})_{m\times n} = \frac{X_{ij} - \bar{X}_j}{S_j} \tag{6}$$

5. Compute the eigenvalues λ and eigenvectors l of the matrix R.
6. Confirm the first k principle components in accord with the regulation that the value of Formula (7) of the matrix R is larger than 85% but smaller than 1. Formula (7) is the formula of the Accumulative ratio of contribution (A.R.C.):

$$\sum_{j=1}^{k} \lambda_j / \sum_{j=1}^{n} r_{jj} \tag{7}$$

7. Calculate the index value Z with Formula (8) which is made up of the first k principle components and form a new characteristic image matrix. It can reflect the general extracting characteristics of the original image.

$$Z=LX. \tag{8}$$

4 Results

Simulated experiments have been made by KPCA (the environment of the experiments is Matlab7.0). The following are the results of the experiments:

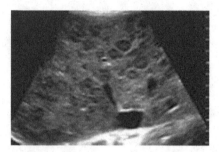

Fig. 1. The original B-SCAN ultrasound image of liver cancer (Diffuse nodular hepatic cancer)

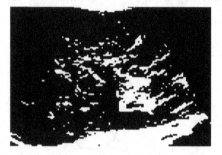

Fig. 2. The Fig.1's characteristic extracted by KPCA (97.48% (from Table 1) of the black areas stands for the distribution of the nodules of hepatic cancer and the white areas reveal the face of the liver is uneven)

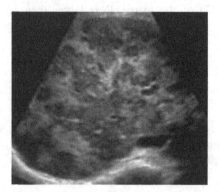

Fig. 3. The original B-SCAN ultrasound image of liver cancer (Multiple hepatocellular carcinomas)

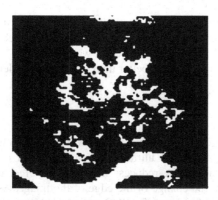

Fig. 4. The Fig.3's characteristic extracted by KPCA (99.46% (from Table 1) of the black areas stands for the distribution of the nodules of hepatic cancer and the white areas reveal the face of the liver is uneven)

Fig. 5. The results of the characteristic of the Fig.1 extracted by 4 levels wavelets transform (much of the characteristics of the liver cancer are dropped and much noise is reserved)

The figures showed that the effect using KPCA is much better than using wavelets. Most of liver cancer focus information had been caught when the characteristics of original images were extracted by using KPCA. But the results by using 4 levels wavelets had lost much useful information.

The first 3 Kernel Principle Components ($l_i, i = 1,2,3$, KPC) of Fig.1 which have been extracted by KPCA are listed in Table 1. Every KPC ($l_i, i = 1,2,3$) is a vector

Table 1. Kernel Principle Components of the figures

KPC	Fig.1				Fig.1		
l_1	0.4998	0.2445	0.2004	0.1517	0.4998	0.2445	0.2004
l_2	0.8178	0.3832	0.1212	0.1023	0.8178	0.3832	0.1212
l_3	0.8428	0.2198	0.1995	0.1162	0.8428	0.2198	0.1995
A.R.C.	97.48%				117.63%		
A.R.C of Fig.2	99.46%				117.95%		

and its elements represent the contribution to the original images. A.R.C which calculated by Formula (7) can reveal what percentage of the general characteristics is preserved. As to A.R.C. of Fig.1, the KPC, when having 4 elements, can reflect 97.48% of the original image, and is better than when it has 3 elements.

5 Limitation

Though the effect of KPCA is much better than wavelets when it is applied to extract characteristics from the B-SCAN ultrasound image of liver cancer, KPCA had its deficiencies: One is that KPCA reduces the precision of characteristic extracting because it is sensitive to the change of the edge of the image. As it can be seen from the Table 1, the abnormal values of A.R.C are much larger than 1 when 3 of the eigenvectors are extracted because of the edge noise of the image. The other is that there is no all around test of KPCA as there are no enough image samples. There will be some improvement in KPCA in next study.

6 Conclusion

As it can be seen from the depiction above, KPCA can reveal the distribution of the cancer cells of the B-SCAN ultrasound image of liver cancer on a large scale. Over 95% of the liver cancer areas can be found accurately and clearly by using KPCA. And it can efficiently resist the confusion of noise.

Acknowledgments. Thank to Mr. Zhang for providing the B-SCAN ultrasound image of liver cancer and Xianzhong Tian for discussion of the method and others who help us a lot.

References

1. Yao, M.: Digital Image Processing. China Machine Press (2006)
2. Zhang, Y.: Image processing and analysis. Press of Tsing Hua University (1999)
3. Castleman, K.R.: Digital Image Processing. Press of electronic industry (1998)
4. Chaudhuri, J., Sarkar, B.B., Texture, N.: segmentation using fractal dimension. IEEE-PAMI 17(1), 72–77 (1995)
5. Gupta, L., Sortrakui, T.: A Gaussian-mixture-based image segmentation algorithm. Patern Recognition 31(3), 315–326 (1998)
6. Grasemann, U., Miikkulainen, R.: Effective Image Compression using Evolved Wavelets. In: GECCO 2005, Washington, DC, USA (2005)
7. Sun, Y., Ozawa, S.: Semantic-meaningful Content-based Image Retrieval in Wavelet Domain. In: MIR 2003, Berkeley, California, USA (2003)
8. Bai, X., Jin, J.S., Feng, D.: Segmentation-Based Multilayer Diagnosis Lossless Medical Image. In: Conferences in Research and Practice in Information Technology, Compression Pan-Sydney Area Workshop on Visual Information Processing (VIP 2003), vol. 36, pp. 9–14 (2003)

9. Bordes, N., Hugh, T., Pailthorpe, B.: Semi-Automatic Feature Delineation In Medical Images. In: Conferences in Research and Practice in Information Technology, Australasian Symposium on Information Visualisation, Christchurch, vol. 35 (2004)
10. Yu, J.: Multivariate statistical analysis and application. Press of Zhongshan University (2001)
11. Vapnik, V.: The Nature of Statistical Learning Theory. Springer, New York (1995)
12. Vapnik, V.: Statistical Learning Theory. Wiley, New York (1998)
13. Cristianini, N., Shawe-Taylor, J.: An Introduction to Support Vector Machines and Other Kernel-based Learning Methods. Cambridge University Press, Cambridge (2004)
14. Berger, M.: Nonlinearity and Functional Analysis. Academic Press (1977) Science Press, London (2005)
15. Cristianini, N., Shawe-Taylor, J.: An Introduction to Support Vector Machines and other Kernel-based Learning Methods. Cambridge University Press, Cambridge (2000)
16. Wu, J.: Principle Component Analysis and Application Based on Kernel Function. Systems Engineering 23 (2005)
17. Yairi, T., Machida, K., Fujimaki, R.: An Approach to Spacecraft Anomaly Detection Problem Using Kernel Feature Space. In: KDD 2005 (2005)
18. Kim, K.I., Jung, K., Kim, H.J.: Face recognition using kernel principal components analysis. IEEE Signal Processing Letters (2002)
19. He, G.-h., Jun-ying, G.: Face recognition method based on KPCA and SVM Computer. Engineering and Design 26(5), 1190–1193 (2005)
20. Kim, K.S., Kim, P.K., Song, J.J., Park, Y.C.: Analyzing Blood Cell Image to Distinguish Its Abnormalities. ACM Multimedia (2000)
21. Leventon, M., Grimson, E., Faugeras, O.: Statistical shape influence in geodesic active contours. In: Proc. IEEE Conf. on Computer Vision and Patt. (2000)
22. Ghosh, P., Mitchell, M.: Segmentation of Medical Images Using a Genetic Algorithm. In: GECCO 2006 (2006)

Robust Automatic Segmentation of Cell Nucleus Using Multi-scale Space Level Set Method*

Chaijie Duan, Shanglian Bao, Hongyu Lu, and Jinsong Lu

Beijing Key Lab of Medical Physics and Engineering, Peking University,
Beijing 100871, P.R. China
bao@pku.edu.cn

Abstract. In this paper, we propose a novel scheme for cell nucleus segmentation which is multi-scale space level set method. Under this scheme, all nuclei of interest in a microscopic image can be segmented simultaneously. The procedure includes three stages. Firstly, the mathematical morphology method is used to search seed points to localize interested nuclei. Secondly, based on the distribution of these seed points, a level set function is initialized. Finally, the level set function evolves and eventually stops zero level set contours at the boundaries of nuclei labeled by seed points. The evolution in the last stage is a three phase evolution. In each phase, information of different scale spaces is employed. This method was tested by truthful microscope images of lymphocyte, which proved its robustness and efficiency.

Keywords: multi-scale space, level set, electrostatic field, boundary based segmentation, region based segmentation.

1 Introduction

Various approaches for medical image segmentation based on the level set method have been proposed while few focus on cell nucleus segmentation. Though cell nucleus images have relatively regular shapes, harmonious gray level distribution and are easier segmented, methods for fast and precisely segmenting nuclei simultaneously are still far from clinical application.

1.1 DNA Ploidy Analysis

Pathology diagnosis results are the gold standard for diagnosing the existence of malignant tumors. DNA ploidy is an important parameter in pathology diagnosis. DNA aneuploidy always indicates the existence of malignant tumors. Therefore, DNA ploidy analysis is valuable for pathology diagnosis, evaluating malignancy

* This work partially supported by National Basic Research Subject of China (973 Subject) (No.2006CB705700-05), National Natural Science Foundation of China (No.10527003 and 60672104), Doctor Program Fund (No.20040001003), Joint Research Foundation of Beijing Education Committee (No. SYS100010401) and Beijing Nature Science Foundation Committee 3073019.

X. Gao et al. (Eds.): MIMI 2007, LNCS 4987, pp. 80–88, 2008.

and making treatment plans. This work can be done by doctors manually as well as an automatic computerized analysis system. Doctors are more experienced while the automatic system is more efficient and precise. It is more convenient if an automatic computer aided system is developed to help doctors do pre-filtering and quantitative calculation. A robust and efficient segmenting approach is used to segment cell nuclei is of a vital impact on the performance of such a system.

1.2 Cell Nucleus Segmentation

The simplest way to segment cell nuclei is by making use of gray level information and segmenting an image into white object and black background with a couple of gray level thresholds. This method is very fast, but does not perform well. It always includes irrelevant regions whose gray level is similar with cell nuclei's and can not separate nuclei and cytoplasm correctly.

Recently, many researches have focused on applying geometric models to medical image segmentation. Comparing with traditional boundary/surface based and region based segmentation models, geometric models take advantage of both boundary/surface information and region information which makes the segmenting results more reliable [1,2].

Geometric models further branch out into the active contour or snake method and the level set method. Some work on cell nucleus segmentation is based on snake model improved image force [3] or new curve evolution methods [4] to make the segmentation more effective. The former work also integrated a new image force based on electrostatic field into snake model, called eSnake [5].

Based on shape characters and gray level distribution, we propose a new multi-scale space level set method for cell nucleus segmentation. This method includes three evolution stages, in which level set function evolves according to information of different scale spaces respectively. Edge and region information used in each stage guarantees zero level set contours move fast toward expected boundaries in large scale space and stop at expected boundaries precisely in local small scale space. Information of average nuclei intensity is used as well as the electrostatic field referred above.

2 Image Preprocessing

Clinically, cell nuclei of interest in a microscopic image have to be segmented simultaneously. Most studies gave the results of single object segmentation. Though level set method is able to segment multi-objects by use of only one level set function based on its topology flexibility, an arbitrarily initialized level set function always leads to a long convergence time and is vulnerable to noise while evolving.

In order to improve this condition, some pre-processing work is needed before segmenting. As a result of the pre-processing, a group of seed points representing nuclei of interest are produced. First, two gray level thresholds are selected and nuclei whose gray level are within the thresholds are labeled as white. All the other regions containing cytoplasm, unrelated cells, impurities, etc. are colored black. Then, mathematical morphologic erosion is performed to split partly overlapped

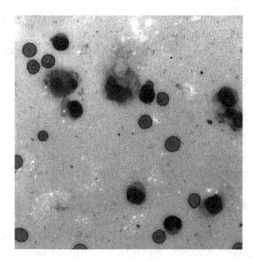

Fig. 1. Raw microscopic image of lymphocyte

nucleus regions with a disk operator. This disk move through out the white regions. If any pixel under the disk is black, then the pixel under the central point of the disk is converted to black. We choose proper iteration time to ensure connective regions are totally separated. After erosion, white regions become smaller seed points of the original nuclei. These seed points maintain shape characteristics of the original nuclei. Since there are some nuclei with abnormal shapes induced by reasons other than pathology, they have no correspondence with malignant tumor and have to be eliminated. Hit-Miss operator is used here to meet this goal. The Hit-Miss operator only preserves seed points whose shape approximates roundness and changes only in size within a rational range and eliminates any other seed. A similar mathematic morphology method was used in [3], but it did not use Hit-Miss operation to eliminated nuclei with abnormal shapes. Then, zero level set contours, also called frontline, are initialized as separated circles around seed points. Radius of these circles is same and close to average radius of nuclei of interest. Fig. 1 shows an example of a raw microscopic image of lymphocyte and fig. 2 illustrates the initialized zero level set contours around seed points.

3 General Multi-scale Space Level Set Model for Cell Nucleus Segmentation

The multi-scale space was mentioned in our former work [6], in which we introduced a general level set method in multi-scale space. This method is described in the equation below

$$\frac{\partial \phi}{\partial t} = \alpha k_I \left| \nabla \phi \right| - \beta \kappa \left| \nabla \phi \right| - \gamma \mathbf{E} \cdot \nabla \phi \ . \tag{1}$$

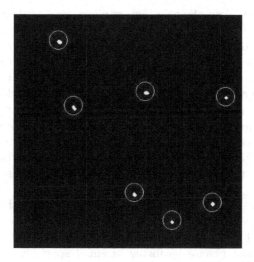

Fig. 2. Example of preprocessing with seed points and initialized frontline

In equation (1), ϕ is level set function and t is time step. $\frac{\partial \phi}{\partial t}$ is added artificially to evolve level set function ϕ. On the right hand of this equation, there are three terms. The first term αk_I has the same effect as balloon force in snake model which is used to inflate or deflate the active contours. The second term $\beta \kappa$ is a smoothing parameter, where κ is the curvature at each point. $\gamma \mathbf{E}$ is a velocity expressed by the electrostatic field $\mathbf{E}$.

The first two terms are common in most level set functions. The electrostatic field $\mathbf{E}$ was first proposed in our eSnake model [5]. In this model, we first performed edge detection on the original image and derived the gradient image. Then we made the assumption that there was a template plane above the gradient image, the image plane and each pixel on the image plane was an electric-charge with electric quantity directly proportional to its gray value. Therefore, all pixels together produced an electrostatic potential on the template plane. By calculating the first-order derivatives of the potential, we obtained the distribution of electrostatic field $\mathbf{E}$ on the template plane.

Thus we proved that the position on the template plane where $\mathbf{E}$ declined to zero indicated the edge point. Test results showed that the closer the template plane was to the image plane, the more the image edges were accurately localized. If the edge of an object had a high gradient value, then the active contours were able to be pulled toward and eventually stopped at the edge. Cell nuclei have distinct gray level from any other part in images and their gradient value on edge is high. Therefore, electrostatic field $\mathbf{E}$ in equation (1) makes frontline converge at the edges of cell nuclei.

Consider the parameter k_I again. $k_I = 1/\left(1 + \left|\nabla I_E^h\right|\right)$ decreases to zero in the high gradient region too. $\left|\nabla I_E^h\right|$ represents the modulus of the image gradient. E in $\left|\nabla I_E^h\right|$ indicates the image is smoothed by using electrostatic field. h is the distance between template plane and image plane. k_I is used to stop inflating or deflating frontline at boundaries.

In equation (1), different values of α, β, γ enable an image to be segmented in different scale spaces. Typically, nonzero value of α is used to segment images in a large scale space. The frontline is evolving fast until arrives at the high gradient edges. Nonzero value of γ makes the electrostatic field available. Since electrostatic field intensity produced by an electric-charge attenuates very fast as the distance increasing, its influence is constrained within a small region. On the other hand, electrostatic field at a single point on template plane is decided by several charges around it on image plane, which weakens the effect of noises. Therefore, the electrostatic field is used to do precise segmentation in a small scale space.

The general multi-scale space level set method was tested using simulation images as well as real medical images. Most of them demonstrated the robustness and efficiency of this method. Since this method combines fast searching in large scale space and precise localizing in small space, it boosts segmenting speed while keeping the precision. The general model was also applied to digital microscopic images containing lymphocytes. Three segmenting procedures with different parameters were performed one after another automatically. All the procedures were based on preprocessed gradient images. In the first stage, we set $\alpha < 0$, $\beta > 0$, $\gamma > 0$ and made the electrostatic field dominate the evolvement. By resetting the electrostatic field to point to the outside of the nucleus equal to zero, the frontline stopped at or moved inside the high gradient boundaries of nuclei in the end. Then, we decreased α and set γ equal to zero. After several iterations, the frontline moved toward and stopped at the high gradient boundaries quickly.

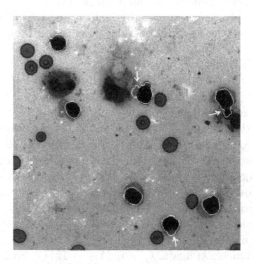

Fig. 3. Leakages occurred when segment nucleus using general multi-scale space level set model

At the last stage, we set $\alpha = 0$, $\beta = 0$, $\gamma > 0$. The frontline adjusted its position and further improved segmentation precision.

Generally, the procedure discussed above works well. Nevertheless, on condition that the gradient of boundary between nucleus and cytoplasm is too weak or weaker than it is between cytoplasm and background, leakage occurs. One example shows in Fig. 3. White arrows indicate where the leakage happened.

4   Improved Multi-scale Space Level Set Method for Cell Nuclei Segmentation

4.1   Region Based Energy

Repeated experiments indicate that the leakages occurred to a significant quantity of cell nuclei. This is partly because the general model only depends on information from the gradient image. The frontline leaks out nucleus boundaries of weaker gradient and is even further attracted by the boundary gradient of cytoplasm.

To resolve this problem, we attempted to use the gradient image as well as raw image. Even though the gradient of nucleus boundary is weaker, nucleus is distinct in average gray level from any other region. An energy generated from average gray level of nucleus was desired.

The most used level set model based on regional gray level information is the Mumford-Shah method [7]. This model performs well if the image consists of regions of approximative constant gray level respectively. In our case, only the nucleus regions are considered and have a constant gray level distinct from other regions. Application of the Mumford-Shah model directly is time consuming and does not perform well. A simplified model is needed.

In our three stage segmenting procedure, only the second stage segments images in large scale space. Since regional information is defined in large scale space, it is only used at the second stage. As a result of the first stage, the frontline has moved inside or stopped at the nucleus boundaries at the beginning of the second stage. Therefore, the only request to the new term is pulling the frontline back if it leaked out of the nuclei. The new energy is defined as (2), a term included in the Mumford-Shah method

$$E_{in}(\phi, c_{in}) = \int_{\Omega} |I(x,y) - I_{in}|^2 H(\phi)\, dxdy \; . \tag{2}$$

The Euler-Lagrange equation of Eq. (2) is Eq. (3)

$$\frac{\partial \phi}{\partial t} = -\delta(\phi)[I(x,y) - I_{in}]^2 \; . \tag{3}$$

$\frac{\partial \phi}{\partial t}$ is artificially added as in Eq. (1). The expression $I_{in} = \frac{\int_{\Omega} I(x,y)H(\phi)dxdy}{\int_{\Omega} H(\phi)dxdy}$ is the average gray level of the cell nuclei and Ω represents the image region in 2-D space. $H(\phi)$ is Heaviside function.

Add (3) to the general model with a weight parameter λ, we have

$$\frac{\partial \phi}{\partial t} = \alpha k_I |\nabla \phi| - \beta \kappa |\nabla \phi| - \gamma \mathbf{E} \cdot \nabla \phi - \lambda \delta (\phi) (I - I_{in})^2 \; . \tag{4}$$

4.2 Implementation of Improved Model

The improved model is implemented using the narrow band method with a distance template [6]. A 19×19 matrix is constructed. The values of elements within a disk record the distances between themselves and the central element of the matrix. The central element then moves along the frontline point by point to construct or reinitiate level set function within the narrow band. It is very efficient for saving distance computing time.

Based on the narrow band re-initialization scheme, it is easier to define velocities on nonzero level set. We calculate velocities of all level sets as well as the zero level set in a narrow band using Eq. (4) directly and found that it did work.

To further improve the computing efficiency, we modified (3) and (4) to (5) and (6)

$$\frac{\partial \phi}{\partial t} = -[I(x, y) - I_{in}]^2 \; . \tag{5}$$

$$\frac{\partial \phi}{\partial t} = \alpha k_I |\nabla \phi| - \beta \kappa |\nabla \phi| - \gamma \mathbf{E} \cdot \nabla \phi - \lambda (I - I_{in})^2 \; . \tag{6}$$

The average gray level of nuclei is re-expressed as $I_{in} = \frac{\int_{inside(c)} I(x,y) dx dy}{\int_{inside(c)} dx dy}$, and inside(c) represents regions inside frontline where $\phi < 0$. c is frontline where $\phi = 0$. Simplified model, although is much faster without calculating $H(\phi)$ and $\delta(\phi)$, may induce some new problems discussed later.

4.3 Experiments and Results

The improved multi-scale space level set method was tested using realistic digital microscopic images of lymphocyte. The robustness and efficiency of such method were demonstrated. Fig. 4 is an example. In Fig. 4, only the nuclei whose size and shape met our requests were picked out and segmented. We used the same raw image in Fig. 4 as in Fig. 3. The improvements are obvious. The white arrows point to positions where leakage happened in Fig. 3. In Fig. 4, all nuclei were well segmented. Parameters in the improved model with three stages are respectively: $\alpha = -0.5, \beta = 0, \gamma = 3, \lambda = 0$ in the first stage, $\alpha = -6, \beta = 0, \gamma = 0, \lambda = -0.005$ in the second stage and $\alpha = 0, \beta = -0.5, \gamma = 1, \lambda = 0$ in the third stage.

This shows that the improved method resolves the leaking problem. The new added term takes advantage of regional information of nucleus gray level and compensates the defects of edge based general model. The whole procedures were done within 2 second on Borland C++ platform with CPU speed 2.0 GHz and 1 GB RAM.

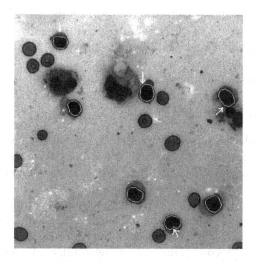

Fig. 4. Improved multi-scale space level set model applied to nuclei segmentation

5 Discussion

The general multi-scale space level set method applied to segmenting cell nucleus works well in most experiments. The formation of the initial level set function is very important. Since the electrostatic field is effective only in regions nearby, if initial zero level set contours are far from the nucleus boundaries, the level set function should not evolve correctly in the electrostatic field. Mathematical morphology is a good way to localize the initial contours by producing seed points. It takes advantage of topology flexibility of level set method. Besides, initializing contours near the final boundaries makes the contours converge very fast.

If we chose proper iteration number, zero level set contours, and the frontline, general model gives correct segmenting results. However, if iteration numbers increased, the frontline may leak out of weak gradient boundaries, which indicates that the general model does not give stable results. This problem is resolved as we introduced an energy expression based on regional gray level of nuclei. This improved model has been demonstrated to be a good solution to the leaking problem. It first pulls frontline inside nuclei, then, inflates it with restriction that the region energy E_{in} is minimized. Since the frontline is moving from inside to outside, once it steps out of the nuclei, E_{in} increases and it is pulled back. The third stage is a small scale space operation, and it uses more local information which ensures the convergence of the frontline to the true boundary.

The final Eq. (6) is simplified and its validity was only deonstrated by cell images. The reason is that all simplifications aim at the cell nucleus segmentation exclusively. Experiments show that, although, electrostatic field calculating is relatively time consuming, the procedures are still fast enough as a whole for clinical application.

A defect induced by the simplification happens in the second stage. Because of the absence of $\delta\left(\phi\right)$, the E_{in} is effective through out the narrow band which leads to an earlier energy increased. As a consequence, the frontline stops evolving earlier as well. The segmented nuclei should be slightly smaller. Whether it has impact on the automatic diagnosis results is still unknown.

6   Conclusion

A general multi-scale space level set method was applied to cell nucleus images, which uses information in different scale spaces and thus can segment regions of interest fast and precisely. We, for the first time, applied this method to digital microscopic images of lymphocyte. After producing seed points of all cell nuclei of interest and initializing zero level set contours, the frontline, around seed points, the general model can segment all useful nuclei simultaneously. The segmenting results are correct for most nuclei if the stained smear was well prepared. However, problem occurs on condition that the gradient of nucleus boundaries is not strong enough to stop the moving frontline correctly. To solve this problem, an improved method is proposed. This method inherits all good properties of the general model and resolves the leakage problem by introducing region based energy. Simplifying the improved model aimed at cell nucleus segmentation further cuts down computing time. Advanced works are expected to validate the reliability of this model in clinic.

Acknowledgments. The authors would like to acknowledge Zhang Yibao, of the Peking University Health Science Center, for improving the general style of the English.

References

1. Suri, J.S., Singh, S., Reden, L.: Computer Vision and Pattern Recognition Techniques for 2-D and 3-D MR Cerebral Cortical Segmentation (Part I): A State-of-the-Art Review. Pattern Analysis and Applications 5, 46–76 (2002)
2. Suri, J.S., Singh, S., Reden, L.: Fusion of Region and Boundary/Surface-Based Computer Vision and Pattern Recognition Techniques for 2-D and 3-D MR Cerebral Cortical Segmentation (Part-II): A State-of-the-Art Review. Pattern Analysis and Applications 5, 77–98 (2002)
3. Hu, M., Ping, X., Ding, Y.: Automated Cell Nucleus Segmentation Using Improved Snake. In: 2004 International Conference on Image Processing
4. Wu, T., Stockhausena, J., Meyer-Ebrechta, D., Bocking, A.: Robust automatic coregistration, segmentation, and classification of cell nuclei in multimodal cytopathological microscopic images. Computerized Medical Imaging and Graphics 28, 87–98 (2004)
5. Lu, H., Yuan, K., Bao, S., Zu, D., Duan, C.: An ESnake Model for Medical Image Segmentation. Progress in Natural Science 15, 424–429 (2005)
6. Lu, H.: Studies and Applications of Modeling Techniques in Active Contours for Medical Image Segmentation. PHD thesis Peking University (2006)
7. Chan, T., Vese, L.: Active contours without edges. IEEE Transaction on Image Processing 10, 266–277 (2001)

Principal Geodesic Analysis for the Study of Nonlinear Minimum Description Length

Zihua Su, Tryphon Lambrou, and Andrew Todd-Pokropek

Department of Medical Physics and Bioengineering
Malet Place Engineering Building
University College London, London, UK, WC1E 6BT
{z.su,tlambrou,atoddpok}@medphys.ucl.ac.uk
http://cmic.cs.ucl.ac.uk/staff/zinhua_su/

Abstract. The essential goal for Statistical Shape Model (SSM) is to describe and extract the shape variations from the landmarks cloud. A standard technique for such variation extraction is by using Principal Component Analysis (PCA). However, PCA assumes that variations are linear in Euclidean vector space, which is not true or insufficient on many medical data. Therefore, we developed a new Geodesic Active Shape (GAS) mode by using Principal Geodesic Analysis (PGA) as an alternative of PCA. The new GAS model is combined with Minimum Description Length approach to find correspondence points across datasets automatically. The results are compared between original MDL and our proposed GAS MDL approach by using the measure of Specificity. Our preliminary results showed that our proposed GAS model achieved better scores on both datasets. Therefore, we conclude that our GAS model can capture shape variations reasonably more specifically than the original Active Shape Model (ASM). Further, analysis on the study of facial profiles dataset showed that our GAS model did not encounter the so-called "Pile Up" problem, whereas original MDL did.

Keywords: Principal Geodesic Analysis, Minimum Description Length, Nonlinear Statistical Shape Model, Correspondence Problem.

1 Introduction

Statistical Shape Model (SSM) emerged as an important tool for image processing, which is incorporated into applications such as: image segmentation, surface registration, and morphological analysis, etc [1-3]. Recently, ASM [4] has become a popular tool for analyzing these problems. However two problems remain in the ASM. The first problem is how to identify landmarks automatically, which has been studied by many different researchers [5-7]. The state of the art technique for tackling this landmark identification problem is Minimum Description Length (MDL), which uses information theory to measure the description length of a shape model and the model that has the minimum description length holds the right correspondence. This MDL method has been applied to real clinical problems successfully. For example, software has been built to help diagnose heart infarction from cardiac scintigrams and

X. Gao et al. (Eds.): MIMI 2007, LNCS 4987, pp. 89–98, 2008.

is also used to diagnose Parkinson's disease in DaTSCAN images [8]. The second problem for ASM is that it uses Principal Component Analysis (PCA) to pick up the main axes of the landmarks cloud, and model the first few main axes. However this linear approximation will not always hold right in real medical datasets, in which case non-linear variations normally exist, such as bending fingers, soft tissue deformations, etc. Recently, different approaches have been implemented to work as an alternative of PCA. Wang et.al. [9] added additional artificial matrix to the eigen-matrix extracted from the training set. In this way, they argued that more global accurate variations were captured. Su et.al. [10] incorporate Markov Random Fields (MRF) to facilitate points neighborhood relations and used Independent Component Analysis (ICA) as an alternative of PCA to pick up the variations within the training set. Though more accurate results have been achieved by the above approaches, still the parameterized variations are in a linear Euclidean vector space. We also noted that kernel PCA [11] has become a popular method for nonlinear feature decomposition, but none explicit nonlinear shape model was presented.

We propose a non-linear shape model by introducing Principal Geodesic Analysis (PGA) [12] into Point Distribution Model (PDM) and facilitate the building of SSM problem by incorporating MDL into out approach. In section 2, we will review the details of PGA, ASM and MDL. Experimental results are shown in section3. The GAS model based MDL approach and original MDL were applied to several datasets, further analysis was performed by comparing Specificity between the two methods. Moreover, two algorithms are performed on complicated dataset to test model's ability to fight the problem "Pile Up". In the last section, a brief summary and conclusion were given.

2 Geodesic Shape Model

For building a Geodesic Active Shape model (GAS), four concepts have to be clarified which are Intrinsic Mean, Non-linear Variation, Geodesic Subspace and Projection. To make these concepts easier to understand, we will first review the original ASM.

2.1 Active Shape Model

Given a set of training examples with landmarks on the boundary, we can build a statistical shape model easily. In a 2D case, each shape boundary information is represented by concatenating n landmarks points into a $2n$ element vector and the new shape can then be represented by

$$\phi = \overline{\phi} + Vb \tag{1}$$

Where $\left(\overline{\phi}\right)$ is the Euclidean mean of the training examples V is the eigen-vectors captured by PCA and b is a weighting vector for shape parameters. From Eq.(1), we can see that ASM assumes shape variations as linear translations. However, in many cases real medical data have complicated nonlinear variations like thickness, blending or twisting which a linear model can not handle easily. Next, we are going to unveil the four important concepts of Geodesic Shape Model which are Intrinsic Mean, Nonlinear Variation, Geodesic Subspace and Projection.

2.2 Intrinsic Mean

Like in ASM, all dataset will be aligned according to the mean shape. In nonlinear shape model, we use the concept of Intrinsic Mean to substitute the Euclidean mean in ASM. The definition is as follows: Given a set of shape landmark vectors, the intrinsic mean μ on the manifold M can be formulated as:

$$\mu = \arg\min_{x \in M} \sum_{i=1}^{N} d(x, x_i)^2 . \tag{2}$$

As we can see from Eq.(2), the intrinsic mean is given by minimizing the sum of "distances" between shapes in training set and the potential mean shape. Different from the notation in ASM, the distance in nonlinear shape model is calculated in Riemannian space. Computing the Intrinsic Mean involves solving the problem of minimizing the Eq.(2), the validity of this minimum is proved by Fletcher *et.al.* in [13]. Pseudo code is given in below to show how to calculate it efficiently.

$$\mu_o = \frac{1}{n}\sum_{i=1}^{n}\Phi(x_i)$$ Do

$$\Delta\mu = \frac{1}{n}\sum_{i=1}^{n}\left(\log_{\mu_j}(x_i)\right)$$ $$\mu_{j+1} = \mu_j\Delta\mu$$

While $\|\Delta\mu\| > \theta$; θ is a small positive constant.

2.3 Nonlinear Variation

Given a set of points $x_1, \ldots, x_n$ on a complete, connected manifold M , the definition of sample variance will be as follows:

$$\sigma^2 = \varepsilon\left[d(\mu, x)^2\right]. \tag{3}$$

We can see that the variance of the data is equal to the expected value of the squared Riemannian distance from the intrinsic mean. By introducing the Riemannian Exponential Map and Riemannian Log Map concepts as in [13], we can extend Eq.(3) to:

$$\sigma^2 = \frac{1}{n}\sum_{i=1}^{n} d(\mu, x_i)^2 = \frac{1}{n}\sum_{i=1}^{n} \left\| \log_\mu (x_i) \right\|^2 . \tag{4}$$

For securing the positivity of x_i, translation has to be used as follows:

Algorithm for making sure of the positivity

Input: $x_1,...,x_n \in M$ Output: $x_1',...,x_n' \in M$

Do: $templ_i = \mathrm{Pr}\,ocrustes(x_i)$; Procrustes Alignment

$temp2_i = Centralization(templ_i)$; Centralization to mean

$x_i' = temp2_i + \theta$; θ is a small positive constant

While $i < n$

2.4 Geodesic Subspace

In ASM, PCA describes the notion of sub-manifolds as a linear subspace in Euclidean space. A geodesic is a curve that is the shortest path between points. In PGA, we use geodesic to define the sub-manifolds and it is natural to define a geodesic as one dimensional subspace. It is worth noticing that if N is a sub-manifold of manifold M, geodesics of N are not necessarily geodesics of M. For example, the sphere S^2 is a sub-manifold of S^3, but its geodesics are great circles, while geodesics of S^3 are straight lines. The illustrations of PCA in linear space and PGA in curved space can be seen in Fig.1.

Fig. 1 shows different results when applying PCA and PGA to perform feature extraction. We can see that by using Geodesics, PGA can deal with curved space and capture nonlinear deformation without losing too much information while PCA can only do approximations of nonlinear variations.

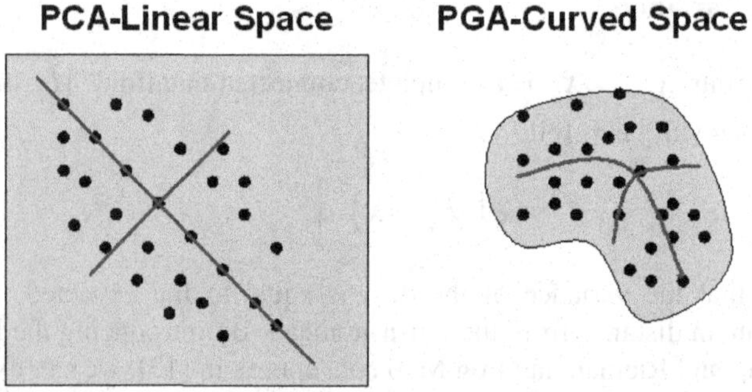

PCA-Linear Space   **PGA-Curved Space**

Fig. 1. On the left, an illustration of PCA in Euclidean space is shown; red orthogonal lines represent eigen-vectors captured by PCA. On the right, an example of PGA analysis on curved space is shown; red lines are geodesics picked up by PGA.

2.5 Projection

In Euclidean space, projection is intuitive, however in Riemannian space, the projection of a point x in manifold M onto sub-manifold N can be defined as follows:

$$\Phi(x) = \operatorname*{arg\,min}_{\substack{x \in M \\ y \in N, N \in M}} d(x, y)^2 .$$ (5)

As a minimization process, there is no guarantee that the projection of a point exists or it is unique. However, by limiting to a small enough neighborhoods around the intrinsic mean, a unique projection can be assured.

2.6 Calculating Geodesic Active Shape Model

We are now ready to define the Geodesics Active Shape (GAS) Model for data $x_1, \ldots, x_n$ on a connected Riemannian manifold M. Our goal, analogous to PCA, is to find a sequence of nested geodesic sub-manifolds that maximized the projected variance of the data. These sub-manifolds are captured by the PGA. So, the principal geodesic sub-manifolds are first constructed by an orthogonal basis of tangent vectors. Then the linear PCA is performed in this tangent space. Therefore, we give out the GAS model as follows:

$$\phi = \mu \exp(Pb) .$$ (6)

Where ϕ is a new shape, μ is the intrinsic mean shape from the training set. It is worthy to be noticed that when b is equal to zero, the new shape is actually the intrinsic mean shape. For making a comparison between ASM and GAS, we build the two shape models from a dataset composed of 18 hand contours marked by an expert. The result is shown in Fig. 2 by moving the first two weighting components between $-3\sqrt{\lambda_i}$ to $3\sqrt{\lambda_i}$.

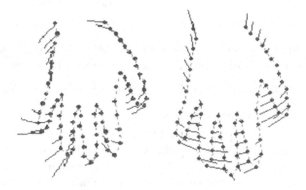

Fig. 2. On the left Shows the GAS mode; on the right shows the ASM. Shown is the mean shape with red marks; the whiskers emanating from the marks indicate five standard deviations of the first principal components. It can be observed that, though not that obvious, in the finger tip area, the Gas model capture the curved variations.

From the two models we can see that, the ASM assume the variations to be linear combinations and GAS model will have both curved and straight variations. For more quantitative analysis on both models, we need to introduce Specificity which will be unveiled in the next section.

2.7 Minimum Description Length

The so called "correspondence problem" has been widely studied. The problem involves how to identify the correspondence points across the datasets. Davies *et.al.* [7] pose the problem into a learning process, thus good shape properties can be achieved by choosing a well defined objective function. They choose an information theory based algorithm by minimizing the description length of the training set. In this paper, we adopt the lasted version of MDL from [14], which is as follows:

$$Description\ Length = \sum L_m$$
$$L_m = 1 + \log\left(\lambda_m / \lambda_{cut}\right)\ for\lambda_m \geq \lambda_{cut} \tag{7}$$
$$L_m = \lambda_m / \lambda_{cut} \qquad\qquad for\lambda_m < \lambda_{cut}$$

Where the cost function is as simple as a combination of λs, and λ_{cut} is a constant evaluated by the resolution of images. In experiment we make it 0.3 which correspondences to a cut-off at 0.3 pixels for the shapes with original radius 100 pixels. An efficient optimization algorithm was adopted from Ericsson [15]. By finding the gradient of cost function, Ericsson uses some more efficient numerical algorithm such as Conjugate Gradient. The gradient is given as follows:

$$\frac{\partial \lambda_k}{\partial \theta_{mn}} = 2s_k u_{mk} V_K \frac{\partial \phi_m}{\partial \theta_{mn}}, \quad \frac{\partial DL}{\partial \theta_{mn}} = \sum_{\lambda_k \geq \lambda_c} \frac{1}{\lambda_k} \frac{\partial \lambda_k}{\partial \theta_{mn}} + \sum_{\lambda_k < \lambda_c} \frac{1}{\lambda_c} \frac{\partial \lambda_k}{\partial \theta_{mn}} \tag{8}$$

Here s, u and V are the outputs of Single Value Decomposition (SVD) applied onto the shape covariance matrix, for example, the SVD of shape $\left(\phi\right)$ gives $\phi = USV^T$ [14]. If ϕ is zero centered, V will correspond to P in Eq.(1) and the diagonal of $S^T S$ gives the eigen-values λ_k.

In addition, due to a minor pitfall of the MDL, in some cases the cost function will be trapped in a "meaningless" local or globally minimum. Different researchers have reported this problem in [7, 14, 15]. When the cost function was trapped in a "meaningless" minimum, points along the boundary will pile up into some congested area and therefore can't describe the rest of the shapes. In this way, the cost function attains a meaningless lower value. Some remedy can be added to the cost function. One way is to add more curvature based additional term to the main cost function, the other way is to use a master example which means one of the examples was maker by an expert and the points on it will not be moved during optimization. In the experiments, the original MDL met this "pile up" problem even though one master example is incorporated. However our proposed approach solved this problem without changing the frame of MDL.

3 Experiments

In this section, we will show the definition of Specificity which was used to evaluate the model's ability to capture accurate and specific variations. Two experiments are conducted which are dataset composed of femurs and facial profile silhouettes. In either experiment ASM based MDL and GAS based MDL are implemented and applied onto the datasets.

3.1 Specificity

Due to lack of ground truth, it is very difficult to measure the accuracy of variations captured by different approaches. In this part, a "Benchmark" Comparison criteria is introduced here, which is Specificity [16]. Specificity is the ability to measure if the model can generate instances of the objects that are close to those in the training set. We selected the weighting parameters randomly in the range between $-3\sqrt{\lambda}$ to $3\sqrt{\lambda}$. The Specificity and its error level are given as follows:

$$S(\Theta) = \frac{1}{N} \sum_{j=1}^{N} \left| \phi_j(\Theta) - \phi_j' \right|, \ \sigma_{S(\Theta)} = \frac{\sigma}{\sqrt{n_s - 1}} \qquad (9)$$

Where x_j are shape examples generated by the model, x_j' is the closest shape in the training set to x_j, σ is the sample standard deviation of $S(\Theta)$, Θ is number of mode, n_s is the number of samples we generated and N in our case is 100000.

3.2 Comparison Results

In order to validate our proposed algorithm, our experiments are conducted on two datasets examining the Specificity Ability. The first dataset is composed of 32 contours of femurs with 65 marks, and 9 nodes. The second dataset is composed of 22 silhouettes of faces with 65 marks, and 9 nodes. In either experiment ASM based MDL and GAS based MDL are implemented and applied on the datasets.

From this experiment we can observe that GAS MDL find the correspondence in a seemingly same manner, and GAS model are more specific than ASM. So we can conclude that GAS model can capture variations reasonable more specific than ASM.

In the second experiment, we are going to validate the algorithm on the dataset of facial profiles. When applying the ASM MDL to the dataset, the algorithm met the problem so called "Pile up" (see Fig. 4). So, an external term added to the ASM MDL

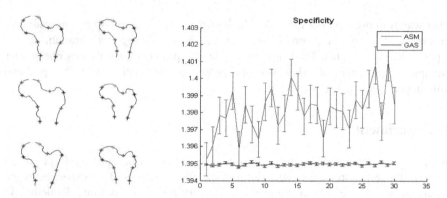

Fig. 3. On the left Shows the correspondence found by GAS MDL model; on the right shows the Specificity comparison between ASM MDL and GAS MDL. We can observe that GAS achieved lower normalized error value on Specificity than original MDL did.

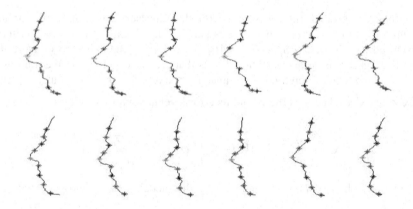

Fig. 4. On the top, results of ASM MDL analysis of silhouettes contours. Here 6 examples are shown, they are one step between MDL finally converged (Blue is level one, green is level two, black is level three and red is level four). It can be seen that the points at the bottom of facial profiles tried to pile up. On the bottom, results of GAS MDL are shown; it didn't encounter the pile up problem.

to make sure a valid convergence and again the comparison is performed between ASM MDL and GAS MDL on Specificity in Fig. 5.

Similar to the previous experiment, our proposed GAS model achieved lower value on the measurement of Specificity. Therefore we conclude that GAS model can convey more accurate variations than ASM and in its application to the dataset of facial profiles, the GAS MDL did not encountered the so called "run away" problem, but original ASM MDL did.

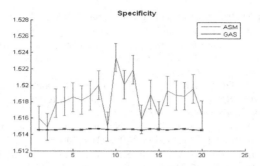

Fig. 5. Results of Specificity Analysis of silhouette contours between ASM and GAS. The notation is same as Figure 3. It can be seen that our proposed GAS achieves lower values in most of Θ ; therefore our GAS is more specific than ASM.

4 Conclusion and Future Work

In this paper, an in depth analysis of PGA, a novel geodesic shape model and its application to MDL have been presented. From the initial results performed on the two datasets, we can conclude that GAS model can capture variations reasonable more specific and the model can deal with nonlinear shape variations. On its application to the dataset of facial profiles, the original MDL was trapped in a meaningless local minimum even when the one master example was used, but GAS MDL did not. Therefore, we conclude that dealing with complicated shape forms, GAS MDL has more potential ability to fight the "Pile up" problem.

In the next stage of research, we are going to validate our algorithm on more 2D datasets with complicated shape forms. Extension to 3D datasets is undergoing and we have attained some encouraging initial results.

References

1. Gerig, G., Styner, M.: Shape verse Size: Improved Understanding of the Morphology of Brain Structures. Medical Image Computing and Computer Assisted Intervention, 24–32 (2001)
2. Chui, H., Rangarajan, A.: A new algorithm for non-rigid point matching. In: Proceeding IEEE Conference Computer Vision Pattern Recognition, pp. 44–51 (2000)
3. Walker, M.A., Highley, J.R., Esiri, M.M., McDonald, B., Roberts, H.C., Evans, S.P., Crow, T.J.: Neuronal populations and volumes of the hippocampus and its subfields in schizophrenia. Am.J.Psychiatry, 821–828 (2002)
4. Cootes, T.F., Taylor, C.J., Cooper, D., Graham, J.: Training models of shape from sets of examples. In: 3rd British Machine Vision Conference, pp. 9–18 (1992)
5. Hill, A., Taylor, C.J.: Automatic landmark generation for point distribution models. In: 5th British Machine Vision Conference, pp. 429–438 (1994)
6. Kotcheff, A.C.W., Taylor, C.J.: Automatic construction of eigenshape models by direct optimization. Medical Image Analysis, 303–314 (1998)
7. Davies, R.H., Cottes, T.F., Taylor, C.J.: A minimum description length Approach to statistical shape modeling. IEEE Transaction Medical Imageing, 525–537 (2002)

8. Ericsson, A.: Automatic Shape Modeling and Applications in Medical Imaging, Doctoral dissertation. Centre for Mathematical Sciences, Lund University (2003)
9. Wang, Y., Staib, L.H.: Boundary finding with correspondence using statistical shape models. In: Proceedings of IEEE Conference on Computer Vision and Pattern Recognition, pp. 338–345 (1998)
10. Su, Z., Lambrou, T., Todd-Pokropek, A.: Independent Component Analysis Based Active Shape Model with Spatial Relations for Finding Correspondence. Medical Image Understanding and Analysis, 46–50 (2006)
11. Schölkopf, B., Smola, A., Müller, K.-R.: Nonlinear component analysis as a kernel eigenvalue problem. Neural Computation, 1299–1319 (1998)
12. Fletcher, P.T., Lu, C., Pizer, S.M., Joshi, S.: Statistics of Shape via Principal Geodesic Analysis on Lie Groups, pp. 95–100 (2003)
13. Fletcher, P.T., Lu, C., Pizer, S.M., Joshi, S.: Principal geodesic analysis for the study of nonlinear statistics of shape, pp. 995–1005 (2004)
14. Thodberg, H.H.: A Minimum Description length Approach to statistical shape modeling. LNCS, pp. 525–537 (2003)
15. Ericsson, A., Karlsson, J.: Minimizing the Description Length using steepes descent. In: Proceeding British Machine Vision Conference, pp. 93–102 (2003)
16. Davies, R.H.: Learning Shape: Optimal Models for Analysing Natural Variability, Doctoral Dissertation. University of Manchester (2003)

Learning a Frequency–Based Weighting for Medical Image Classification

Tobias Gass[1], Adrien Depeursinge[2], Antoine Geissbuhler[2],
and Henning Müller[2]

[1] Lehrstuhl für Informatik 6, RWTH Aachen, Germany
`gass@informatik.rwth-aachen.de`
[2] Medical Informatics, University and Hospitals of Geneva, Switzerland
`henning.mueller@sim.hcuge.ch`

Abstract. This article describes the use of a frequency–based weighting developed for image retrieval to perform automatic annotation of images (medical and non–medical). The techniques applied are based on a simple *tf/idf* (term frequency, inverse document frequency) weighting scheme of GIFT (GNU Image Finding Tool), which is augmented by feature weights extracted from training data. The additional weights represent a measure of discrimination by taking into account the number of occurrences of the features in pairs of images of the same class or in pairs of images from different classes. The approach is fit to the image classification task by pruning parts of the training data. Further investigations were performed showing that weightings lead to significantly worse classification quality in certain feature domains. A classifier using a mixture of *tf/idf* weighted scoring, learned feature weights, and regular Euclidean distance gave best results using only the simple features. Using the aspect–ratio of images as feature improved results significantly.

1 Introduction

Since the amount and importance of visual data in many domains rises each year it is of great interest to find efficient means to seek for visual information. Content–based image retrieval (CBIR)[1,2] has therefore been one of the most active research areas in computer science over the last 15 years. In medicine the amount of data produced is extremely important. The total amount of cardiology image data produced in the Geneva University Hospital, for example, was around 1 TB in 2002, which is impressive considering it is only one subsection of the data produced at the hospital in general [3]. Radiology produced over 60'000 images per day in 2006. CBIR usually deals with the problem to find images similar to a query consisting of one or more images (Query By Example, QBE). In the medical domain with an electronic multimedia patient record this can help to find similar cases. Using original medical DICOM (Digital Imaging and COmmunication in Medicine)[1] files for data analysis can become an important

---

[1] `http://medical.nema.org/`

X. Gao et al. (Eds.): MIMI 2007, LNCS 4987, pp. 99–108, 2008.
© Springer-Verlag Berlin Heidelberg 2008

aid in diagnosis and treatment. The GNU Image Finding Tool (GIFT)[2] [4] was developed at the University of Geneva and is suited for these tasks because it treats visual data in the same way as textual data. This makes it easy to incorporate visual and textual features in a single processing step. Nevertheless, it is interesting to compare the performance of an information–retrieval based system such as GIFT, which uses very simple generic visual features, to other CBIR systems such as FIRE[3] (Flexible Image Retrieval Engine) [5], which is built to be flexible in means of available features and distance measures. The ImageCLEF[4] evaluation campaign [6,7] provides a platform for such a comparison, containing tasks in retrieval and classification of images in both the medical and non–medical domains. In this paper, we present various approaches to improve classification performance with GIFT by keeping the simple feature space and learning frequency–based feature weights from the available training data.

2   Methods

The methods described in this paper rely heavily on those used in GIFT. The learning approaches applied are based on algorithms published in [8] using the idea to translate the market basket analysis problem to image retrieval.

2.1   Databases

Two different databases from the ImageCLEF 2006 automatic annotation tasks were used to evaluate classification performance.

IRMA. The IRMA (Image Retrieval in Medical Applications, [9]) database of medical images was created at the hospitals of the RWTH Aachen. It consists of 11'000 x–ray pictures of several parts of the human body. Each image is annotated with the label of one out of 116 classes. In the ImageCLEF medical automatic annotation task, 1'000 of these images without class label had to be classified using the 10'000 images with supplied label as training data. Size of the classes varies strongly. A great difficulty is the strong visual similarity between some classes. Since availability of computation power during the experiments was low, a set with 1'000 images was used for system optimisation.

LTU. The LTU (LookThatUp) database, which was provided by the company LookThatUp[5], consists of images of a wide range of objects such as ashtrays or computer–equipment. A subset of 14'015 images of 21 classes was used for the non–medical automatic annotation task of the ImageCLEF2006 competition. 1'000 images served as an unlabelled test set for the evaluation. All experiments

---

[2] http://www.gnu.org/software/gift/
[3] http://www-i6.informatik.rwth-aachen.de/ deselaers/fire.html
[4] http://www.imageclef.org/
[5] http://www.ltutech.com

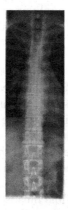

Fig. 1. Example x-ray of the spine

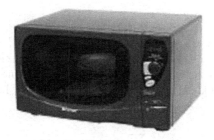

Fig. 2. Example picture of class "oven"

on the LTU database were performed by using the settings derived from experiments with the IRMA–database without any optimisation. This was done to show the ability to generalise from the derived results. In general, the non–medical automatic annotation task is hard due to the strong visual dissimilarities within classes.

2.2 Features Used

GIFT uses four groups of features, which are described in more detail in [4]:

- A global color histogram, which is based on the HSV (Hue, Saturation, Value) color space and quantised into 18 hues, 3 saturations, 3 values and usually 4 levels of grey.
- Local color blocks. Each image is recursively partitioned into 4 blocks of equal size, and each block is represented by its mode color.
- A global texture histogram of the responses to Gabor filters of 3 scales and 4 directions, which are quantised into 10 bins with the lowest one being discarded.

- Local Gabor block features by applying the filters mentioned above to the smallest blocks created by the recursive partition and using the same quantisation into bins.

This results in 84'362 possible features where each image contains around 1'500. The images in the IRMA database are not coloured and thus the number of possible features is reduced. Because of this and as a color histogram is usually an effective feature, we decided to increase the grey level features by extracting also 8, 16 and 32 levels, resulting in a higher–dimensional space. Such changes in feature space have frequently been used in the medGIFT[6] project. The GIFT uses this extension of the color space for both the color block features and the color histogram. This may not be the best approach, since similarity for color blocks with only four different possible bins is low. Hence, a separation of color spaces was tested, only using the enlarged color space for the color histogram features and not for the color block features.

2.3   GIFT Scoring

Several weighting schemes are implemented in GIFT. The basic one used in this paper is the *term frequency/inverted document frequency(tf/idf)* weighting, which is well known from text retrieval. Given a query image q and a possible result image k, a score is calculated as the sum of all weights of features which are occurring in k.

$$\text{score}_{kq} = \sum_j (\text{feature weight}_j) \tag{1}$$

The weight of each feature is computed by dividing the term frequency(tf) of the feature by the squared logarithm of the inverted collection frequency(cf).

$$\text{feature weight}_j = tj_j * \log^2(1/(cf_j)) \tag{2}$$

This results in giving features frequent in the collection a lower weight. These features do not discriminate images very well from each other. An example for such a feature is black background being present in many medical images. This weighting applies only to the block features. For histogram features a generalised histogram intersection is used to compute a similarity score [10].

The strategy described above does not use much of the information contained in the training data, only the feature frequencies are exploited and not the class memberships of the images. For optimising the retrieval of relevant images, learning from user *relevance feedback* was presented in [8]. In this article we use the described weighting approaches and add several learning strategies to optimise results for the classification task, where class membership of the training data is known.

---

[6] http://www.sim.hcuge.ch/medgift/

Learning Strategies. The original learning approach presented in [8] was to analyse log files of system use and find *pairs* of images that were marked together in the query process. Frequencies can be computed of how often each feature occurs in pairs of images. A weight can then be calculated by using the information whether or not the images in the pair were both marked as *relevant* or whether one was marked *relevant* and the other as *notrelevant*. This results in desired and non–desired cooccurence of features.

In this paper, we train weights more focused on classification. This means that user interaction is not regarded but rather relevance data on class membership of images by looking at the class labels of the training data. Each result image for a query is marked as relevant if the class matches that of the query image and non–relevant otherwise. This allows for a more focused weighting than what real users would do with relevance feedback. We then applied several strategies for extracting pairs of images for the queries. In a first approach, each possible pair of images occurring together at least once is considered relevant. This yields very good results for image retrieval in general [8].

In the second approach we aim at discriminating positive and negative results in a more direct way. To do so, only the best positive and the worst negative result of a query are taken into account when computing pairs of marked images.

In a third approach, we prune all queries which seemed *too easy*. This means that if the first N results were already positive, we omitted the entire query from further evaluation. Everything else follows the basic approach. This is based on ideas similar to Support Vector Machines (SVM), where only information on the class boundaries is taken into account. It assumes that all images that are in the middle of the class would be classified correctly anyways.

Computation of Additional Feature Weights. For each image pair detected, we calculate the features they have in common and whether the image pair was positive (both images in the same class) or negative (images in different classes). This results in positive and negative cooccurence on a feature level. We used two ways to compute an additional weighting factor for the features:

- Basic Frequency : In this weighting scheme, each feature is weighted by the number of occurrences in pairs where both images are in the same class, normalised by the number of occurrences of the feature in all pairs.

$$\text{factor}_j = \frac{|\{f_j | f_j \in I_a \wedge f_j \in I_b \wedge (I_a \to I_b)_+\}|}{|\{f_j | f_j \in I_a \wedge f_j \in I_b \wedge ((I_a \to I_b)_+ \vee (I_a \to I_b)_-)\}|} \quad (3)$$

In the formula, f_j is a feature j, I_a and I_b are two images and $(I_a \to I_b)_{+/-}$ denotes that I_a and I_b were marked together positively (+) or negatively (-).
- Weighted Probabilistic :

$$\text{factor}_j = 1 + (2 * \frac{pp}{|\{(I_a \to I_b)_+\}|}) - \frac{np}{|\{(I_a \to I_b)_-\}|} \quad (4)$$

Here, pp is the probability that the feature j is important for correct classification, whereas np denotes the opposite.

The additional factors calculated in this way are simply multiplied with the already existing weights using tf/idf for the calculation of similarity scores for all the test images.

2.4 Other Scoring Methods

During the experiments it became obvious that the frequency–based feature weights combined with the scoring method did not improve classification performance as much as hoped. Since GIFT uses four types of features it was necessary to have a more detailed idea of how the methods perform on each group of features. To achieve this, tests were performed where a single feature group was evaluated in GIFT. Experiments with Euclidean distance instead of the GIFT scoring were also attempted. In the latter case we experimented with applying the learned feature weights to the distances, which worked surprisingly well.

2.5 Classification

With the similarity scores computed for each image, a simple 5–Nearest neighbour algorithm was used to classify unlabelled test data. Each vote was weighted by the similarity score achieved. The selection of 5-NN was based on manual tests performed in a first stage, where between 1 and 10 images were regarded with sometimes varying results.

3 Experimental Results

All optimisations were done on the IRMA database. Due to the constraints in available computational power partly on small, disjunct subsets as training and test data. The given error rates were obtained by applying the tested methods to the automatic–annotation tasks of the ImageCLEF2006 competition.

3.1 Classification on the IRMA Database

The medical image annotation task was organised for the second time in 2006, after a first test in 2005. To augment the complexity the number of classes was raised from 60 to 116. 10'000 images were made available as training data and 1'000 images had to be classified.

Enhancing the Color Space. The baseline results of GIFT can be seen in Table 1. They show that a larger number of grey levels does not help, as error rates increase.

Frequency–Based Learned Feature Weights. In Table 2, the results of the GIFT using the learning approaches described above can be seen. Surprisingly, the effect of learning is small in comparison to the good results obtained for retrieval. The only method improving the error rate was the frequency–based weighting combined with best/worst pruning of the queries.

We also combined eight grey levels with the described techniques but the results were worse. Interestingly, the probabilistic weighting was not as much affected by the selections of relevant results as the frequency–based weighting.

Table 1. Error rates on the IRMA database using a varying number of grey levels

Number of grey levels	Error rate
4	32,0%
8	32,1%
16	34,9%
32	37,8%

Table 2. Error rates using various weighting strategies and 4 grey levels. S_1 corresponds to using the naive strategy, S_2 to pruning the queries found too easy, and S_3 means only using the best positive and worst negative result of each query.

Used strategy	Frequency weighting	Probabilistic weighting
S_1	35,3%	32,4%
S_2	33,2%	32,5%
S_3	31,7%	32,2%

Classification on Single Feature Groups. In these experiments we classified the data by using each feature group separately. The varying weighting strategies were performed. The probabilistically learned feature weights were omitted because of inferior performance in earlier experiments. It turns out that performance varies greatly, so a classification with mixed scoring methods seems most viable (see Table 3. If the classification in GIFT was performed without any weighting whatsoever, the error rate increased from 32% to 34%, so a more detailed approach is necessary.

Mixed Scoring. It is interesting to see how the GIFT scoring method performs in comparison to standard metric–based similarity measures. The first results were interesting as a simple Euclidean–distance–based 5–NN outperformed the GIFT by decreasing the error rate to 29.8%. At this point, several experiments on small test and training sets were conducted in which GIFT scoring, Euclidean distance(L2), and other feature weightings were tested. The methods with the best results on these subsets were then used, improving the error rate significantly to 27.5%. This score was achieved with the scoring method/weighting approach described in Table 4.

Table 3. Error rates on the four feature groups using several weighting approaches

Feature group	unweighted baseline	with tf/idf	learned weights	tf/idf+learned weights
Color block	36,6%	39,6%	35,1%	40,4%
Color hist	74,5%	–	73,8%	–
Gabor block	56,3%	42,3%	50.0%	45,4%
Gabor hist	53,1%	–	51.8%	–

Table 4. Best setup for classification

Feature group	scoring method	learned feature weights
Color block	L2	–
Color hist	GIFT tf/idf	–
Gabor Block	GIFT Histogram Intersection	used
Gabor hist	L2	used

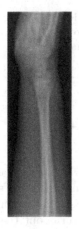
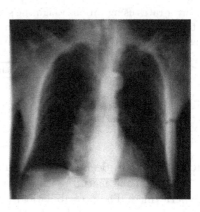

Fig. 3. X–rays of a leg and the chest, with different aspect ratios

Aspect Ratio. In the medical image domain and particularly for x–rays contained in the IRMA database, the aspect ratio of an image is highly correlated to the content of the image. This seems logical since x–rays are performed to show only the region of interest. Bones from the arm, for example, have a significantly different form than a chest. This leads to the idea to use the aspect ratio as a fifth feature group and include it into classification (Figure 3). This approach again improved the classification error rate on the best setup we used from 27,5% to 26.4%.

3.2 Classification on the LTU Database

The non–medical automatic annotation task consisted of 14'035 training images from 21 classes selected from a total set of more than 200 classes and over 100'000 images. The entire dataset was regarded as too difficult. Subsets such as *computer equipment* were formed, mainly with images crawled from the web with a large variety of contained objects. The task remained hard with only three research groups finally submitting results. The content of the images was regarded as extremely heterogeneous even for the same class. Without using any of the described learning methods and a simple 5–nearest–neighbour classifier, the GIFT had an error rate of 91,7% (by chance voting

Table 5. Error rates on the LTU database using various strategies

Method used	Error rate
baseline	91,7%
with learned feature weights	90,5%
with mixed scoring	88,3%
classifier combination	89%

would have 95% and would only be slightly worse). Using the learning method with best/worst pruning and the frequency–based weighting described above the error rate decreased to 90,5%. We also applied the mixed scoring method derived from the former experiments and achieved an error rate of 88.3%. A combination of available results could not further improve the classification performance (see Table 5).

4 Interpretation

The results show that the approach with the simple visual features in GIFT is not perfectly suited for image classification. GIFT uses four groups of global and local features, with just two similarity measures (histogram– and non–histogram features). It is, due to the good generalisation of the methods to more than one database, obvious that color and texture features have to be treated differently. Regarding the results it seems that color features frequent in the collection are still necessary to discriminate classes from each other. This can be due to very large classes that have many features in common and misclassifying some of these images can be more costly than loosing performance on very small classes. If these features get reduced in weight too much, the performance decreases. On the other hand, texture features, which occur often throughout the training data are carrying less discriminative information and thus perform better when they are weighted accordingly.

5 Conclusions and Future Work

In this article, we have shown the possibilities to use a frequency–based weighting scheme developed for image retrieval in a classification context. The performance of these weights depends on the features they are applied to, where color features seem to be less weighable or learnable than texture features. In general, the performance of the derived methods is still lower than other CBIR systems available. This results mostly from the simple feature set used that does not take into account small shifts or changes in size of the object in the image. Pre–treatment of images to remove background might be one solution. Another solution is the use of salient features for retrieval.

Acknowledgements

This work was partially supported by the Swiss National Science Foundation (Grant 205321-109304/1). The IRMA database is courtesy of Dr. Thomas M. Deserno, Department of Medical Informatics, RWTH Aachen, Germany.

References

1. Smeulders, A.W.M., Worring, M., Santini, S., Gupta, A., Jain, R.: Content-based image retrieval at the end of the early years. IEEE Transactions on Pattern Analysis and Machine Intelligence 22(12), 1349–1380 (2000)
2. Eakins, J.P., Graham, M.E.: content–based image retrieval. Technical Report JTAP–039, JISC Technology Application Program, Newcastle upon Tyne (2000)
3. Müller, H., Michoux, N., Bandon, D., Geissbuhler, A.: A review of content–based image retrieval systems in medicine – clinical benefits and future directions. International Journal of Medical Informatics 73, 1–23 (2004)
4. Squire, D.M., Müller, W., Müller, H., Pun, T.: Content–based query of image databases: inspirations from text retrieval. In: Ersboll, B.K., Johansen, P. (eds.) Pattern Recognition Letters (Selected Papers from The 11th Scandinavian Conference on Image Analysis SCIA 1999, vol. 21, pp. 1193–1198 (2000)
5. Deselaers, T., Weyand, T., Keysers, D., Macherey, W., Ney, H.: FIRE in Image-CLEF 2005: Combining content-based image retrieval with textual information retrieval. In: Peters, C., Gey, F.C., Gonzalo, J., Müller, H., Jones, G.J.F., Kluck, M., Magnini, B., de Rijke, M., Giampiccolo, D. (eds.) CLEF 2005. LNCS, vol. 4022, pp. 652–661. Springer, Heidelberg (2006)
6. Clough, P., Grubinger, M., Deselaers, T., Hanbury, A., Müller, H.: Overview of the ImageCLEF 2006 photo retrieval and object annotation tasks. In: Peters, C., Clough, P., Gey, F.C., Karlgren, J., Magnini, B., Oard, D.W., de Rijke, M., Stempfhuber, M. (eds.) CLEF 2006. LNCS, vol. 4730, pp. 579–594. Springer, Heidelberg (to appear 2007)
7. Müller, H., Deselaers, T., Lehmann, T.M., Clough, P., Eugene, K., Hersh, W.: Overview of the imageclefmed 2006 medical retrieval and medical annotation tasks. In: Peters, C., Clough, P., Gey, F.C., Karlgren, J., Magnini, B., Oard, D.W., de Rijke, M., Stempfhuber, M. (eds.) CLEF 2006. LNCS, vol. 4730, Springer, Heidelberg (to appear 2007)
8. Müller, H., Squire, D.M., Pun, T.: Learning from user behavior in image retrieval: Application of the market basket analysis. International Journal of Computer Vision (Special Issue on Content–Based Image Retrieval) 56(1–2), 65–77 (2004)
9. Lehmann, T.M., Güld, M.O., Thies, C., Fischer, B., Spitzer, K., Keysers, D., Ney, H., Kohnen, M., Schubert, H., Wein, B.B.: Content–based image retrieval in medical applications. Methods of Information in Medicine 43, 354–361 (2004)
10. Swain, M.J., Ballard, D.H.: Color indexing. International Journal of Computer Vision 7, 11–32 (1991)

Greek-English Cross Language Retrieval of Medical Information

E. Kotsonis, T.Z. Kalamboukis, A. Gkanogiannis, and S. Eliakis

Department of Informatics
Athens University of Economics and Business
Athens, Greece
tzk@aueb.gr

Abstract. Health information systems on the web basically support the English language. To access high-quality online health information it is frequently a barrier for non-English speakers or speakers of English as a foreign language. In this work we present a cross-language retrieval system to support Greek users in the medical domain, overcome the language barrier. We have performed a case study on the impact of stemming in the cross lingual retrieval in association with dictionary based query translation techniques. Finally, we conclude with results from a preliminary evaluation of the Greek-English CLIR prototype.

1 Introduction

Cross-language information retrieval (CLIR) is a subfield of information retrieval dealing with retrieving information written in a language different from the language of the users query. Today search engines retrieve documents written in the same language as the query. Cross-language retrieval supports users of multilingual document collections by allowing them to submit queries in their own language, and retrieve documents in any of the languages covered by the retrieval system. CLIR systems can be used by people with good reading skills in a second language but poor skills in writing and therefore these users cannot compose a query that will fulfill their information need as they could do in their mother language.

Cross-language and monolingual retrieval functionality can certainly be provided by a single system. An effective monolingual retrieval is actually the core of a cross-lingual retrieval system [1]. Indeed when we search for documents written in a foreign language, we must choose between two primal approaches: either to translate the documents of the target language, or to translate the queries. In both cases the problem is reduced to the monolingual retrieval. However, both directions of translation have their weaknesses: translating large document collections could be, computationally, an impractical task and short queries on the other side introduce uncertainty in their translations. Furthermore query translation imposes a kind of cost, which must be paid at the most challenging time - when a search engine is trying to optimize response time for a large number of

X. Gao et al. (Eds.): MIMI 2007, LNCS 4987, pp. 109–117, 2008.

nearly simultaneous queries. Thus we are seeking for a simple and fast algorithm to translate the queries.

It is a well-known fact that information retrieval is not equally difficult for each language [2]. For example, the morphological analysis of the documents may be considered as minor for languages like English compared to languages like Greek with a rich inflectional and derivational system. The plural inflection of the English noun which, apart few exceptions, is very simple (add -s) while in Modern Greek there are 41 different inflectional suffixes. Also there are different forms of the written Greek language: such forms include classical Greek and Modern Greek. In this work we examine Modern Greek texts in the domain of medicine. This is actually a mixed language of modern with puristic Greek. It must be mentioned here that in any CLIR or monolingual retrieval system dealing in a language with a rich inflectional and derivational system stemming plays an important role on the performance.

The major approaches for CLIR include the use of bilingual dictionaries [3,4], parallel collections [5] and comparable collections [6] or some kind of combination of these. In this work we address the problem of disambiguation when dictionary-based techniques are used for the translation. In particular we present a case study on the impact of stemming in the complexity of a word-by-word translation algorithm with look-ups to bilingual dictionaries.

In the rest of this work we present the architecture of the CLIR system, the translation module and results from the OHSUMED database, a subset of the MEDLINE database. Finally we conclude on the performance of the algorithms used and extensions are proposed for future implementation.

2 System Architecture

The proposed system contains two subsystems: a multilingual subsystem, for retrieving bilingual documents (a collection of scientific articles in medicine available in the Greek web) and a cross language subsystem, which provides only the interface to the MEDLINE database using the PubMed search engine. The PubMed search engine[1] is maintained by the US National Center for Biotechnology Information and provides public access to the MEDLINE database over the web. The interface performs all the analysis of the query before its submission to the database, that is stop-words removal, stemming, automatic translation and disambiguation as well as procedures for query expansion. The system's architecture is presented in figure 1.

As far as the Greek database is concerned the Lucene search engine is used, an information retrieval system developed by Apache [2]. Lucene, supports many types of preprocessing, scoring, indexing, and retrieval models and supports several retrieval models, including the standard vector space model. To enhance the retrieval we have incorporated a Greek stemmer as well as a list of the most frequently used words (stopwords).

---

[1] http://www.ncbi.nlm.gov/entrez/query.fcgi?db=pubmed
[2] http://lucene.apache.org

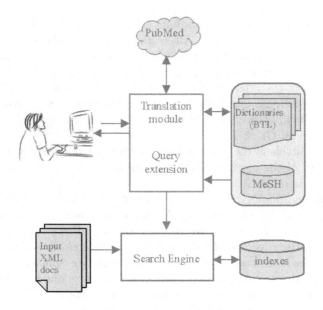

Fig. 1. CLIR, System's architecture

The Greek document collection contains bilingual articles in the medical domain, which are either entirely in English or in Greek, or they can use both languages with abstracts and references written in English. To ensure proper indexing of these documents using our standard architecture of Lucene, all documents are in UTF-8 format. The documents were indexed automatically using the TF*IDF weighting scheme [7]. Indexing includes stop-word removal, consulting a stopword list, stemming for the remaining tokens and weight estimation of terms, defined by $w(t, d)$

$$w(t, d) = TF(t, d) * log_2 \left(\frac{N}{DF(t)} \right) \tag{1}$$

where $TF(t, d)$ is the number of occurrences of term t in the document d, $DF(t)$ is the number of documents in the collection that contain the term t and N is the total number of documents in the collection.

All the documents are in XML format. The structured data are used to filter the retrieved documents by the year of publication, and the thematic topic.

The user submits queries in natural language and has the choice to see the results from the Greek or the English database. Each document title in the ranked list of the results is followed by the best passage of the document containing query words.

3   Dictionary Based Query Translation

In a CLIR system, users may be supported either to reformulate the query in order to choose the appropriate translations of the query terms, or to provide a fully automated query translation unit. This last task introduces uncertainty due to the small size of the query. Although machine translation techniques are the state of the art in translation theyt are far from perfect and certainly not fast enough to be used in an online retrieval system. Dictionary-based approaches have been used in the literature for several languages in the past [4,8].

For the translation a Greek-English bilingual dictionary was used, consisting of about 40,000 fully inflected words or phrases. The dictionary was constructed by merging several Greek-English dictionaries (Bilingual Term Lists) and glossaries freely available in the web. Although we are not in a position to guarantee for the validity of the resulting dictionary we used these resources as the base for translation in our CLIR system.

Due to the morphological complexity of the Greek language, we expect the dictionary to have limited coverage. In order to improve on the coverage, a stem-based dictionary was derived from the original. However, although stemming improves the coverage of the dictionary introduces an additional level of uncertainty since more words with different meanings are conflated into the same stem. Thus in our case we face two levels of uncertainty: one introduced by the stemming process; and one due to the translation of words with more than one possible translation.

In what follows we have experimented with three algorithms for automatic query translation based on dictionary look-ups:

1. **Word by word translation:** In the word-based scenario, all the possible translations of a word remain in the translated query. Words of the target language that are present in the original query remain unchanged. For the experiments the stemmer described in [2] was used. We shall refer to this as stemmer-1. At this stage an investigation of the impact of the morphological normalization (stemming) on retrieval effectiveness was carried out, by testing a more conservative, based strictly on grammar rules, stemmer [9]. The experimental results presented in the next section show a significant improvement of the new stemmer (stemmer-2) in the case of the simple word-by-word translation algorithm.

2. **Word by word translation and disambiguation:** To reduce ambiguity due to stemming a filtering step is applied that selects the most appropriate translation. A given Greek word, g, first is stemmed to g' and then translated using the dictionary, see figure 2. Suppose

$$T(g') = \{(e_1, g_1), (e_2, g_2), \ldots, (e_k, g_k)\} \tag{2}$$

is the set of all possible translations where by the pair (e_i, g_i) we denote a couple of an English word or phrase with its corresponding translation into Greek. Our filter function selects as the most appropriate translation, e_i, the one with minimum Levenstein distance $(\min \|g - g_i\|)$ between the original word g and g_i. Other distance measures based on n-grams have been tested but not reported in the present work. In table 1 we present two examples of translating the queries No 8 and No 73 of the OHSUMED database.

3. **Phrase based translation:** Accurate translation demands larger units. Other studies [3] have shown that phrases are a natural way of refining queries. In the phrase based translation an approach is proposed that uses phrases from dictionary as fundamental units for translation of the query. All the phrases in the dictionary that are present in the query are sorted by their size in ascending order and then substituted by their translation counterparts starting from the largest one. The size of a dictionary entry equals to the number of words it contains. To achieve this goal the dictionary was first indexed using the Lucene search engine. For a query Q, the dictionary was searched to find an entry, say Pr, that best matches with Q using the similarity metric

$$sim\,(Pr, Q) = \frac{|Pr \cap Q|}{|Pr|} \tag{3}$$

By $|Pr|$ we denote the number of words of a dictionary entry. From the answers we keep only those with $sim\,(Pr, Q) = 1$. In that case it holds that $Pr \subseteq Q$. However, the similarity function does not ensure that the terms reserve their order inside the phrase and the query. To ensure that words inside Pr and Q have the same order an additional parsing of the query is needed.

From the experimental results it is evident that translation by phrases outperforms all other dictionary-based techniques. Indeed many of the medical terms in the dictionary are compound terms.

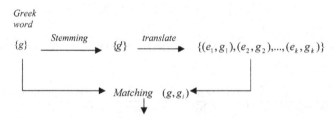

Fig. 2. Filtering of the most appropriate translation

4   Experimental Results

To test the performance of the algorithms proposed we utilized the **OHSUMED** test database[3], a subset of the MEDLINE database, extracted for the monolingual retrieval research [10]. This database is accompanied by a collection of 106 English language queries. We have used the corrected versions of these queries. For all but 5 queries, relevant document subsets are known. We use the 233,445 documents subset that contains abstracts and MeSH phrases for each document.

---

[3] ftp://medir.ohsu.edu/pub/ohsumed

Table 1. Translation of the OHSUMED No.8 and No.73 queries

	Query No.8	Query No.73
Original English	*work-up of hypertension in patient with horseshoe kidney*	*portal hypertension and varices, management with TIPS procedure*
Query translated by an expert	Διαγνωστικές εξετάσεις για υπέρταση σε ασθενή με πεταλοειδή νεφρό.	Πυλαία υπέρταση και κιρσοί οισοφάγου, αντιμετώπιση με διασφαγιτιδική ενδοηπατική πυλαιοσυστηματική παράκαμψη.
Word by World translation	diagnosis diagnostics diagnostic examination survey examination interrogation test hypertension supreme superlative disease weak patient illness sickness complain asthenia patients inpatient slim kidneys nephron kidney kidneys kidney renal nephritis nephron	portal hypertension supreme superlative varix varicose vein varicose veins esophagitis esophagus oesophagus portosystemic by pass
Word by World translation and disambiguation	diagnostic examination hypertension patient slim weak inpatient kidney	portal hypertension varicose veins oesophagus esophagus portosystemic by pass
Phrase Based Translation	workup hypertension inpatient patient weak slim kidney	portal hypertension varicose veins esophagus oesophagus faced with portosystemic by pass

Table 2. Average precision at the top-k retrieved documents with and without stemming

Top Retrieved Docs	English Queries	No stemming			Using stemming		
		WbW Translation	WbW and Disambiguation	Phrase Based Translation	WbW Translation	WbW and Disambiguation	Phrase Based Translation
5	0.3623	0.1283	0.1283	0.1509	0.1811	0.2264	0.2340
10	0.3142	0.1189	0.1189	0.1406	0.1689	0.2170	0.2198
20	0.2660	0.1090	0.1090	0.1288	0.1434	0.1797	0.1788
100	0.1419	0.0526	0.0526	0.0662	0.0775	0.0944	0.0970
200	0.1002	0.0362	0.0362	0.0471	0.0553	0.0650	0.0692

For our cross language experiments, a fluently English speaking medical doctor has translated the 106 queries first into Greek. The Greek queries are then translated back into English by our automatic methods.

Table 3. Average precision at the top-k retrieved documents from two different stemmers

		AvgPr(%) Word by Word Translation		
Top Retrieved Docs	English Queries	Stemmer-1	Stemmer-2	Improvement
5	36.23	18.11	20.00	5%
10	31.42	16.89	19.34	7.8%
20	26.60	14.34	16.70	8.8%
100	14.19	7.75	9.07	9.3%
200	10.02	5.53	6.19	6.6%

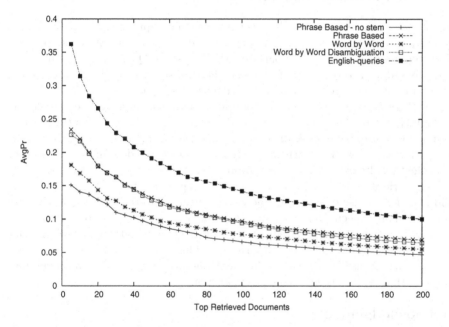

Fig. 3. Average precision plot with respect to the top-k retrieved documents

For the evaluation of the performance the well-known measure of precision was used on the top retrieved documents. Precision is defined by [7]:

$$Precision = \frac{Number\ of\ relevant\ documents\ retrieved}{Number\ of\ documents\ retrieved} \quad (4)$$

In tables 2 and 3 we present values of the averaged precision for the top-k ranked documents over all the queries. The performance of the cross language retrieval is evaluated against the same system running in a monolingual mode (English collection English queries), which serves as the base line of our evaluation. Figure 3 presents visually the performance of the algorithms.

In table 3 results are presented from the word-by-word translation method with the two stemmers mentioned above. From these results it is evident that stemmer-2 performs best in the case of word-by-word translation. In the other two cases, (phrase-based translation and word by word with disambiguation) both stemmers perform equivalently. This sounds reasonable since the disambiguation step removes the uncertaintly introduced by the use of an aggressive stemmer while when larger units are used in the translation, like phrases, the ambiguity is kept to the minimum.

According to the results it is apparent that phrase-based retrieval is best performing achieving a performance between 65%-70% of the corresponding monolingual retrieval.

5   Conclusions-Extensions

The main issue addressed here is the evaluation of an approach to remove disambiguation introduced by the stemming. According to our results it is apparent that stemming is an important part on a CLIR system. Query words are morphologically reduced to their root forms and then substituted by their counterparts in the target language through the dictionary. To reduce the ambiguity due to morphology we have introduced a double translation filter and to reduce the ambiguity due to the translation we used phrases as basic units for translation. Although we are making use of resources freely available in the web, the resulting performance of the algorithms tested is quite fair and comparable to other published results from counterpart approaches.

The retrieval model we have described at its present state is the simplest one and it makes no use of semantic knowledge of terms. Certainly the effectiveness of retrieval on a specific domain, such as medicine, can be improved when domain knowledge is used. Such knowledge may contain synonymous terms and phrases, broader or narrower terms, related terms etc. This is an ongoing research, and we are currently translating a part of the MeSH metathesaurus in the cardiovascular domain, that will be used for query expansion.

Acknowledgements

We thank Dr. D. Soulis for his excellent job of translating the OHSUMED-database queries into Greek.

This work was partially funded by EU, ASIA ICT/TIME project and partially by the Greek Secretariat of Research and Technology, Image, Speech and Language Processing, Action 3.3, MedAS project.

References

1. Hollink, V., Kamps, J., Monz, C., de Rijke, M.: Monolingual document retrieval for european languages. Information Retrieval 7, 33–52 (2004)
2. Kalamboukis, T.: Suffix stripping with modern greek. Program 29(3), 313–321 (1995)

3. Ballesteros, L., Croft, W.: Phrasal translation and query expansion techniques for cross-language information retrieval. In: Proceedings of the 20th ACM SIGIR Conference, pp. 84–91 (1997)
4. Hull, D., Grefenstette, G.: Querying across languages: A dictionary–based approach to multilingual information retrieval. In: H.P., F., D., H., P., S., R., W.(eds.) Proceedings of the 19th International Conference on Research and Development in Information Retrieval (ACM SIG/IR 1996), pp. 49–57 (1996)
5. Dumais, S., Letsche, T., Littman, M., Landauer, T.: Automatic cross–language retrieval using latent semantic indexing. In: Hull, D., Oard, D. (eds.) 1997 AAAI Symposium on Cross–Language Text and Speech Retrieval (1997), http://www.clis.umd.edu/dlrg/filter/sss/papers/dumais.ps
6. Sheridan, P., Wechsler, M., Schauble, P.: Cross language speech retrieval. In: Belkin, N., Narasimhalu, A., Willett, P. (eds.) Proceedings of the 20th International Conference on Research and Development in Information Retrieval (ACM SIGIR 1997), pp. 99–109 (1997)
7. Salton, G., Wu, H., Yu, C.: Measurement of term importance in automatic indexing. J. Am. Soc. Inf. Sci. 32, 175–186 (1981)
8. Pirkola, A., Hedlund, T., Keskustalo, H., Jarvelin, K.: Dictionary-based cross-language information retrieval: Problems, methods, and research findings. Information Retrieval 4, 209–230 (2001)
9. Holton, D., Mackridge, P., Filippaki-Warburton, E.: Greek Grammar. Patakis Editions (2006)
10. Hersh, W., Buckley, C., Leone, T., Hickam, D.: Ohsumed: An interactive retrieval evaluation and new large test collection for research. In: Croft, B., van Rijsbergen, C. (eds.) Proceedings of the 17th Annual International Conference on Research and Development in Information Retrieval (ACM SIG/IR 1994), pp. 192–200 (1994)
11. Ballesteros, L., Croft, W.: Dictionary methods for cross-lingual information retrieval. In: 7th Conference and Workshop on Database and Expert Systems Applications, pp. 791–801 (1996), http://ciir.cs.umass.edu/info/psfiles/irpubs/ir.html

Interest Point Based Medical Image Retrieval

Xia Zheng[1], MingQuan Zhou[1,2], and XingCe Wang[2]

[1]State Key Laboratory of Cognitive Neuroscience and Learning,
Beijing Normal University, Beijng, P.R. China
[2]College of Information Science and Technology,
Beijing Normal University, Beijng, P.R. China
xiasbee@sina.com.cn

Abstract. The technology of medical image retrieval in picture archiving and communication systems (PACS) is of great importance. A shape prior algorithm retrieval based on interest point is presented in this paper. Firstly, according to the formulaic composition of a medical image, a Harris point detector is improved to extract some interest points in images. Secondly, by combining invariants for each point and an edge type histogram, the feature vector for matching is constructed. Finally, a strategy for matching vectors is implemented to retrieve medical images. The test results prove the efficiency of this approach.

Keywords: medical image retrieval, interest point, shape type histogram.

1 Introduction

The technology of medical image retrieval in picture archiving and communication systems (PACS) is of great importance. Imaging systems and image archives have often been described as an important economic and clinical factor in the hospital environment [1-3]. The fundamental retrieval method is to exploit some features such as color, texture and shape, which can be extracted by a machine automatically. Today, with the increasing number of medical images, the retrieval systems should be designed as an effective and efficient tool for user browsing and navigating in medical image databases. In order to obtain good results, segmentation is an important step in some methods. The images then can be segmented into several regions. The query is implemented by features matching, which are extracted from regions. Carson et al. [4] employed a so called "blobworld" representation which is based on segmentation using EM algorithms combined color and texture features. In NETRA [5], images are segmented into homogeneous regions using a technique called "edge flow".

However the result of segmentation depends on the content of the medical image. Completely automated segmentation of images is an unsolved problem. Even in fairly specialized domains, automated segmentation causes many problems and is often not easy to be realized. Therefore many researchers seek different solutions. Applying some salient points to solve the problem is a new trend. These points have special properties which can make them stand out in comparison to their neighboring points. They are often also called interest points. Considering medical images have a formulaic

X. Gao et al. (Eds.): MIMI 2007, LNCS 4987, pp. 118–124, 2008.

composition for each modality and anatomic region, a new retrieval method based on some interest points is proposed to query medical images without global image descriptors. The remainder of this paper is organized as follows. In section 2, works related to point detection are introduced and an improved Harris point detector applied in this work is described. Section 3 provides information on direction information acquisition and details how they are represented. Matching strategy and results are presented in Section 4. Finally, Section 5 concludes the paper.

2 Interest Point Detection

The initial step is to collect images. The collection contained a large number of monochrome images, such as x-rays and CT scans, with very specific layout. The patients are positioned very precisely to show the area under investigation at the centre of the image. A neuroimage database composed of clinical volumetric CT images is used.

We are interested in using gray-level image attributes which are invariant with respect to a group of transformations such as the orthogonal and affine transforms. It is necessary to consider invariants up to the third order to obtain good characterization of the gray-level images. As a matter of fact, these invariants are difficult to estimate in a stable fashion. In our work, the first order derivatives and other information are used to obtain similar good results. In order to obtaining a precise and stable first order detector, an improved Harris point detector is chosen.

The Harris point detector introduced in [6] is a popular interest point detector due to its strong invariance to: rotation, scale, illumination variation and image noise. It is calculated based on a second moment matrix M describing the gradient distribution in the local neighborhood of a point. The Harris operator can be defined by positive local extrema of the following operator:

$$C_H(M) = Det(M) - K * Trace^2(M) \, , \quad K = 0.04 \qquad (1)$$

where the constant K indicates the slope of the "zero line". A basic extension of the intensity based M is defined as [7]:

$$M = \begin{bmatrix} R_x^2 + G_x^2 + B_x^2 & R_x R_y + G_x G_y + B_x B_y \\ R_x R_y + G_x G_y + B_x B_y & R_y^2 + G_y^2 + B_y^2 \end{bmatrix} \qquad (2)$$

where i_x and i_y ($i \in \{R,G,B\}$) are first order. Subscripts x and y indicate directions. In practice, Gaussian smoothing is needed as preprocessing to reduce the noise. Due to the nature of medical image, for each color plane $\{R,G,B\}$, the gray-value of each pixel is re-expressed. So the matrix M is adapted as follows:

$$M = \begin{bmatrix} i_x^2 & i_x i_y \\ i_x i_y & i_y^2 \end{bmatrix} \tag{3}$$

where i represents the intensity value. Our concrete approach to extract the interest points is described as follows:

- Reduce noise of the medical image with a Gaussian filter. Isolated noise points and small structures are filtered out.
- Image is divided into many regions. The number of the regions is related to the complexity of image. Multiresolution quadtree can be applied.
- For each region, Eq. (3) based on an improved Harris point detector is used to get interest points, and the constant K is adjusted after many experiments.

Fig.1 is an example of our work on interest point extraction. As shown, these points in the images contain sufficient information.

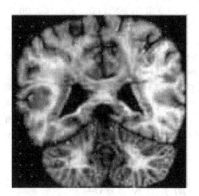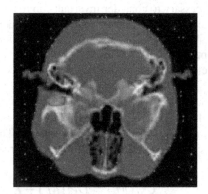

Fig. 1. The interest points extracted and visualized on two medical images

3   Feature Vectors Construction

As the gradient information is robust against variation, it is used to characterize selected interest points. Each point is expressed in a vector I .

$$I = (i, \| \nabla i \|^2) \tag{4}$$

Eq. (4) is robust to scale and viewpoint changes, considering computation for several Gaussian sizes. It can also be made robust to the main illumination transformations with image normalization. In order to enhance the representation ability of I , it is extended with other information. As we can see, the shape of the medical image is obvious and it is helpful to the whole retrieval process. Then I can be combined with the shape feature.

In our work, edge type histograms represent shape information. There are four types of edge .Each one denotes one direction (0°, 45°, 90°, 135°). The different edge detectors are defined as Fig.2.

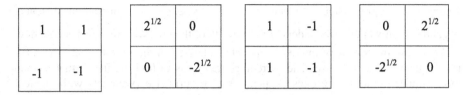

Fig. 2. Four types of edge detector

Using the interest point as the target pixel, a 4×4 window is opened, which is a 4-connectivity. These edge detectors work on it. In further study, instead of using 4-connectivity, we choose an 8-connectivity (or an 8-neighborhood) where horizontal, vertical and diagonal directions are allowed, since in a 4-connectivity, only vertical and horizontal directions may be followed. Therefore, the interest points become the central pixel in the local region, and the number of edge type increases. Every edge type histogram is calculated as shape information. Each interest point is expressed in an n–dimensional space T .

$$T = (t_1, t_2, \cdots, t_n) \tag{5}$$

where n is the number of edge type. T and I combine to make the feature vector of every interest point.

4   Matching and Results

When a feature vector is achieved, the matching method consists of comparing each feature vector of the first image with its counterpart in the second image in order to find the points which look the most similar. To compute the likeness of two vectors, we complete following steps.

We can easily compute the likeness of gray-value. To get the likeness of edge type histogram, Eq.(6) is applied.

$$D(T^i, T^j) = \sum_{k=1}^{n} |t_k^i - t_k^j| \tag{6}$$

Synthesizing the two comparing methods using Eq.(7), S corresponds to matching the results of two vectors.

$$S = \frac{w_I D_I + w_T D_T}{w_I + w_T} \tag{7}$$

where D_I is gray-value distance, and D_T is edge type histogram distance. w_I and w_T are weights which denote the priority of the gray feature and shape feature.

After building a base of interest points characterized in the vector space, we index the medical image database. The searching strategy is to find the image that has the most similar points to the ones in query. We performed experiments with medical images from patients. The results show that traditional retrieval methods are time consuming and limited by only using one feature. Its performance can not solve the scale and viewpoint changes. But the interest point based retrieval process, we proposed in this paper, is simple and robust to changes. It can give results not only with simple shapes, but also with complex shapes.

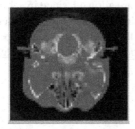

Fig. 3. Target image

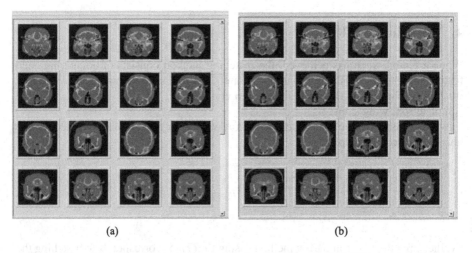

(a)   (b)

Fig. 4. The retrieval results. (a) Using simple shape based method. (b)Using our method.

As we can see, Fig.3 is a target medical image. Fig.4 (a) is the result of an experiment using a simple shape feature to retrieve images. Although most similar images are retrieved, there are some missing images with similar features. Compared with (a), Fig.4 (b) is the result of the proposed retrieval process in this paper. It is obvious that more images are found. The similarity of these images is very high.

Fig.5 is a query example in our PACS. In the system, the retrieval approaches are classified into four main types. The color based one focuses on color images. Many medical images with complex surfaces can be retrieved using texture based methods. In order to query the images with notable shape, the third type is used. The fourth type is to combine two or three features to complete the retrieval needs. In short, it is difficult to find one specific method that can solve the retrieval problems for all different types. Our work is to seek the most suitable one for each.

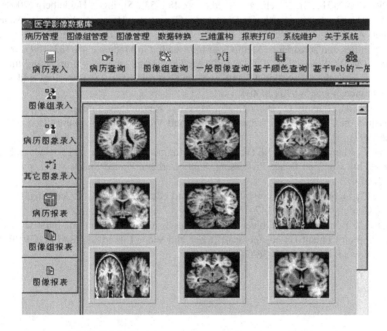

Fig. 5. Medical image query window of our PACS

5   Conclusion

In this paper, we have defined a new point based retrieval method for medical images. First we use an improved Harris point detector to extract interest points in every region. We have shown that adding these invariants gives sufficient information against variation to consider only the first order invariants. Secondly, each point is characterized and a feature vector is constructed. The feature vector is extended by applying a shape feature (edge type histogram). Finally we index the medical image database and implement the technique for medical image matching on this differential characterization, which works robustly and rapidly. Indeed, experimental results show the relevance of our approach and the percentage of correct matches is high, approximately 97.8%.Using this matching scheme, a large number of images can be matched rapidly. The achieved results prove that the method can be successfully used for medical image retrieval based on an object or region.

Acknowledgements. We would like to acknowledge the helpful discussions with Professor GuoHua Geng. The work was supported in part by an NSFC grant (No.60573179).

References

1. Greenes, R.A., Brinkley, J.F.: Imaging systems in Medical Informatics: Computer Applications in Healthcare, ch.14, 2nd edn., pp. 485–538. Springer, Heidelberg (2000)
2. Kulikowski, C., Ammenwerth, E., Bohne, A., Ganser, K., Haux, R., Knaup, P., Maier, C., Michel, A., Singer, R., Wol, A.C.: Medical imaging informatics and medical informatics: Opportunities and constraints. Methods of Information in Medicine 41, 183–189 (2002)
3. Vannier, M.W., Staab, E.V., Clarke, L.C.: Medical image archives - present and future. In: Proceedings of the International Conference on Computer-Assisted Radiology and Surgery, Paris, France, pp. 565–570 (2000)
4. Greenspan, H., Carson, C., Belongie, S., Malik, J.: Region-based image querying. In: IEEE Workshop on Content-based Access of Image and Video Libraries, Puerto Rico, pp. 42–49 (June 1997)
5. Ma, W.Y., Manjunath, B.S.: NETRA: a toolbox for navigating large image database. In: Proc. of IEEE Int. Conf. on Image Processing, Santa Barbara, United States, vol. 1, pp. 568–571 (1997)
6. Harris, C., Stephens, M.: A combined corner and edge detector. In: Proceedings 4th Alvey Visual Conference, UK, pp. 147–151 (1988)
7. Gouet, V., Boujemaa, N.: Object-based queries using color points of interest. In: IEEE Workshop on Content-Based Access of Image and Video Libraries (CBAIVL/CVPR 2001), Kauai, Hawaii, USA, pp. 30–36 (2001)

Texture Analysis Using Modified Computational Model of Grating Cells in Content-Based Medical Image Retrieval

Gang Zhang[1, 2], Z.M. Ma[1], Zhiping Cai[1], and Hailong Wang[1]

[1] College of Information Science and Engineering, Northeastern University
3-11 Wenhua Road, Shenyang, Liaoning 110004, China
mazongmin@ise.neu.edu.cn
[2] School of Software Engineering, Shenyang University of Technology
No. 58 Xinghua South Street, Tiexi District, Shenyang, 110004, China

Abstract. In neuroscience, grating cells in areas V1 and V2 of the visual cortex of monkeys can respond vigorously to a grating of bars of appropriate orientation, position and periodicity. Computational models of grating cells have been proposed and used to make texture analysis for medical images. To improve the matching precision, the computation models of grating cells were applied to the responses of simple cells and not for the pixel values of the input image. In this paper, the computational models of grating cells is modified to express uncertain information. Multi-valued logic is introduced into the computation of the responses of the grating subunit. Texture pattern is computed by means of the modified computational model of grating cells. Experiments show that the content-based medical image retrieval system using the modified computational model of grating cells has good performance.

Keywords: Grating cells, computational model of grating cells, texture analysis, content-based medical image retrieval.

1 Introduction

In the last two decades, a digital medical imaging revolution has transformed medicine. Technologies such as Computerized Tomography (CT) and Magnetic Resonance Imaging (MRI) have radically changed the way that physicians diagnose and treat diseases [1]. With the development of medical imaging technology and multimedia technology, there has been an exponentially increasing trend in the amount of medical image storage [2]. It is clear that early text-based image retrieval (TBIR) cannot meet the need of image expression and image retrieval. Under such as a circumstance, content-based medical image retrieval (CBMIR) has received a much attention. Also different anatomical parts as well as normal and abnormal states of the same anatomical parts can have different textures. So texture analysis is one of the most important research topics in CBMIR. The discovery of orientation-selective cells in the primary visual cortex of monkeys almost 40 years ago and the fact that most of the neurons in this part of the brain are of this type triggered a wave of research activity aimed at a

X. Gao et al. (Eds.): MIMI 2007, LNCS 4987, pp. 125–132, 2008.

more precise, quantitative description of the functional behavior of such cells [3]. Some computational models of orientation-selective visual neurons such as simple cells, complex cells, grating cells and so on have been proposed. In addition, some computational models that simulate the principle of operation of these cells (e.g., Gabor filters) have been proposed [4]. In recent years, researchers have applied these computational models, especially Gabor filters, for texture analysis in content-based medical image retrieval.

Grating cells respond vigorously to a grating of bars of appropriate orientation, position and periodicity. In contrast to other orientation-selective cells, grating cells respond very weakly or not at all to single bars, i.e., the bars which are isolated and do not form part of a grating [4]. However, current computational models of grating cells use two-valued logic, which limits its expression on uncertain information during feature expression.

In this paper, a modified computational model of grating cells is introduced into content-based medical image retrieval. Multi-valued logic is applied in the computational model of grating cells. Texture pattern is computed by means of the modified computational models of grating cells.

The rest of the paper is organized as follows: Section 2 reviews related work, Section 3 presents the modified computational model of grating cells, Section 4 investigates the feature representation and similarity measurement, Section 5 gives the simulation and performance analyses, and Section 6 concludes this paper.

2 Related Work

The physiological and pathological information of human organs is visually quite different and doctors can rely on different imaging knowledge for clinical diagnosis. Therefore, medical image databases are employed to store medical images of different anatomical parts. CBMIR are mainly aimed at specific anatomical parts [5, 6]. In [5], a method of texture analysis for CT images of hepatocellular carcinoma and liver cysts was proposed, which was used in computer-aided diagnostic system for focal liver lesions. Spatial and second-order probabilistic texture features were applied for image feature representation and Bayes classifiers were developed for image classification. In [6], a method of adaptive enhancement for unsupervised segmentation of three-dimensional MRI brain images was proposed. In their method, three brain tissues are of interest, CerebroSpinal Fluid (CSF), Grey Matter (GM) and White Matter (WM). Minimum error global thresholding is used to segment the three-dimensional MRI brain image. A spatial-feature-based fuzzy C-Means (FCM) clustering was used for a locally adaptive enhancement and segmentation with 3-D clustering-result-weighted median and average filters.

Different anatomical parts as well as the normal and abnormal states of the same anatomical parts can have different textures. So the texture analysis methods can be used for studies of the characterization of anatomical parts. In recent years, texture analysis methods based on multi-resolution, multi-channel (e.g., Gabor wavelet transform) and fuzzy logic have received much attention [7, 8]. In [7], a Gabor wavelet transform, which combines the wavelet transform method with the theory of directed filter, is used for texture analysis. This method builds a mathematical model for the rotate invariant texture analysis based on the research results in psychophysiology. However, this method directly uses the texture features extracted from the Gabor-wavelet. As a result, it takes a long time to compute the texture feature vector, which affects the efficiency of retrieval systems directly. In [8], a texture analysis method that uses statistical methods and fuzzy logic was proposed. In their method, a fuzzy set of dominant directions was introduced into the texture feature expression and similarity measurement. Experiments show that this method improves the retrieval performance of system efficiency.

Researchers have simulated a human's observation on scenery to extract low-level visual features, for a long time. Several computational models of orientation-selective visual neurons, such as simple cells, complex cells, grating cells and so on, have been proposed. These models provide valuable information for the extraction and representation of image features (especially medical image features) [9, 10]. In [9], simple cells were modeled by linear filters followed by half-wave rectification. Their orientation and spatial frequency selectivity can be explained by the specific kind of linear filtering involved. In [10], complex cells were modeled by three stages, which are linear filtering, half-wave rectification and local spatial summation. In [4], grating cells were modeled by two stages. In the first stage, the responses of so-called grating subunits were computed by using as input the responses of centre-on and centre-off simple cells with symmetric receptive fields. In the second stage, the responses of the grating subunits of a given preferred orientation and periodicity were summed together within a certain area in order to compute the response of a grating cell. However, two-valued logic was use for the computational model of grating cells in [4]. Consequently the computational model cannot express uncertain information.

3 Modified Computational Models of Grating Cells

Grating cells are found in the same cortical area (V1) as simple and complex cells and similarly to simple and complex cells show orientation selectivity. The computational model of grating cells uses the responses of simple cells as input and the simple cells are modeled by a family of two-dimensional Gabor functions as follows:

$$G(x, y) = \frac{1}{2\pi\delta_x\delta_y}\exp(-\frac{1}{2}(\frac{x^2}{\delta_x^2} + \frac{\gamma^2 y^2}{\delta_y^2}))\exp(-2\pi i\frac{x}{\lambda} + \varphi) \tag{1}$$

We hope that the information in the position (x, y) of a light impulse in the visual field can be strengthened when the Gabor function is acted on the (x, y) central symmetry area. So we use the real part of the Gabor function above, which is denoted as follows:

$$G(x, y) = \frac{1}{2\pi\delta_x\delta_y}\exp(-\frac{1}{2}(\frac{x^2}{\delta_x^2} + \frac{\gamma^2 y^2}{\delta_y^2}))\cos(2\pi\frac{x}{\lambda} + \varphi) \tag{2}$$

Here the parameters δ_x and δ_y denote the standard deviation of the Gaussian factor, which are used to determine the size of the receptive field. The parameter λ denotes the wavelength and $1/\lambda$ denotes the spatial frequency of the harmonic factor $\cos(2\pi x/\lambda+\varphi)$. Here δ_x/λ and δ_y/λ are used to determine the spatial frequency bandwidth of the simple cells along x and y direction. Usually, $\delta_x/\lambda = 0.56$ and $\delta_y/\lambda = 0.56$. The parameter γ denotes the spatial aspect ratio and is used to determine the eccentricity of the receptive field ellipse. Generally the parameter γ has a range from 0.23 to 0.92 [11]. The parameter φ denotes the phase offset in the argument of the harmonic factor $\cos(2\pi fx+\varphi)$ and is used to determine the symmetry of the function $G(x, y)$. In [12], $G(x, y)$ is symmetric for $\varphi = 0$ and $\varphi = \pi$ with respect to the center of the receptive field. It is shown in [4] that a cell with a symmetric receptive field reacts strongly (but not exclusively) to a bar which coincides in direction, width and polarity with the central lobe of the receptive field.

The parameters x and y are denoted as follows:

$$x = (x' - \xi)\cos\theta - (y' - \eta)\sin\theta \text{ and } y = (x' - \xi)\sin\theta + (y' - \eta)\cos\theta \quad (3)$$

Here the arguments x' and y' specify the position of a light impulse in the visual field, and ξ and η specify the centre of a receptive field within the visual field. The argument θ is the direction, in which the Gabor filters perform and specifies the orientation of the normal to the parallel excitatory and inhibitory stripe zones.

3.1 Response of a Simple Cell

If a luminance distribution image is $f(x, y)$ of size M×N, the response R of a simple cell in the visual field Ω is denoted as follows.

$$R = \begin{cases} X(\dfrac{R_1/R_2 * C_1}{R_1/R_2 + C_2}) = \begin{cases} 0 & 0 & G'(x,y) = 0 \\ 0 & \dfrac{R_1/R_2 * C_1}{R_1/R_2 + C_2} < 0 \\ \dfrac{R_1/R_2 * C_1}{R_1/R_2 + C_2} & \dfrac{R_1/R_2 * C_1}{R_1/R_2 + C_2} \geq 0 \end{cases} & G'(x,y) <> 0 \end{cases} \quad (4)$$

Here the parameters C_1 and C_2 are the maximum response level and the semi-saturation constant, respectively. The parameters R_1 and R_2 are denoted as follows:

$$R_1 = \sum_x\sum_y(\sum_s\sum_t f(x-s, y-t)G(s,t)) \quad (5)$$

$$R_2 = \sum_x\sum_y(\sum_s\sum_t f(x-s, y-t)G'(s,t)) \quad (6)$$

Here the parameters s and t are the Gabor filter mask size variables. The function $G'(x, y)$ can be denoted as follows.

$$G'(x, y) = \frac{1}{2\pi\delta_x\delta_y}\exp(-\frac{1}{2}(\frac{x^2}{\delta_x^2} + \frac{\gamma^2 y^2}{\delta_y^2}))$$ (7)

3.2 Modified Computational Model of Grating Cells

The modified computational model in this paper still consists of two stages. In the first stage, multi-valued logic is introduced to quantize the uncertain information. In the second stage, fuzzy values of responses of grating subunits are used to compute the response of a grating cell.

Suppose that a grating subunit of three bars is a segment of length 3λ passing through point (ξ,η) in orientation θ. The segment is divided in the intervals of length $\lambda/2$ and the maximum activity of one sort of simple cell, centre-on or centre-off, is determined in each interval. The point (ξ,η) is selected as the center and each interval is marked with a value in $\{-3, -2, -1, 0, 1, 2\}$. The results are shown in Fig1.

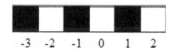

-3   -2   -1   0   1   2

Fig. 1. Grating subunit of three bars

It can be found from Fig. 1 that the subunit of a grating cell is activated if centre-on and centre-off cells of the same preferred orientation θ and spatial frequency $1/\lambda$ are alternately activated in the intervals of length $\lambda/2$ along a line segment of length 3λ centered on point (ξ,η) and passing in direction θ. However, it cannot be determined by the method in [4] that whether or not a grating cell can be activated if adjacent centre-on and centre-off have adjacent responses. In the paper, multi-valued logic is introduced into the computational model of the grating cell to address this problem.

Suppose that the center of the visual field is (ξ',η') and the position of grating subunit is (ξ,η). If $n = \{-3, -1, 1\}$, the parameter φ in formula (2) is 0. If $n = \{-2, 0, 2\}$, the parameter φ in formula (2) is π. The centre-on and centre-off can be computed with the formula as follows:

$$M(n) = \max\{R \mid \xi',\eta': n\frac{\lambda}{2}\cos\theta \le (\xi'-\xi) < (n+1)\frac{\lambda}{2}\cos\theta, n\frac{\lambda}{2}\sin\theta \le (\eta'-\eta) < (n+1)\frac{\lambda}{2}\sin\theta\}$$ (8)

Having been normalized, $M(n)$ can be denoted as follows:

$$M'(n) = \frac{M(n)}{\max\{M(n) \mid n = -3\cdots2\}}$$ (9)

The response of a grating subunit can be computed as follows.

$$Q = \begin{cases} 1 & \forall n, n \in [-3,1], |M'(n) - M'(n+1)| < L_1 \\ 1 - \min\{|M'(n) - M'(n+1)|\} & \forall n, n \in [-3,1], L_1 < M'(n) - M'(n+1)| < L_2 \end{cases} \quad (10)$$

Here the parameter L_1 denotes the maximum threshold width that a human can distinguish between the difference $M'(n)$ and $M'(n+1)$, and L_2 denotes the minimum threshold width that human can distinguish the similarity between $M'(n)$ and $M'(n+1)$. If $|M'(n)-M'(n+1)|$ is between L_1 and L_2, fuzzy values that are 1-$\min\{|M'(n)-M'(n+1)|\}$ are used to express the response of the grating subunit.

In the second stage of the model, the response of a grating cell is computed by the weighted summation of the responses of the grating subunits. Furthermore, the sum of grating subunits with orientation θ and $\theta+\pi$ is used so that the model is made symmetric for opposite directions. The response of a grating cell can be denoted as follows:

$$G(\theta) = \sum_{\xi'}\sum_{\eta'} \exp(-\frac{(\xi - \xi')^2 + (\eta - \eta')^2}{2(\beta\delta^2)})(Q(\theta) + Q(\theta + \pi)) \quad (11)$$

Here the parameter β determines the size of the area over which the effective summation takes place. A value of $\beta = 5$ results in a good approximation of the spatial summation properties of grating cells and $\theta \in [0,\pi)$.

4   Feature Representation and Similarity Measurement

This paper uses responses of the modified computational model of grating cells for texture features of a medical image. The texture feature vector can be denoted as follows:

$$F = \{G(\theta) \mid \text{dominance}(\theta) \in [0, \pi)\} \quad (12)$$

Here dominance (θ) denotes the dominant directions between 0 and π.

Let F_1 be the texture feature vector of an image in the medical image database and F_2 the texture feature vector of the sample image. Then the similarity measurement can be expressed as follows:

$$S = (\sum_{i=1}^{n}(F_1(i) - F_2(i))^2)^{\frac{1}{2}} \quad (13)$$

Here the parameter n is the amount of the elements in F. To evaluate the performance of a retrieval system which uses the method given above, two parameters, which are precision and recall, are introduced.

Definition 1. Assume that N and N' denote the numbers of the retrieved items and the retrieved correlated items, respectively. Then N'/N is called precision.

Definition 2. Let N'' and N' denote the numbers of the correlated items and the retrieved correlated items, respectively. Then N'/N'' is called recall.
Precision and recall may be 1.

5 Simulation and Performance Analyses

We select two groups of test sets in which each group consists of 100 medical images. The elements in the first group of test sets come from a chest CT image database. We select 25 images from the same chest CT image database and divide each image into 4 sub-images. The second group of test sets is made up of the sub-images.

We use the method in [4] and the method proposed in this paper to compute the texture feature vector for the first group of test sets, respectively. We also use the similarity measurement proposed in this paper to compute the similarity between each image of the image database and the sample image. We use the precision and the recall to measure retrieval performance. Experiments show that when the method in [4] is used, the precision is 70% and the recall is 75%. However, when the method proposed in this paper is used, the precision and the recall are 79% and is 90%, respectively. Now we focus on the second group of the test sets. Then the precision is 82% and the recall is 85% if the method in [4] is used, while the precision is 90% and the recall is 95% if the method proposed in this paper is used.

6 Conclusion

Texture analysis is one of the most important research topics in content-based medical image retrieval. However, current texture analysis methods respond not only to texture pattern, but also to non-texture pattern and even the pattern that is not perceived as texture at all. In neuroscience, the computational model of grating cells has been proposed to respond to the texture pattern only. In this paper, the computational model of grating cells is modified and multi-value logic is introduced to express uncertain information. According to the response of the modified computational model of grating cells, a texture feature vector is built and used for the similarity measurement between medical images. Experiments show that the method proposed in this paper improves the retrieval performance effectively.

Acknowledgments. The authors wish to thank the anonymous referees for their valuable comments and suggestions, which improved the technical content and the presentation of the paper. This work is supported by the Program for New Century Excellent Talents in University (NCET-05-0288).

References

1. Müller, H., Michoux, N., Bandon, D., Geissbuhler, A.: A Review of Content-based Image Retrieval Systems in Medical Applications – Clinical Benefits and Future Directions. International Journal of Medical Informatics 73, 1–23 (2004)
2. Greenspan, H., Pinhas, A.T.: Medical Image Categorization and Retrieval for PACS Using the GMM-KL Framework. IEEE Transactions on Information Technology in BioMedicine 11, 190–202 (2007)
3. Hubel, D.H., Wiesel, T.N.: Sequence Regularity and Geometry of Orientation Columns in the Monkey Striate Cortex. Journal of Comparative Neurology 158, 267–293 (1974)
4. Petkov, N., Kruizinga, P.: Computational Models of Visual Neurons Specialized in the Detection of Periodic and Aperiodic Oriented Visual Stimuli: Bar and Grating Cells. Biological Cybernetics 76, 83–96 (1997)
5. Smutek, D., Shimizu, A., Kobatake, H., Nawano, S., Tesar, L.: Texture Analysis of Hepatocellular Carcinoma and Liver Cysts in CT Images. In: Hamza, M.H. (ed.) Proceedings of the 24th IASTED international conference on Signal processing, pattern recognition, and applications, vol. 520, pp. 56–59. ACTA Press, CA (2006)
6. Xue, J.H., Aleksandra, P., Wilfried, P., Etienne, K., Van De Walle, R., Ignace, L.: An Integrated Method of Adaptive Enhancement for Unsupervised Segmentation of MRI Brain Images. Pattern Recognition Letters 24, 2549–2560 (2003)
7. Arivazhagan, S., Ganesan, L.: Texture Classification Using Wavelet Transform. Pattern Recognition Letters 24, 1513–1521 (2003)
8. Zhang, G., Ma, Z.M., Cai, Z.P.: Directed Filter for Dominant Direction Fuzzy Set in Content-based Image Retrieval. In: Proceedings of the 22nd ACM Symposium on Applied Computing (SAC 2007), pp. 76–77. ACM Press, Seoul, Korea (2007)
9. Movshon, J.A., Thompson, I.D., Tolhurst, D.J.: Spatial Summation in the Receptive Fields of Simple Cells in the Cat's Striate Cortex. J. Physiol. 283, 53–77 (1978)
10. Movshon, J.A., Thompson, I.D., Tolhurst, D.J.: Receptive Field Organisation of Complete Cells in the Cat's Striate Cortex. J. Physiol. 283, 79–99 (1978)
11. Jones, J.P., Palmer, L.A.: An Evaluation of the Two-dimensional Gabor Filter Model of Simple Receptive Fields in Cat Striate Cortex. J. Neurophysiology 58, 1233–1258 (1987)
12. Burr, D.C., Morrone, M.C., Spinelli, D.: Evidence for Edge and Bar Detectors in Human Vision. Vision Res. 29, 419–431 (1989)

A New Solution to Changes of Business Entities in Hospital Information Systems

Zhijun Rong[1], Jinsong Xiao[2], and Binbin Dan[1]

[1] Department of Industrial Engineering, Wuhan University of Science and Technology,
Wuhan 430074, China
[2] Shanghai ESosi Company
rongzhijun@263.net

Abstract. A Hospital information system (HIS) has been proposed to respond to some challenges of the complex business process in a hospital. The business processes undergo constant change and the HIS needs to swiftly adapt to reflect these changes. This paper proposes an approach, which is used to define services and solutions for hospital applications according to the business-entity changes in the hospital business processes. The objective of this approach is to minimize the effect of business requirement changes on the system development. Focusing on the transition from the process-oriented to the application-oriented perspectives, some central development considerations are also presented, which can be used to guide the design of service-based interoperability and illustrate these aspects with examples from our current work. This solution will improve the robustness and extensibility of HIS.

1   Introduction

Hospitals are complex entities which depend on specialized information communicates throughout the organization via communication networks. Management of the collection, analysis, use, and communication of health related information is considered the most important public health service. Yet the operation of hospitals presents considerable challenges to effective information flow. Hospital information system (HIS) can provide the solution to the integration of clinical as well as financial and administrative applications. There is an extensive and exponentially growing body of literature on the development, application and implementation of HIS that supports clinical patient care and hospital services [1-3]. Although HIS is a technique that has been proven useful for managing information and improving performance in hospitals, one inherent problem with the enterprise software development process is that it suffers from a lack of agility to match the pace at which the business needs to change in order to keep up with the market trends and competition. Adaptation to new requirements, multiple medical cultures and integration with existing systems is difficult in a constantly changing health environment [4-5]. There are also growing demands to coordinate or automate various processes, to find common descriptions and ways to execute them via electronic transactions supporting seamless quality care for

X. Gao et al. (Eds.): MIMI 2007, LNCS 4987, pp. 133–140, 2008.
© Springer-Verlag Berlin Heidelberg 2008

the patients [6-8]. HIS has been limited by the lack of a flexible and extensible programming environment that supports complex and variable business requirements. It is required to migrate from a specific to a compatible architecture and meet different business requirements. Central challenges for HIS development include lack of reconfigurable platforms and reuse technologies. Reconfigurable platforms can be very effective for lowering development costs because they allow the reuse of architectural resources across a variety of applications. Reuse technologies can improve the system development with the approaches of architecture, database and schema design in detail. There are many ways for IT solutions that directly satisfy business requirements and needs such as business-driven development (BDD), schema evolution, business rule management (BRM), universal framework for variable business requirements. Since the application systems have individual features, we need not only the global mechanism but also the concrete approach to business-entity changes in specific application field.

This paper is concerned with the implementation of a hospital information system (HIS) to automate hospital processes. During the development of HIS, the business requirements are variable that cause the problems effecting the whole project development quality and cycle. This paper proposes a new solution to entity changes in HIS in order to improve the extensibility and robustness of HIS. Our purpose here is to describe the method as it was implemented in a practical HIS. The rest of this paper is organized as follows. In Section 2, we present the current approaches to entity changes based on distributed architecture and analyze the business entity data in multi-tier HIS. Section 3 describes our solution. The experience and a case study are presented in Section 4. Finally, Section 5 concludes the paper.

2   Business Entity in Multi-tier HIS

Currently the application of a HIS is extended greatly both in depth and scope. However, it's a common problem that a HIS becomes harder and harder to be maintained. HIS is a typical distributed application across a network because client and data store resources are usually located on different computers [9]. According to the application requirement, system framework and application integration for a HIS which is the multi-tier application architecture based on browser/web application server/transaction server/database as shown in Fig 1. Business appearance tier provides the application service interface for the user interface. Business rule tier realizes and describes the detailed business request. Data access tier determines the stored procedures and SQL (Sequential Query Language) operation according to the business entities. Data access logic component implements CRUD (Create, Retrieve, Update, and Delete) operation on database tables. Based on this architecture, the data access tier needs not to know which database will be accessed that makes the solution proposed in this paper reality. A HIS consists of a series of corresponding modules including doctor workstations, nurse workstations, medicine management system and clinical treatment systems. It supports the healthcare, financial, clinical information exchange and share between hospitals departments and patient information services based on Web. The information package can be divided into three sections: index section; content section and additional section. In fact, the information is the carriers of the business entities. We take a medical order as example. The index section of a medical order consists of patient ID, bed No, department code, doctor ID etc. The content section consists of medicine, specification, taking frequencies etc. The additional section can be defined by the clients. It consists of time requirement such as order execution time, pre-execution time set and pre-finish time set. Different hospitals have different organization structures and cultures that cause the business process complex and changeable. A critical challenge faced by the developer of HIS is to define the information properly in order to achieve the interactions between systems and hospitals. There are many information body structures in different hospitals. Even in a hospital, the client requirements for the information body will be different at different time. HIS has close relationship with business process as well as business rules. Business rules should continuously be adjusted according to the varying situation of hospital in order to meet the request under new situation and keep high efficiency and production. For any change of business rules should cause the modification of resource code, which often need the help from development team. It is definitely a long period from business change to modification by developing team after the necessary intercommunion between users and developers [10]. Business rules management technologies try to separate and externalize business rules from the application code. The rule engine is developed to separate and deploy business rules furthermore it will increase the system development cost. A business entity represents a "thing" handled or used by business workers [11]. The realization of workflow is based on the cooperation of business entities. Therefore the design of business entities is the key to the system development. Figure 1 shows the business entity data flow in HIS.

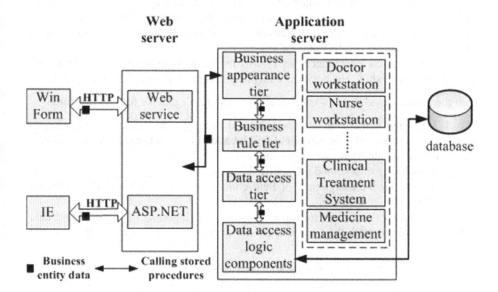

Fig. 1. Business entity data flow in HIS

3 Solution Implementation

It is very important to understand that solutions to business entity change during application system development might be a systematic engineering. Traditional applications and architectures are not able to keep up with business innovation, primarily because the processes are not adaptable to business needs. Though many research works proposed different technologies helping enterprise achieve business flexibility through IT by modeling the business processes that collectively define the way the business executes, the more attention has been paid to the final results rather than the implementation process. As aforementioned, the solutions such as BDD, BRM etc presented a mechanism that needs to be devised by which IT efforts are interlocked with business strategy and requirements through an execution framework that is standardized, well understood, and can be executed repeatedly and successfully. The establishment of standard mechanism, business model, business rule engine will be hard needing supports of developers and business clients and more time and capital. In fact, the application system needs more reliable and direct methods which can realize the agility and extensibility during the development process. The approach described as follows is executable and reliable to HIS development. The approach strategies are:

1. The index information should be designed as independent field in the relational database. The content and additional information in the message body should be designed as high volume character fields.

2. The format of high volume character fields with 2000 length can be designed according with clinical document architecture (CDA) level one in health-level 7 (HL7).

3. The data call tier implements the database operation by calling the stored procedures. It accepts the business entity from the callers such as business rule tier and business appearance tier, thereafter develops the dataset from database into business entity and returns the results to the callers.

4. The business appearance tier returns the business entity to the client fronts. The client fronts exhibit the business entity according to the different requirements.

If the clients raised the new requirements, we should make the following efforts:

1. If the new contents need to be exhibited and input independently, the business entity will be modified. The new field will be added to its schema document. Otherwise, the business entity remains unchanged.

2. The client fronts should be modified.

3. To modify the assignment of field comments in database without modifying the table structure in database.

4. To modify the stored procedures of getting and inputting in order to make data input in accordance with the assignments and records in accordance with the business entity.

Obviously, neither the global development strategies will be affected at the database level nor the middle tiers such as business rule tier, data access tier and data access components will be changed with our solution strategies. Only the interface tier, end front interface and database tier and stored procedures will be modified. It will improve the robustness and extensibility of HIS. The HIS development proves the solution efficient.

4 Case Study

We use an example to describe our approach. There is a medical order transmission between clinical treatment system and doctor workstation. The medical order entity is described by XML schema:

```
<xs:element name="Medical order in hospital"
xmlns:xs="http://www.w3.org/2001/XMLSchema">

    <xs:complexType>

      <xs:sequence>
<!—index information-->

<xs:element name="patient ID" type="xs:string" minOc-
curs="0" />

<xs:element name="in-hospital ID" type="xs:string" mi-
nOccurs="0" />

      ......

<xs:element name="inspection item code"
type="xs:string" minOccurs="0" />

<!—medical information-->

<xs:element name="patient name" type="xs:string" minOc-
curs="0" />

<xs:element name="patient sex" type="xs:string" minOc-
curs="0" />

      ......

<xs:element name="time requirement" type="xs:string"
minOccurs="0" />

<!—Additional information-->

<xs:element name="appointing time" type="xs:string" mi-
nOccurs="0" />

<xs:element name="sampling time" type="xs:string" mi-
nOccurs="0" />

      </xs:sequence>

    </xs:complexType>

</xs:element>
```

In the database, we use the following script to establish medical order table corresponding to the entity.

```
create table medical order table

(

    patient ID                        VARCHAR2(100),
```

......

```
department                      VARCHAR2(100),
medical information             VARCHAR2(2000),
additional information          VARCHAR2(2000)
)
```

The data format of medical information is assigned as:

```
"<patient_name>Patient name</patient_name>
<patient_sex>Patient sex</patient_sex>
......
<time_info>Time requirement</time_info>"•
```

The data format of additional information is assigned as:

```
"<booking_time>Booking time</booking_time>
<sampling_time>Sampling time</sampling_time>"
```

We use SQL query with a function when achieving the stored procedure of record-set.

```
select patient id,
  in-hospital id,
  ......
  inspection item code,
  getXmlField(medical inforamtion ,'patient_name '),
  ......
  getXmlField((medical inforamtion,'time_info '),
getXmlField(additional information,' appointing_time'),
  getXmlField(additional information,' sampling_time ')
from medical_order_in_hospital
```

The function getXmlField is in charge of returning the value of specific node from XML character string. It has two parameters. One is the assigned XML character string; the other is the path of needed node. When clients need to add the information about sampling such as sampling location, sample type, sampling way etc, we can modify the medical information of entity as:

```
<!—medical information-->

<xs:element name="patient name" type="xs:string" minOc-
curs="0" />

<xs:element name=" patient sex " type="xs:string" mi-
nOccurs="0" />

......
```

```
<xs:element name="sample type" type="xs:string" minOc-
curs="0" />

<xs:element name="sampling way" type="xs:string" minOc-
curs="0" />
```

The assignment of data format of medical information should be modified. The sample_info field will be added. Its form is as follows:

```
"<patient_name>patient name</patient_name>

......

<time_info>time requirement</time_info>

<sample_info>

    <sampling_part>sampling location</sampling_part>

    <sample_type>sample type</sample_type>

    <collect_way>sampling way</collect_way>

</sample_info>"•
```

We modify the SQL query during the stored procedure as:

```
select patient id,

    ......

    getXmlField(medical information,'patient_name '),

    getXmlField((medical information,'patient_age '),

    ......

getXmlField(additional information,' appointing_time'),

    getXmlField(additional information,' sampling_time ')

from medical_order_in_hospital
```

The structures of healthcare information including the medical records, patient information and medical orders, vary frequently. The structure changes will affect the database schema and make the midlayer that means the application server illustrated in Fig.1.unstable. The application server is very important to the stability of whole system. The approach presented above can provide a solution to this problem.

5   Conclusions

This paper is by no means an effort to cover system design with a high-level mechanism or framework but gives the sequence of steps of our solution in detail. The challenges of the business and IT relationship functioning in hospitals are huge, particularly in terms of application system adapting to the business requirements. Furthermore, the core requirement of HIS like extensibility, adaptability and integration influence the design of system architecture. The development of HIS is based on the solving the complex relationship between business and IT. We have presented a new solution to business entity change to meet these core requirements while HL7 is implemented as integration standard. This approach can provide a changeable solution to the existing problems and enhance the effectiveness of HIS. This paper provided a practical understanding of the essential tenets of business-entity data between multi-tiers of HIS. Additionally, it explained how to execute a solution through various work activities that align the final IT solution with business needs. Companies now understand the inherent advantages of an approach that takes them toward asset-based, business-centric IT solutions. It is hoped that this paper has provided useful insights into business-centric HIS, a solution that is practical and reliable to HIS development.

Acknowledgement

This research has been supported and financed by the Science and Technology Development Foundation of Wuhan University of Science and Technology under Grant No.2005XY16.

References

1. Huang, E.-W., Hsiao, S.H., Liou, D.M.: Design and implementation of a Web-based HL7 message generation and validation system. International Journal of Medical Informatics 58, 49–58 (2003)
2. Hutchison, A., Moser, M., Kaiserswerth, M., Schade, A.: Electronic data interchange for hospital. IEEE Comput. Mag. 34, 28–34 (1996)
3. Dixon, M., Cook, S., Read, B.: Implications of WWW technologies for exchanging medical records. J. Inform. Prim. Care 9, 2–9 (1999)
4. Van de Velde, R.: Framework for a clinical information system. Int. J. Med. Inf. 57, 57–72 (2000)
5. Archetypes, B.T.: Constraint-based Domain Models for Future-proof Information Systems. In: Baclawski, K., Kilov, H. (eds.) Eleventh OOPSLA workshop on behavioral semantics (2002)
6. Chappell, D.: Enterprise Service Bus. O'Reilly Publishing, CA (2004)
7. OMG Hospital Domain Task Force. CORBAmed Roadmap, Version 2.0 (draft). OMG Document CORBAmed/2000-05-01(2000)
8. Wangler, B., Ahlfeldt, R.-M., Perjons, E.: Process Oriented Information Systems Architectures in Hospital. Health Informatics Journal 4, 253–265 (2003)
9. Rong, Z., Xiao, J., Feng, J.: Development of hospital information system based on.Net platform. In: Sangwan, R., Qing, M. (eds.) Proceedings of IEEE international conference on service operation and logistics, and informatics, pp. 250–253 (2006)
10. Li, H., Xue, M., Ying, Y.: A web-based and integrated hospital information system. In: Proceedings of the IDEAS workshop on medical information systems: the digital hospital, pp. 157–162 (2004)
11. Mitra, T.: Business driven development (2006), http://www. ibm.com/ developerworks/ cn/ webservices/ws-bdd/

A Software Client for Wi-Fi Based Real-Time Location Tracking of Patients

Xing Liu[1], Abhijit Sen[1], Johannes Bauer[2], and Christian Zitzmann[2]

[1] Kwantlen University College, Surrey, BC, Canada
[2] University of Applied Sciences, Regensburg, Germany
xing.liu@kwantlen.ca

Abstract. More and more healthcare personnel are using computer networks and wireless enabled PDAs (personal digital assistants) in their daily work. This leads to the vision of smart environments with location-based knowledge and information services in healthcare facilities. Location tracking of healthcare workers and patients naturally facilitates the realization of such visions. It is also useful in enhancing the safety of the residents in a nursing facility. This paper introduces the authors' efforts in applying wireless technology to track the locations of residents in nursing homes. A software client is developed for an industrial location tracking product. The design and implementation of the software client are discussed in this paper. Test results are also reported.

Keywords: Wireless technology, position and location tracking, healthcare applications, software development.

1 Introduction

Recent advances in wireless technologies have made organizations increasingly mobile. According to [1], characteristics of a mobile organization are: dispersed geographically as well as in its workforce, flexible, adaptive and agile. Wireless technology, by its very nature, can help organizations achieve such mobility. Among the mobility attributes wireless technology brings into organizations, wireless location tracking plays an important role. Firstly, wireless tracking technology facilitates location based knowledge and information sharing. One example is the supply of patient information to nurses via their PDAs based on the room a patient is in, such as allergies and drugs prescribed. Other examples are nursing facility management (such as asset tracking) and facility efficiency improvement (such as wirelessly tracking the patients, automatically record the time they need in visiting each hospital office so that managers can come up better schedules for the doctors). Knowing where people are at any given time and being able to communicate with them are critical for location-based knowledge and information services.

Secondly, wireless tracking technology enhances the safety of the employees and residents in a mobile organization. For example, in nursing homes, knowing the locations of some of its residents/patients is important, especially if those residents are mentally or physically ill. There have been reports in the news that residents went lost

X. Gao et al. (Eds.): MIMI 2007, LNCS 4987, pp. 141–150, 2008.
© Springer-Verlag Berlin Heidelberg 2008

in nursing homes and later found dead [2]. Similar accidents also occurred in hospitals [3][4]. Workers in nursing homes have noticed that residents could fall asleep anywhere in the premises. It is also possible for them to be locked outside the premises so they catch cold or freeze to death. Many measures have been taken to prevent residents from getting into areas they are not supposed to access within premises and from getting out the premises. However, research indicates that accidents are still happening.

Thirdly, wireless location tracking technology has made location based rescue possible in a mobile organization. This is particularly important for patients with heart diseases. No matter where a patient is in the nursing premise, if there is an emergency, the patient only needs to press a button on the wireless device to send a request for help. The request can contain the important information about the patient together with his or her location. The traditional information collecting process by a phone operator (no matter how short time it requires) will no longer be necessary.

Investigations conducted in the local communities indicated that location tracking and monitoring systems will be helpful for their nursing facilities. However, such systems have not been implemented. A location tracking system will not only add another level of safety protection in nursing homes, but also increase the efficiencies of nursing home management because often it takes time to find the whereabouts of some residents and equipments. For residents who are also Alzheimer patients, indoor location monitoring becomes even more important.

Indoor wireless location tracking has been an active research topic. Important pioneer work can be found in [5] where a system named RADAR was introduced. Some novel location algorithms were proposed in [6]. In [7], a wireless LAN based location determination system called Horus was introduced. The system was aiming to have high accuracy and low computational requirements. More recent work [8] shows interesting ideas for ensuring reliable identification of location-tracked human objects by combining biological attributes such as body odors and body temperatures into its Remote Personal Tracking System (RPTS).

Currently the authors are working on applying wireless location tracking technologies to healthcare and solving problems originated from the applications. The authors researched the market for wireless products that can be used for monitoring the locations of indoor mobile objects. GPS was the one the authors looked at first. However, it was found that GPS was not suitable for the applications because of its poor indoor coverage. Standard RFID products were also considered. However, the authors found that RFID products required expensive proprietary hardware. They work in special frequency bands. Substantial investment is needed in setting up the infrastructure for RFID. The third type of products the authors found on the market was Wi-Fi based location tracking systems. These products can work effectively with ranges up to hundreds of meters. Hardware is readily available off the shelves and is inexpensive. These products can make use of the existing computer network infrastructure in organizations. Only moderate efforts are required to have such systems installed.

Wi-Fi based wireless networks have been widely accepted. More and more such networks are being deployed in company offices, universities and colleges, libraries, hospitals and other facilities. Although Wi-Fi networks are predominantly used for data transfer and communication, there is growing interest in using Wi-Fi networks for positioning and tracking of assets and human beings to improve efficiency and safety. Wi-Fi networks use radio technologies IEEE 802.11b/g/a to provide secure, reliable and fast wireless connectivity. A Wi-Fi network can be used to connect computers to each other, to the Internet, and to wired networks (which use IEEE 802.3 or Ethernet). Wi-Fi networks operate in the unlicensed 2.4 and 5 GHz radio bands, with mega bits per second data rates [9].

There are several Wi-Fi based products on the market, such as the ERTLS (Ekahau Real-Time Location System) from Ekahau [10] and the AeroScout Visibility System from AeroScout [11]. Ekahau's product is relatively inexpensive. It has a Java based software development kit (SDK) for customized development. For this reason, the authors decided to purchase the Wi-Fi based development kit from Ekahau. The kit consists of the Ekahau Position Engine software, a Java SDK, and several wearable Wi-Fi tags. However, the current Ekahau SDK has some drawbacks. The first drawback is that the only way to access and display location data is to use a software named "Manager" provided by Ekahau. However, the Manager software was designed for calibrating the Position Engine, not as a general application client. It is used to record signal samples and establish a position model. Its user interface (UI) was more suitable for technical users. For practitioners such as nurses, the Manager's user interface is complex and has many unnecessary features. On the other hand, the Manager source code is not available so it is impossible to simplify it. The second drawback of the Ekahau SDK is that real-time location data cannot be saved in a general-purpose database management system. Thirdly, the Manager software does not provide support for communication with devices such as video cameras and audio equipment. If these customized functionalities are to be provided by Ekahau, it will be very costly, even if Ekahau is ever willing to provide such customizations.

Development was carried out to come up with a software client that overcomes the above drawbacks. The development work of the first stage is reported in this paper. The contributions of this paper are as follows: (1) Design and implementation of a platform-neutral, simple and easy to use software client that works with the Ekahau Position Engine and Ekahau Wi-Fi tags; (2) Applications of the software client in real-life environments. (3) Establishment of a software platform that serves as a foundation for future extensions such as general database capabilities, audio/visual capabilities, and interfacing actuator hardware and software from different vendors.

This paper is organized as follows. Section 2 gives an overview of the Ekahau positioning system. Section 3 introduces the design of the software client. Section 4 discusses the implementation of the software client and the tracking system. Section 5 provides the test results. Future work and the conclusion are provided in Section 6 and Section 7 respectively.

2   Overview of the Ekahau Location Tracking System

The Ekahau location tracking system [10] consists of two functional components: the Ekahau Real-Time Location System (ERTLS) and the Ekahau Wi-Fi tags. ERTLS is a software system based on radio frequency technologies. It continually monitors and reports real-time locations of tracked objects. The ERTLS system operates over the standard 802.11b/g wireless networks and uses no proprietary hardware infrastructure. Ekahau Wi-Fi tags form part of the location tracking system. The tags can be attached to any mobile objects or assets allowing real-time tracking of them in any standard Wi-Fi network.

There are four software components in the Ekahau Real-Time Location System (ERTLS) software package. The first component is the Ekahau Client which is a program that runs on a client device (laptop PC, PDA, and Wi-Fi tag, etc.). Client devices require it to communicate with the Position Engine. The second component is the Ekahau Positioning Engine (EPE). The EPE is a Java-based server that runs on a PC. It calculates and reports the tag location coordinates (x, y, floor) and tracking features to client applications within a Wi-Fi network (802.11b/g) coverage area. The EPE software was designed to work with any off-the-shelf standard Wi-Fi access points. The third component is the Ekahau Manager. This is an application program which can record sample location data for calibrating a positioning model. The model is then used to estimate the locations of the client devices being tracked. The manager can also analyze wireless signals and display the location of each tracked wireless client device. The last component is the Ekahau Application Framework and SDK which provide tools and programming interface for user developed applications that utilize the EPE location information.

3 Client Software Design

The location tracking software client is developed using the Ekahau SDK and works with the Ekahau Position Engine. The relationship between the software client and the Ekahau Position Engine is shown in Fig. 1.

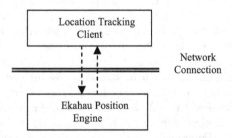

Fig. 1. Client software for location tracking

The Ekahau Position Engine is a stand-alone software application. It can be installed on a server (local or remote). In a Microsoft Windows environment it runs as a service. The location tracking software client communicates with the Position Engine via a network connection so it can be installed on any computing device as long as the device has a network connection to the server where the Position Engine is installed. It is the Position Engine that collects location data and other information from the wireless tags. The tags send their location data and status information to the Position Engine through the wireless access points which are placed all over the monitored environment. The developed software client is expected to receive the location data and other status information from the Position Engine, save the data in a general database, visually present the data to the user and activate other devices (such as door lock, video camera, or alarm). Location data can be further processed in the software client if necessary.

The network connection between the software client and the server can be wired or wireless. If it is wireless, the connection is Wi-Fi based in this work.

3.1 Graphic User Interface (GUI) of the Software Client

Simplicity is the main consideration when the software client was designed. This is because the graphical user interface is intended for healthcare workers who may not have had extensive technical training on computer and software. The authors expected the UI to contain only essential information and to be very straightforward to use. The authors also had it in mind that the software client might be installed in hand-held devices such as PDAs or Smart Phones in the future. The user interface has only a few items to choose from which provide the most essential information. The most important information is location - a healthcare worker should be able to use the software client to find out where a patient or colleague is. The information provided includes: floor number or area name and the estimated x- and y- locations which are displayed on a map. The interface also has a list which shows the names of all the people being tracked. A healthcare worker should be able to choose a floor map to visually locate a person.

It is reasonable for each floor in a building to have a separate map. However, the areas on a map should not be too small so they are clearly visible. Therefore, if a floor is too large in area, more than one map can be used for the floor. As a minimum, the software client's GUI should have a window to show a floor map with the locations of the patients displayed on the map. User interface controls are provided for a healthcare worker to choose the floor of his or her interest to view.

A healthcare worker should also be able to choose a specific person to monitor. User interface controls are provided for this. The software client provides information for the person's name, the floor level or area name where the person is located, the signal status for the tag the person carries, and the tag's battery status (percent charge remaining). If necessary, the IP address and MAC address of the tag can also be displayed (not implemented in this work). Fig. 2 shows the GUI layout of the software client.

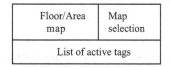

Fig. 2. The GUI of the client software

3.2 Software Design

The main Java classes used in the software client are shown in Fig. 3:

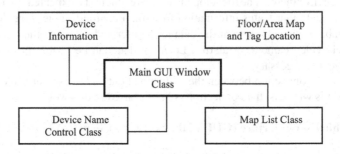

Fig. 3. Java classes of the client software

The following is a brief description of the main Java classes used:

- *Main GUI Window Class*: This class is the main GUI of the client. It provides access to all the other functions. It maintains a connection to the Position Engine. It creates the software objects representing the tags. It holds the instances of all classes used for tag positioning, device handling, and tag name processing. It also keeps the main GUI updated.
- *Floor/Area Map and Tag Location Class*: This class displays the map of a floor or an area, as well as the positions of the tags being tracked which are located on the floor or the area. This class also checks the status of a tag and displays it on the map.
- *Map List Class*: This class keeps a list of all the maps registered with the Position Engine. When a map is selected from this list, it is displayed on the Floor/Area Map window.
- *Device Information Class*: This class holds the information about a tag or a general wireless device (for example, a laptop computer). The information includes the name of the device, the battery/signal status, the IP address and the MAC address of the device, etc.
- *Device Name Control Class*: This class enables a healthcare worker to change the displayed tag name to the real name of a patient.

The above classes help with retrieving the device and location information from the Position Engine and display it to the user. The retrieved location and other data are not saved in any general-purpose database systems in this work. The database development part is going to be reported separately.

4 Location Tracking System Implementation

The classes of the software client were implemented using Java. The software was developed using JBuilder 2005 together with the Ekahau Java SDK.

The software runs on a Dell Latitude D510 laptop computer with a 1.6GHz processor. In this work, the Ekahau Position Engine was also installed on the same computer as the software client. Therefore in this case, the server which the Position Engine is running on is the local host. The software client contacts the local host to get the services provided by the Position Engine.

To be able to track the locations of the tags, the area needs to be covered with wireless signals. Based on Ekahau's recommendation, each location to be tracked should be covered by signals from at least three wireless access points (better five). The tags, the access points (except the dummy ones) and the Position Engine all need to be on the same wireless local area network (WLAN). Dummy access points that are not part of the WLAN are helpful in improving location accuracy. The WLAN in this work consists of a D-Link DI-624 Airplus Xtreme G wireless router, four D-Link Airplus G wireless DWL-G700AP access points, the tags, and the server laptop computer. The devices obtain their IP addresses dynamically from the router (or they can be programmed manually). The access points and the router are arranged in such a way that in all locations of the test area, five access point signals can be detected. The DI-624 router and the DWL-G700AP access point with the original omni-directional antenna can reach over 100 meters indoor and 400 meters in open space according to DLink's specifications (tests indicate that effective coverage when the environment has walls and furniture etc can only be about 40 meters).

5 Test Results

Experiments were conducted to test the software client developed. In general, five steps need to be followed in order to deploy an Ekahau based location tracking system. The steps are: 1) *Hardware installation*. The router is placed at a location where it could communicate with all access points reliably (ideally, with LOS - line of sight). The router and the access points should be placed in such way that they cover the entire area of interest, but not cause the so-called symmetric errors (such errors occur when two locations have similar signal measurements due to improper placement of access points). The access points should be placed high enough so that moving objects such as walking people do not cause too much interference to the calibrated environment. 2) *Site survey*. This step is used to ensure that the required number of wireless signals exist at all the locations to be tracked and they are sufficiently strong. The authors used the Ekahau Manager in this step. The laptop with the Manager installed was carried around the test area and the number of signals at each location and their strengths were visually inspected. 3) *Create position model using the Ekahau Manager*. The position model is required by the Position Engine to estimate the locations of the tags. Essentially, a number of sample signals are recorded for each location to be tracked. The Position Engine compares the signal data from the tags against the recorded samples in the position model to figure out the locations when tracking is in operation. The locations sampled should be those where the patients and other people have the possibility to access. In nursing homes, these should include laundry rooms, washrooms, storage areas, and outdoor activity areas by the nursing premises, etc. This step also involves the registration of the map files with the Position Engine and the scale of the actual physical measurements of the areas with the image pixels on a map. When the position model is ready, it is saved for the Position Engine to use. 4) *Deployment*. The Position Engine is installed on a server computer together with the position model. The Position Engine is ready to provide location data when requested by the software client. 5) *Test*. The actual tests were conducted on the third floor of a classroom building in one of the campuses of the authors' institution. The test area size is 58 feet x 61.8 feet = 3584.4 square feet. Several classrooms and a hallway were selected for the tests. The authors also tested the system locally in a real nursing home. However, for publication purposes, a classroom based map is used here.

When the client software is running, it displays a GUI as depicted in the screen capture in Fig.4.

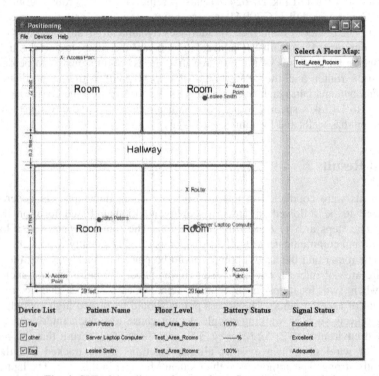

Fig. 4. GUI of the client software after a floor map was loaded

The GUI in Fig.4 shows the map area (top-left), the information area for the active devices and tags (lower bottom area), and the map selection list (top-right). A user can see from the bottom area which devices are being tracked. The devices can be general wireless laptop computers or wireless tags. The lower bottom area also shows the area or floor a device is on, how good its signal reception is, and how much battery the device has left. From the Floor Map dropdown list, the nurse can select a map to view. The selected map is displayed in the top-left map area. In Fig.4, the server computer which had the Position Engine installed was in the same room as the router. The two tags were carried by patient John Peters and patient Leslee Smith, who were in two different rooms. Fig.4 also shows the locations of the access points used in the WLAN.

During the test, it was noticed that if the authors were only interested in which room a patient was in, then for the given test area, only one sample point was needed for each room. The system was able to find out the room or area with very high accuracy. During the many test runs, there was rarely any error in the estimated room or area (over 90% of the time the estimation was correct). However, it was much harder to pinpoint the location of a tag in a room. The errors frequently went beyond 6 feet and sometimes they were even greater than 10 feet. Taking more sample points in a room improved the accuracy. However, the predicted locations were not very stable due to the interferences. It was also observed that the system worked better in residential homes where the walls were mostly wood. For classrooms with concrete walls, the system did not work as well. The other observation was that sometimes the tags seemed to lose connections to the WLAN, and the authors had to reboot the tags or refresh the wireless network connections manually. The authors are aware that Ekahau are producing new tags and a new version of the Position Engine has been released. The authors hope these problems can be solved when these new products are used by the software client.

6 Future Work

The software client can be enhanced to include advanced functions that can be used in a real healthcare environment. The current software client is simple and versatile enough to be used on desktop PCs, laptop computers, as well as PDAs or Smartphones. If the authors are more interested in a powerful system and the system is mainly intended for PCs, then many functions can be added to the software client, such as support for a general database system. The database capability will enable the software client to record the location history of some critical patients. These data will be useful for search and rescue operations if a patient does disappear and in the meantime the wireless device attached to the patient malfunctions (last location is saved). Alarm, audio, video and instant messaging capabilities can also be added to the software client. The client can also be used to drive hardware devices such as door locks. Current development and tests were all based on PCs. Research will be carried to explore the possibility of using the software client in PDAs which will enable the nurses to locate patients anywhere and any time.

7 Conclusion

The authors have developed a simple and easy-to-use software client based on a commercial product and have investigated its applications in real-life environments. The software client is designed for nursing facilities. It can predict the room or area where a patient is located with high accuracy. This can add extra safety to nursing homes and improve their management efficiency. The wireless tracking capability also facilitates location based information and service which renders mobile organizations into smart environments.

Acknowledgement

The authors would like to thank Kwantlen University College's Research and Scholarship Office, Deans Arthur Coren and Wayne Tebb of the School of Business, vice-president Gorden Lee, colleagues Mehdi Talwerdi and Chris Leung, Braydon Short and Werner Pauls of Langley Lodge for their invaluable support.

References

1. Liebowitz, J.: Developing knowledge and learning strategies in mobile organizations. International Journal of Mobile Learning and Organisation 1, 5–14 (2007)
2. Alzheimer's Patient Found Dead on Roof. The Miami Herald and The Associated Press (September 1, 2006)
3. Missing patient found dead on hospital premises after a week, Helsingin Sanomat (International Edition) (November 28, 2001)
4. Missing patient found dead in Dublin, Irish Health (December 19, 2000)
5. Bahl, P., Padmanabhan, V.N.: Radar: An In-Building RF-Based User Location and Tracking System. In: INFOCOM-2000, Tel-Aviv, Israel, vol. 2, pp. 775–784 (2000)
6. Gwon, Y., Jain, R., Kawahara, T.: Robust Indoor Location Estimation of Stationary and Mobile Users. In: INFOCOM 2004, Hong Kong, vol. 2, pp. 1032–1043 (2004)
7. Youssef, M., Agrawala, A.: The Horus WLAN Location Determination System. In: Proceedings of the Third International Conference on Mobile Systems, Applications, and Services (MobiSys 2005), Seattle, WA, USA (June 2005)
8. Yahya, A.A., Iskandarani, M.Z.: Remote Personal Tracking System (RPTS). American Journal of Applied Sciences 3, 2147–2150 (2006)
9. WiFi Overview, http://www.wi-fi.org
10. Ekahau Real-Time Location System, http://www.ekahau.com
11. AeroScout Visibility System, http://www.aeroscout.com

Significance of Region of Interest Applied on MRI and CT Images in Teleradiology-Telemedicine

Tariq Javid Ali[1], Pervez Akhtar[1], M. Iqbal Bhatti[2], and M. Abdul Muqeet[2]

[1] National University of Sciences and Technology, Karachi-Campus, Pakistan
{tariqjavid,pervez}@pnec.edu.pk
[2] Sir Syed University of Engineering & Technology, Karachi, Pakistan
{mibhatti,mabdul}@ssuet.edu.pk

Abstract. Within the expanding paradigm of medical imaging in Teleradiology-Telemedicine, there is increasing demand for transmitting diagnostic medical imagery. These are usually rich in radiological contents, especially in slicing modalities, and the associated file sizes are large which must be compressed with minimal file size to minimize transmission time and robustly coded to withstand required network medium. It has been reinforced through extensive research that the diagnostically important regions of medical images, Regions of Interest, must be compressed by lossless or near lossless algorithm, while on the other hand, the background region be compressed with some loss of information but still recognizable using JPEG2000 standard. Applying on MRI and CT scan images achieved different high compression ratios with varying quantization levels analogously reduced transmission time depending on sources of energy, the MAXSHIFT method proved very effective both objectively and subjectively.

1 Introduction

The objectives of teleradiology-telemedicine are to improve access and to enhance overall quality of care at an affordable cost. Improved access and cost savings could be achieved by allowing a doctor to remotely examine patients or to consult with a specialist. This reduces or eliminates the time and expense of travel necessary to bring the patient to the doctor or the doctor to the patient [1]. Quality of care is improved by providing the diagnostically important images. Rigorous research in diagnostic imaging and image compression in teleradiology-telemedicine is gaining prominence all over the world, particularly in developing countries [2]. Engineers are developing technologies and tools, enabling the medical practitioners to provide efficient treatment. From the elaborate medical information, the doctor prefers to focus on certain selected region(s) of interest. Also the doctors are more comfortable with image processing and analysis solutions that offer subjective analysis of medical images more than depending on the objective engineering results alone. Technology assisted, integrated diagnostic methods are of high relevance in this context [3].

A CT scanner, See Fig. 1, uses X-rays, a type of ionizing radiation, to acquire its images, making it a good tool for examining tissue composed of elements of a

X. Gao et al. (Eds.): MIMI 2007, LNCS 4987, pp. 151–159, 2008.
© Springer-Verlag Berlin Heidelberg 2008

relatively higher atomic number than the tissue surrounding them, such as bone and calcifications (calcium based) within the body (carbon based flesh), or of structures (vessels, bowel). MRI, See Fig. 1, on the other hand, uses nonionizing radio frequency (RF) signals to acquire its images and is best suited for non-calcified tissue. For purposes of tumor detection and identification, MRI is generally superior. However, CT usually is more widely available, faster, much less expensive, and may be less likely to require the person to be sedated or anesthetized [4].

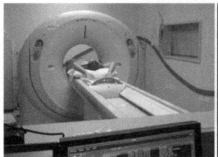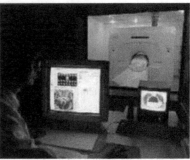

Fig. 1. CT and MRI modalities: (left) Toshiba Aquilion 64 slice CT scanner and (right) Siemens Avanto 1.5T MRI unit.

An 8-bit gray scale image with 512 x 512 pixels requires more than 0.2 MB of storage. If the image can be compressed by 8:1 without any perceptual distortion, the capacity of storage increased 8 times. This is significant for teleradiology-telemedicine scenario due limitations of transmission medium. If we need T units of time to transmit an image, then with 16:1 compression ratio the transmission time will decrease to T/16 units of time.

It has been reinforced through extensive research that the diagnostically important regions of medical images, Regions of Interest, must be compressed by lossless or near lossless algorithm, while on the other hand, the background region be compressed with some loss of information but still recognizable using JPEG2000 standard [5–7]. Applying JPEG2000 ROI coding on MRI and CT scan images achieved different high compression ratios, 16:1 and 8:1 respectively, with varying quantization levels (1/128, 1/64, and 1/32) analogously reduced transmission time depending on sources of energy, the MAXSHIFT method proved very effective both objectively and subjectively.

2 Concepts

In the medical scenario, the region of interest (ROI) is the area of an image, which is of clinical/diagnostic importance to the doctor [8]. Certain image specific features like the uniformity of texture, color, intensity, etc. generally characterize as ROI. Medical images are mostly in gray-scale [9]. The gray scales of an M-bit level image (where M can be 8, 12 or 16 bits) can be represented in the form of bit-planes [10].

2.1 Identifying ROI

Identifying and extracting ROI accurately is very important before coding and compressing the image data for efficient transmission or storage. In different spatial regions and identifying the ROI in the image, it is possible to compress them with different levels of reconstruction quality. This way one could accurately preserve the features needed and transmit those for medical diagnosis or for scientific measurement, while achieving high compression overall by allowing degradation of data in the unimportant regions.

2.2 Lossless Schemes

In medical context the regionally lossless schemes have to be studied more closely. They can be any of the following based on different types of end user/observer or context.

− Visually lossless (non-clinical human observer).
− Diagnostically lossless (clinical-observers, significant degrees of observer dependent variations exist).
− Quantifiably lossless (mostly non-human observer/computer assisted detection).

One important consideration here is that what may be visually lossless or quantifiably lossless may not be diagnostically lossless [11].

2.3 Coding Schemes

Most of the commonly used methods use JPEG2000 algorithm that involves the following important steps [12]. Along with these mentioned below, additional processing related to ROI mask generation and customized coding that suits the user requirement is done.

1. Discrete wavelet transform (DWT) is performed on the tiles or the entire image based on size of the image [13].
2. If the ROI is identified then ROI mask is derived extracting the region indicating the set of coefficients that are required for lossless ROI reconstruction.
3. The wavelet coefficients are quantized as per desired quality of reconstruction.
4. The coefficients that are out of the ROI are scaled up/down by a specific scaling value. If there are more than one ROI, these can be multiply coded with different scaling values.
5. The resulting coefficients are progressively entropy encoded (with the most significant bit planes first). As overhead information, the scaling value assigned to the ROI and ROI mask generation but scales up the background coefficients in order to recreate the original coefficients.

In medical situations during compression phase, lossy schemes are not preferred. To avoid the chance of loosing any diagnostic information, a 32x32 code block size is selected with considering ROI size less than one fourth of the original image. Lossless schemes prove costly with less compression efficiencies and are ineffective in certain application domains. Regionally lossless schemes prove as a valuable/meaningful solution between the completely lossless or lossy ones. In these, lossless coding is done for the ROI and lossy coding to the less significant background image [14].

3 Our Approach

3.1 Some Observations

We develop our approach based on the following observations.

- The doctor prefers to use eyes (subjective decision) to select the region that is of importance through interactive evaluation and manual marking or selection of regions [15, 8].
- The pixels that represent the diagnostically relevant data are of interest to the doctor. These bits need not belong to visually significant data [9].
- The need of higher compression for fast transmission.

3.2 General Scaling and MAXSHIFT Methods

While compressing the medical images it is important to consider ROI masking methods so as to get diagnostically important area as a lossless region. MAXSHIFT method in comparison to general scaling method supports the use of any mask since the decoder does not need to generate the mask, See Fig. 2. Thus, it is possible for the encoder to include an entire subband, that is, the low-low subband, in the ROI mask and thus send a low-resolution version of the background at an early stage of the progressive transmission. This is done by scaling of all quantized transform coefficients of the entire subband. In other words, the user can decide in which subband he will start having ROI and thus, it is not necessary to wait for the whole ROI before receiving any information for the background. However, since the background coefficients are scaled down rather than scaling up ROI coefficients, this will only have the effect that in certain implementations the least significant bitplanes for the background may be lost. The advantage is that the ROI, which is considered to be the most important part of the image, is still optimally treated while the background is allowed to have degraded quality, since it is considered to be less important.

3.3 Transmission Hierarchy

Recent acceptance and deployment of picture archiving and communications system (PACS) [16] in hospitals and the availability of digital imaging and communications in Medicine (DICOM) medical images via PACS is and important building block of telemedicine. Fig. 3 [17] illustrates the extension of a PACS to remote sites using telemedicine.

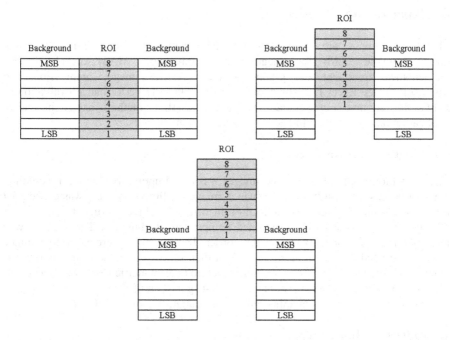

Fig. 2. The MAXSHIFT method: (top left) ROI and background at the same level, (top right) general scaling method, and (bottom) MAXSHIFT method

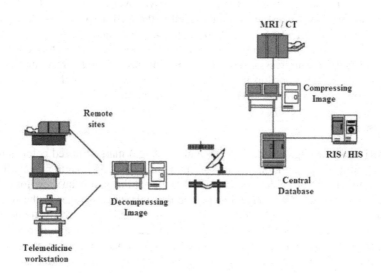

Fig. 3. Transmission hierarchy [17]

4 Experimental Results

MRI and CT images are obtained from a famous national health care institution. We utilize IrfanView [18] for image format conversion, MATLAB [19,20] for mathematical treatment and graphs, JJ2000 [21] for image compression, and Microsoft Office Excel [22] for organizing the data. The performance evaluation of JPEG2000 compression standard using MAXSHIFT method is an individual application on one selected image from each of the modalities.

4.1 Subjective Measurement

The evaluation of the reconstructed images was based upon mixed criteria including: mean opinion score (MOS) [23] for which image quality assessment was carried out by visually comparing the specific ROI of the original and reconstructed images, after the application of the above mentioned compression techniques. The images were presented to six radiologists in a random order. The observers were asked to evaluate the reconstructed images in accordance with their diagnostic value. The ranking was done on an integer scale based on moving picture quality metric (MPQM) model [24] from 1 to 5, that is, 1 (bad), 2 (poor), 3 (fair), 4 (good) and 5 (excellent). An image is ranked as acceptable if it maintains satisfactory diagnostic value (MOS $\geq$ 4).

4.2 Objective Measurement

When reconstructed images to be encoded contain ROI, peak signal to noise ratio (PSNR) is calculated for the ROI alone and over whole image (for the ROI and the background). For all of the ROI experiments a five level DWT is used and all of the coefficients from the lowest level are included in the ROI. Experiment was completed using JJ2000. The effect of JPEG2000 coding on MRI and CT images for lossless compression ratio is presented in Figs. 4 and 5. Compression is performed by means of the JPEG2000 compression standard. The images, at first, are compressed and decompressed at 0.08 bpp up to 4.0 bpp (128:1, 64:1, 32:1, 16:1, 8:1, 4:1 and 2:1 compression ratios) at 1/128, 1/64 and 1/32 quantization levels.

4.3 Discussion

The MRI image in Fig. 4 with ROI (cranial blockage) marked in red color is initially obtained from MRI scan modality and archived in a DICOM imaging database which is later converted to portable gray map (PGM) format through IrfanView for encoding with JJ2000 software. The image then passed through various stages of the JPEG2000 ROI coding algorithm and finally we get a compressed image ready for storage or transmission. The reconstructed image then followed a similar pattern in reverse when a compressed image is received or accessed from archival. A similar process is used for CT image. The size of ROI is less than one fourth for both scenarios and typically about 1/6 of original image.

The superiority of the ROI coding scheme, based on the MAXSHIFT method, over without ROI, can be subjectively and objectively judged at different quantization levels. For MRI image, at 1/128 quantization level achieving a compression ratio of

16:1, subjectively got MOS > 4 and objectively gained up to 20.31 dB, See Figs. 4 and 5. At 1/64 quantization level with same compression ratio, subjectively got MOS ≥ 4 and objectively gained up to 9.31 dB. At 1/32 quantization level with same compression ratio, subjectively got MOS < 4 and objectively show no gain. For CT image, at 1/128 quantization level achieving a compression ratio of 8:1, subjectively got MOS > 4 and objectively gained up to 18.76 dB. At 1/64 quantization level with same compression ratio, subjectively got MOS ≥ 4 and objectively gained up to 6.43 dB. At 1/32 quantization level with same compression ratio, subjectively got MOS <4 and objectively show no gain. Table 1 summarizes both subjective and objective measurements for MRI and CT images at different quantization levels.

Our results show that 16:1 and 8:1 compression ratios on 1/128 quantization level with gains exceeding 18 db appropriate for the MRI and CT images to be reconstructed in lossless settings reducing transmission sixteen and eight times respectively.

Table 1. Subjective and objective measurements at different quantization levels

Image	Quantization (bits)	PSNR (dB)	MOS
	1/128	20.31	> 4
MRI	1/64	09.31	≥ 4
	1/32	00.00	< 4
	1/128	18.76	> 4
CT	1/64	06.43	≥ 4
	1/32	00.00	< 4

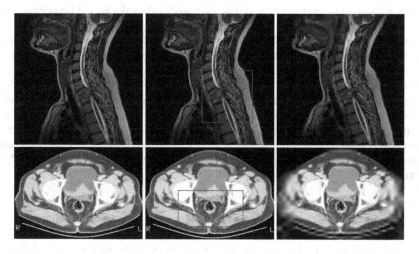

Fig. 4. MRI (top) and CT (bottom) images: original images (top-left) MRI 512x512 and (bottom-left) CT 500x352, (middle-column) images with ROI in red color, and (right-column) reconstructed images from compressed images, with quantization level 1/128 and ratios 16:1 (for MRI) and 8:1 (for CT). Adapted from [25, 26].

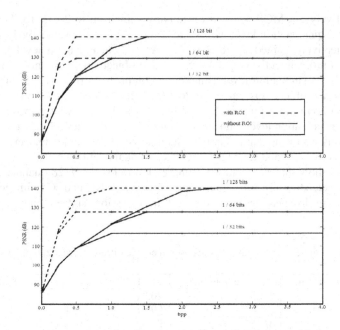

Fig. 5. Objective measures: (top) MRI and (bottom) CT, See Section 4.2 for details

5 Conclusions

Our results of reconstructed medical images quality subjectively and objectively have shown that the application of JPEG2000 standard based on discrete wavelet transform compression technique with ROI coding using MAXSHIFT scaling method proved diagnostically significant in MRI and CT medical imagery and helpful in identifying the diseases zone. A gain exceeded 18 dB at 1/128 quantization level achieved with minimum transmission time through various network medium. The results have shown MRI and CT images compression ratios 16:1 and 8:1 respectively, acceptable, depend on sources of energy, and may be employed for diagnostically lossless transmission in a teleradiology-telemedicine scenario. However, the degree of compression also depend on anatomical structure and complexity of diagnostic information in the image and a suitable level of compression ratio must be considered before archiving clinical images otherwise essential information will be lost.

References

1. Moore, M.: Elements of Success in Telemedicine Projects. Report of a research grant from AT&T Graduate School of Library and Information Science, the University of Texas at Austin (1993)
2. Bedi, B.S.: Standardization Telemedicine: National Initiative in India. In: ATA-2004, Tampa (2004)
3. Grimes, S.: Clinical Engineers: Stewards of Healthcare Technologies. IEEE Engineering in Medicine and Biology Magazine 23(3), 56–58 (2004)
4. Wikipedia: Magnetic Resonance Imaging – Wikipedia, The Free Encyclopedia, http://www.wikipedia.org

5. Boliek, M.: JPEG 2000 Part I Final Committee Draft Version 1.0 (March 2000)
6. Christopoulos, C., Skodras, A., Ebrahimi, T.: The JPEG2000 Still Image Coding System: An Overview. IEEE Transactions on Consumer Electronics 46, 1103–1127 (2000)
7. JPEG2000: Official Website, http://www.jpeg.org/jpeg2000
8. Srinath, M.D.: Image Processing: A Clinical Radiologist Perspective. In: Proceedings of National Conference on Image Processing, Bangalore, India (March 2005)
9. Jayakumar, P.N.: Challenges in Medical Image Processing. In: Proceedings of National Conference on Image Processing, Bangalore, India (2005)
10. ChandraShekar, S.T., Varanasi, G.L.: Region of Interest Coding in Medical Images using Diagnostically Significant Bitplanes. In: Proceedings of Conference on Emerging Aspects of Clinical Data Analysis, Italy (2005)
11. Carrino, J.: Digital Image Quality: A Clinical Perspective. Quality assurance, The Society for Computer Applications in Radiology, Great Falls, VA, pp. 29–37 (2003)
12. Christopoulos, C., Askelf, J., Larsson, M.: Efficient methods for encoding regions of interest in the upcoming JPEG2000 still image coding standard. IEEE Signal Processing Letters 7(9), 247–249 (2000)
13. Burak, S., Tomasi, C., Girod, B., Beaulieu, C.: Medical Image Compression based on Region of Interest with Application to Colon CT images. In: Proceedings of 23rd International Conference of the IEEE Engineering in Medicine and Biology Society, Istanbul, Turkey, pp. 2453–2456 (2001)
14. Varma, K., Bell, A.: JPEG2000 - Choices and Tradeoffs for Encoders. IEEE Signal Processing Magazine 21(6), 70–75 (2004)
15. Kalawsky, R.S.: The Validity of Presence as a Reliable Human Performance Metric in Immersive Environments. In: 3rd International Workshop on Presence, Delft, Netherlands (March 2000)
16. Leotta, D., Kim, Y.: Requirements for picture archiving and communications. IEEE Engineering in Medicine and Biology Magazine 12(1), 62–69 (1993)
17. Akhtar, P., Bhatti, M.I., Ali, T.J., Muqeet, M.A.: Significance of Region of Interest applied on MRI image in Teleradiology-Telemedicine. In: The First International Conference on Bioinformatics and Biomedical Engineering, China, pp. 1331–1334 (2007)
18. Skiljan, I.: Irfanview. Vienna University of Technology (2004)
19. Palm, W.: Introduction to Matlab 7 for Engineers. McGraw-Hill College, New York (2005)
20. Gonzalez, R., Woods, R., Eddins, S.: Digital image processing using Matlab. Pearson Education, Inc., London (2004)
21. Santa-Cruz, D., Grosbois, R., Ebrahimi, T.: JJ2000: The JPEG 2000 reference implementation in Java. In: Proceedings of the First International JPEG 2000 Workshop, Lugano, Switzerland, pp. 46–49 (2003)
22. Bloch, S.: Excel for Engineers and Scientists. Wiley, New York (2000)
23. Kratochvil, T., Simicek, P.: Utilization of MATLAB for Picture Quality Evaluation. Institute of Radio Electronics, Brno University of Technology, Brno
24. Adams, M., Kossentini, F.: Reversible integer-to-integer wavelet transforms for image compression: performance evaluation and analysis. IEEE Transactions on Image Processing 9(6), 1010–1024 (2000)
25. Bhatti, M.I., Akhtar, P., Ali, T.J., Muqeet, M.A.: Implications of JP2K coding standard for MRI image based on a feature of Region of Interest in Telemedicine. In: International Conference on Engineering Education, Coimbra, Portugal, September 2007 (to appear 2007)
26. Akhtar, P., Bhatti, M.I., Ali, T.J., Muqeet, M.A.: Significance of Region of Interest applied on CT image in Teleradiology-Telemedicine. In: 14th International Workshop on Systems, Signals and Image Processing and 6th EURASIP Conference focused on Speech and Image Processing, Multimedia Communications and Services, Maribor, Slovenia, pp. 94–97 (June 2007)

Gender Effect on Functional Networks in Resting Brain

Liang Wang [1, 2], Chaozhe Zhu [2], Yong He [3], Qiuhai Zhong[1], and Yufeng Zang [2]

[1] School of Information Science and Technology,
Beijing Institute of Technology, P.R. China
[2] State Key Laboratory of Cognitive Neuroscience and Learning,
Beijing Normal University, P.R. China
czzhu@bnu.edu.cn
[3] McConnell Brain Imaging Centre, Montreal Neurological Institute,
McGill University, Montreal, QC, Canada H3A 2B4

Abstract. Previous studies have witnessed that complex brain networks have the properties of high global and local efficiency. In this study, we investigated the gender effect on brain functional networks measured using functional magnetic resonance imaging (fMRI). Our experimental results showed that there were no significant difference in global and local efficiency between male and female. However, the gender-related effects on nodal efficiency were found at several brain regions, including the left middle frontal gyrus, right superior temporal gyrus, left middle cingulum gyrus, left hippocampus, right hippocampus, right parahippocampal and left amygdala. These results were compatible with previous findings. To our knowledge, this study provided the first evidence of gender effect on the efficiency of brain functional networks using resting-state fMRI.

Keywords: gender, brain network, efficiency, resting state, functional magnetic resonance imaging (fMRI).

1 Introduction

Gender effects on brain are an important issue in neuroscience. Recently, differences in brain structure and function between males and females have been widely investigated by using neuroimaging techniques. Structural imaging studies have shown gender differences in cortical thickness [1], ratio of gray to white matter [2], regional volume [3]. Functional dimorphisms have been found in emotion [4, 5], vision [6], memory [7, 8], hearing [9, 10], stress [11] and face processing [12]. Functional connectivity has also been used in studies of gender effect on the brain [14, 15]. The brain is a complex network at multiple scales of time and space and supports segregated and integrated information processing [13]. The network efficiency [16, 17], as a novel metric of complex networks, has been applied to investigate anatomical [16] and functional networks [18]. The global efficiency is associated with integrated information processing and measures how well information propagates over the network. The local efficiency, associated with segregated information processing, quantifies how efficiently sub-networks exchange information. The purpose of

X. Gao et al. (Eds.): MIMI 2007, LNCS 4987, pp. 160–168, 2008.
© Springer-Verlag Berlin Heidelberg 2008

the present study was to further investigate the potential gender differences in the efficiency of functional networks in the resting brain.

2 Materials and Methods

2.1 Subjects

A total of twenty healthy human volunteers participated in the experiment: 10 males (21 - 25 years) and 10 age-matched females. All subjects were right-handed and claimed to be no history of head trauma with loss of consciousness, neurological illness, or other severe psychical disease. Written informed consent was obtained from all participants. This study was approved by the Ethics Committee of West China Hospital, Sichuan University.

2.2 Data Acquisition and Pre-processing

All functional images were obtained from a GE 3-T scanner in West China Hospital of Sichuan University. Each subject lay supine with the head snugly fixed by belt and foam pads to reduce the effects of head movement. We acquired 200 volumes with the following parameters: 30 axial slices, thickness/gap = 4.5 / 0 mm, matrix = 64 × 64, repetition time = 2000 ms, echo time = 30 ms, flip angle = 90°, field of view = 220 × 220 mm. Subjects were instructed to keep their eyes closed, relax their minds and remain motionless as much as possible during the EPI data acquisition. The scan lasted for 6.4 min. The first 10 volumes of each subject were discarded to allow for T1 saturation effects, leaving 190 volumes for further analysis.

Image pre-processing was carried out using the SPM5 software package (http://www.fil.ion.ucl.ac.uk/spm) including slice timing, head-movement correction, spatial normalization and resampling (3 mm × 3 mm × 3 mm). Exclusion criteria included maximum displacement in any direction of higher than 1mm and head rotation of higher than 1° and nobody was excluded according to the criteria. Then the fMRI data were temporally filtered (0.0083 ~ 0.15 Hz) [19] by using an ideal rectangle window filter of the AFNI software [20] to remove low-frequency drift and high-frequency physiological noises. The brain was parcellated using the Anatomical Automatic Labeling template [21]. This parcellation divides the brain into 90 anatomical regions (45 in each hemisphere) of interest and the abbreviated regional labels used in this study refer to Achard et al's study [22]. Several sources of spurious variance, including estimated head-motion profiles and the global brain activity were further removed from the mean time series of each region by a multiple linear regression model. The residuals of this regression were then used to substitute for the raw mean time series of the corresponding regions.

2.3 Correlation Matrix and Graph Generation

Pearson's correlation coefficients between the residual time series of each pair of the 90 brain areas were computed to produce a symmetric correlation matrix (i.e., functional connectivity matrix) for each subject. In order to apply graph theoretical analysis to the brain functional networks, the correlation matrix of each subject was converted into a binary graph by considering a threshold, i.e., a wiring cost (See section 2.4 for the definition). The elements of the binary graph will be either 1, if the absolute value of the correlation coefficient exceeds the threshold, or 0, if not. The resulting binary graph is symmetrical and comprised nodes and edges, with each node for one brain region and each edge for one undirected connection. Different threshold values may result in distinct network topologies: high thresholds yield sparser graphs and low thresholds yield denser ones. However, since there is no definitive way currently to select a precise threshold in complex brain networks studies [18], two approaches to the threshold choice were adopted. Firstly, the correlation matrix was thresholded with a wide range of threshold values. Secondly, a conservative threshold with the total number of edges K = 410 was employed, corresponding to a wiring cost 0.1 that has been applied to Achard et al's study [18].

2.4   Cost and Efficiency of Brain Networks

After an undirected graph (i.e., network) had been obtained, several metrics of the graph were worked out to describe the properties of the network. The cost of the graph is defined in (1)

$$C_{cost} = \frac{K}{N(N-1)/2} \tag{1}$$

Where N and K are the total number of nodes and edges in the graph, respectively. $N(N-1)/2$ is the number of all the possible edges in the graph [16, 17]. The cost measures how expensive it is to build a network.

The efficiency of a network G is defined in (2) where $L_{i,j}$ is the shortest length of the path from node i to node j. $E(G)$ measures how well information propagates over the network G.

$$E(G) = \frac{1}{N(N-1)} \sum_{i \neq j \in G} \frac{1}{L_{i,j}} \tag{2}$$

According to the definition, $L_{i,j}$ would be infinite if there is no path between node i and node j, thus contributing nothing to the sum [16, 17]. When the graph G represents a whole network, $E(G)$ measures the global efficiency of the network that quantifies the efficiency of information propagation over it. When considering a subgraph of the whole graph G, such as G_i, which is composed of the nearest neighbors of node i, $/E(G_i)$ indicates the efficiency of the subgraph G_i, measuring how efficient the information is exchanged in the subgraph. The local efficiency of a network G is the average of efficiency over all subgraphs of G and defined in (3)

$$E_{loc} = \frac{1}{N} \sum_{i \in G} E(G_i) \tag{3}$$

Besides the two global metrics, in this study, we also investigated regional nodal efficiency in (4), defined as the inverse of the harmonic mean of the minimum path length between the index node i and all other nodes. $E_{nodal}(i)$ measures the communication efficiency between a node i and all the other nodes in the network [18].

$$E_{nodal}(i) = \frac{1}{N-1} \sum_{j \in G} \frac{1}{L_{i,j}} \tag{4}$$

In this study, the cost was adopted as the threshold to avoid influence from the difference in the correlation level between the males and females. The global and local efficiency were calculated as functions of the cost. It is important to guarantee that the graphs of the two groups have the same cost so that any remaining differences in global and local efficiency between groups reflect differences in graph organization [23].

3 Results

The global and local efficiency, as functions of the cost, were shown in Fig.1 (a) and (b), respectively: female subjects are denoted by black mean and standard error, male subjects by red mean and standard error. As shown in Fig.1, the global and local efficiency of both the males and females increased with the cost value. Though the females had slightly reduced global efficiencies but slightly increased local efficiencies compared with the males, the group differences were not statistically significant.

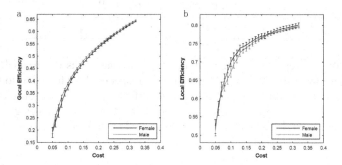

Fig. 1. The (a) global and (b) local efficiency of brain functional networks from all subjects

The nodal efficiency at the cost of 0.1, adjusted for global efficiency, was shown for each of the 90 brain areas in Fig.2. Significantly lower nodal efficiencies of the females were found in several brain areas (space circles) of limbic and paralimbic regions, including hippocampus, parahippocampal gyrus, amygdala, and cingulated gyrus. Significantly increased regions (filled squares) were detected in the frontal and temporal lobe (See Table 1 for details). In Table 1, the positive *t*-scores estimated by two-sample *t* test denoted greater nodal efficiency in males and vice versa. The corresponding *p* values in parentheses denoted the significance level. Abbreviation L and R denoted the left and right hemisphere, respectively.

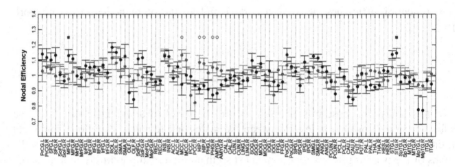

Fig. 2. Effect of gender on nodal efficiency

Table 1. Regions with significant gender difference in the nodal efficiency

Brain Regions	Gender Effects	*t*-scores (*p* value)
Frontal	Middle frontal gyrus, L	-2.79(0.012)
Temporal	Superior temporal gyrus, R	-2.35(0.034)
Limbic/paralimbic	Middle cingulum gyrus, L	2.45(0.024)
	Hippocampus gyrus, L	3.11(0.005)
	Hippocampus gyrus, R	3.32(0.002)
	Parahippocampal gyrus , R	3.17(0.007)
	Amygdala, L	2.73(0.013)

The anatomical representations of brain functional networks of one male and one female subject were shown in Fig. 3 (a) and (b), respectively. The color-coded nodes with larger size indicated the significant gender effect on the regional efficiency, with filled cyan circles and filled red squares indicating lower and higher efficiency in female, respectively. See Table 1 for the color-coded anatomical details.

4 Discussion

Though small-world networks were originally quantified by the clustering coefficient C and the characteristic path length L [24, 25, 26], the formulation required the

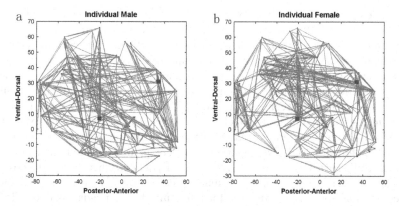

Fig. 3. Anatomical representation of brain functional networks of one male (a) and female (b) subject

graph to be connected, i.e. there exist at least one path connecting any pair of nodes In the case of a higher threshold, possibly resulting in a disconnected graph, the requirement would not be fulfilled since the quantity L would diverge. Therefore, we employed the network efficiency to quantify a whole graph in the study [16, 17]. The metrics of network efficiency can avoid the problem met by the characteristic path length L. Moreover, the efficiency is a more suitable network metric for the brain because the efficiency can characterize parallel information processing which the brain supports [13, 18].

In the current study, we demonstrated, for the first time, the gender effects on the efficiency of brain functional networks. No significant differences in both the global and local efficiency were found between males and females. Previous reports of structural covariance in the human cortex indicated that the patterns of associations identified were remarkably similar between males and females [27]. Our finding was compatible with the previous results. A tendency of gender-related effects was, however, found over the whole range of cost: greater global efficiency in male and greater local efficiency in female, suggesting that the functional networks in males and females exhibited similar function but different architectures. Interestingly, it has been suggested that the gender-differences in problem solving strategies or the neurodevelopment may be associated with gender-specific differences in functional organization of the brain [7].

Except for the comparability described above, we also found gender differences at several regions based on nodal efficiency. Significantly higher nodal efficiencies of the females were detected in the frontal and temporal lobe in this study. Some investigations based on brain morphology reported that some parts of the frontal cortex are bulkier in females than in males [3]. Also, other investigations had been finding anatomical gender differences at the cellular level. For instance, Witelson discovered that females possessed a greater density of neurons in parts of the temporal lobe associated with language processing and comprehension [28]. The existence of the relevant anatomical disparities between males and females may explain the structure difference of brain function networks [29]. Recently, a task-state fMRI study demonstrated greater activity in women than in men in prefrontal and other high-order association cortices [30]. These results were compatible with our findings.

In addition, significantly higher nodal efficiencies of the males were also found in several brain areas of limbic and paralimbic regions, including hippocampus, parahippocampal gyrus, amygdala, and cingulated gyrus. Extensive evidence demonstrated that hippocampus and amygdala differ significantly in their anatomical structure and function between male and female [31]. For example, the amygdala was larger in males than in females [3]. Jackson and others showed that a brief exposure to a stressful learning situation increased the activity of hippocampus in males but decreased in females [32]. The findings were compatible with our investigations. Kilpatrick and others reported that activity of the right hemisphere amygdala covaried with that of other brain regions to a much greater extent in males than it did in females, whereas the reverse was true for left hemisphere amygdala activity [15]. In the present study, greater nodal efficiency was found in only the left amygdala in male. It is seemly inconsistent for amygdala with the current evidence.

The methodological issues need to be addressed. In order to construct functional brain networks, several recent studies used different methods to select a reasonable threshold [18, 22, 23]. As a preliminary study, the adopted threshold was determined based on a recent study on human brain functional networks [18]. Also, the networks we here constructed were unweighted (e.g., independent of spatial scale). In a future study, we would construct continuous weighted brain networks to avoid the threshold issue.

5 Conclusion

To our knowledge, this study provided the first evidence of gender effect on the efficiency of brain functional networks acquired from resting-state fMRI data. Our investigations indicated that there were not significant differences in the global and local efficiency of brain functional networks between male and female. However, the gender effects on nodal efficiency were found at several brain regions. These findings were compatible with previous results, thus enhancing our understanding of the gender-related topological organization of the human brain. Our results suggested that researchers should take into account the gender effects when analyzing their structural functional imaging data from a network perspective.

Acknowledgments

This work was partially supported by the National Key Basic Research and Development Program (973) (Grant No. 2003CB716101) and Natural Science Foundation of China (Grant No. 30500130).

References

1. Luders, E., Narr, K.L., Thompson, P.M., Rex, D.E., Woods, R.P., Deluca, H., Jancke, L., Toga, A.W.: Gender effects on cortical thickness and the influence of scaling. Hum Brain Mapp 27, 314–324 (2006)

2. Allen, J.S., Damasio, H., Grabowski, T.J., Bruss, J., Zhang, W.: Sexual dimorphism and asymmetries in the gray-white composition of the human cerebrum. NeuroImage 18, 880–894 (2003)
3. Goldstein, J.M., Seidman, L.J., Horton, N.J., Makris, N., Kennedy, D.N., Caviness Jr, V.S., Faraone, S.V., Tsuang, M.T.: Normal sexual dimorphism of the adult human brain assessed by in vivo magnetic resonance imaging. Cereb Cortex 11, 490–497 (2001)
4. Canli, T., Desmond, J.E., Zhao, Z., Gabrieli, J.D.E.: Sex differences in the neural basis of emotional memories. PNAS 99, 10789–10794 (2002)
5. Hofer, A., Siedentopf, C.M., Ischebeck, A., Rettenbacher, M.A., Verius, M., Felber, S., Fleischhacker, W.W.: Gender differences in regional cerebral activity during the perception of emotion: A functional MRI study. NeuroImage 32, 854–862 (2006)
6. Klein, S., Smolka, M.N., Wrase, J., Gruesser, S.M., Mann, K., Braus, D.F., Heinz, A.: The Influence of Gender and Emotional Valence of Visual Cues on fMRI Activation in Humans. Pharmacopsychiatry, 191–194 (2003)
7. Speck, O., Ernst, T., Braun, J., Koch, C., Miller, E., Chang, L.: Gender differences in the functional organization of the brain for working memory. Neuroreport 11, 2581–2585 (2000)
8. Garavan, H., Pendergrass, J.C., Ross, T.J., Stein, E.A., Risinger, R.C.: Amygdala response to both positively and negatively valenced stimuli. Neuroreport 12, 2779–2783 (2001)
9. Phillips, M.D., Lurito, J.T., Dzemidzic, M., Lowe, M.J., Wang, Y., Mathews, V.P.: Gender based differences in temporal lobe activation demonstrated using a novel passive listening paradigm. NeuroImage 11, S352 (2000)
10. Kansaku, K., Yamaura, A., Kitazawa, S.: Sex differences in lateralization revealed in the posterior language areas. Cereb Cortex 10, 866–872 (2000)
11. Li, C.-S.R., Kosten, T.R., Sinha, R.: Sex differences in brain activation during stress imagery in abstinent cocaine users: A functional magnetic resonance imaging study. Biological Psychiatry 57, 487–494 (2005)
12. McClure, E.B., Monk, C.S., Nelson, E.E., Zarahn, E., Leibenluft, E., Bilder, R.M., Charney, D.S., Ernst, M., Pine, D.S.: A developmental examination of gender differences in brain engagement during evaluation of threat. Biological Psychiatry 55, 1047–1055 (2004)
13. Bassett, D.S., Bullmore, E.: Small-world brain networks. Neuroscientist 12, 512–523 (2006)
14. Slewa-Younan, S., Gordon, E., Harris, A.W., Haig, A.R., Brown, K.J., Flor-Henry, P., Williams, L.M.: Sex differences in functional connectivity in first-episode and chronic schizophrenia patients. Am J. Psychiatry 161, 1595–1602 (2004)
15. Kilpatrick, L.A., Zald, D.H., Pardo, J.V., Cahill, L.F.: Sex-related differences in amygdala functional connectivity during resting conditions. Neuroimage 30, 452–461 (2006)
16. Latora, V., Marchiori, M.: Efficient behavior of small-world networks. Phys. Rev. Lett. 87, 198701 (2001)
17. Latora, V., Marchiori, M.: Economic small-world behavior in weighted networks. The European Physical Journal B - Condensed Matter and Complex Systems V32, 249–263 (2003)
18. Achard, S., Bullmore, E.: Efficiency and cost of economical brain functional networks. PLoS computational biology 3, e17 (2007)
19. Greicius, M.D., Krasnow, B., Reiss, A.L., Menon, V.: Functional connectivity in the resting brain: a network analysis of the default mode hypothesis. Proc. Natl. Acad. Sci. U S A 100, 253–258 (2003)

20. Cox, R.W.: AFNI: software for analysis and visualization of functional magnetic resonance neuroimages. Comput. Biomed Res. 29, 162–173 (1996)
21. Tzourio-Mazoyer, N., Landeau, B., Papathanassiou, D., Crivello, F., Etard, O., Delcroix, N., Mazoyer, B., Joliot, M.: Automated anatomical labeling of activations in SPM using a macroscopic anatomical parcellation of the MNI MRI single-subject brain. Neuroimage 15, 273–289 (2002)
22. Achard, S., Salvador, R., Whitcher, B., Suckling, J., Bullmore, E.: A resilient, low-frequency, small-world human brain functional network with highly connected association cortical hubs. J. Neurosci. 26, 63–72 (2006)
23. Stam, C.J., Jones, B.F., Nolte, G., Breakspear, M., Scheltens, P.: Small-world networks and functional connectivity in Alzheimer's disease. Cereb Cortex 17, 92–99 (2007)
24. Watts, D.J., Strogatz, S.H.: Collective dynamics of 'small-world' networks. Nature 393, 440–442 (1998)
25. Strogatz, S.H.: Exploring complex networks. Nature 410, 268–276 (2001)
26. Amaral, L.A., Scala, A., Barthelemy, M., Stanley, H.E.: Classes of small-world networks. Proc. Natl. Acad. Sci. U S A 97, 11149–11152 (2000)
27. Mechelli, A., Friston, K.J., Frackowiak, R.S., Price, C.J.: Structural covariance in the human cortex. J. Neurosci. 25, 8303–8310 (2005)
28. Witelson, S.F.: Neural sexual mosaicism: sexual differentiation of the human temporo-parietal region for functional asymmetry. Psychoneuroendocrinology 16, 131–153 (1991)
29. Sporns, O., Tononi, G., Edelman, G.M.: Theoretical neuroanatomy: relating anatomical and functional connectivity in graphs and cortical connection matrices. Cereb Cortex 10, 127–141 (2000)
30. Butler, T., Imperato-McGinley, J., Pan, H., Voyer, D., Cordero, J., Zhu, Y.-S., Stern, E., Silbersweig, D.: Sex differences in mental rotation: Top-down versus bottom-up processing. NeuroImage 32, 445–456 (2006)
31. Cahill, L.: Why sex matters for neuroscience. Nat. Rev. Neurosci. 7, 477–484 (2006)
32. Jackson, E.D., Payne, J.D., Nadel, L., Jacobs, W.J.: Stress differentially modulates fear conditioning in healthy men and women. Biol. Psychiatry 59, 516–522 (2006)

Transferring Whole Blood Time Activity Curve to Plasma in Rodents Using Blood-Cell-Two-Compartment Model

Jih-Shian Lee[1], Kuan-Hao Su[1], Jun-Cheng Lin[1], Ya-Ting Chuang[1],
Ho-Shiang Chueh[1], Ren-Shyan Liu[2,3], Shyh-Jen Wang[2,3], and Jyh-Cheng Chen[1,4]

[1] Dept. of Biomedical Imaging & Radiological Sciences, National Yang-Ming University,
Taipei, Taiwan
[2] National PET/Cyclotron Center, Taipei Veterans General Hospital, Taipei, Taiwan
[3] National Yang-Ming University Medical School, Taipei, Taiwan
[4] Department of Education and Research, Taipei City Hospital, Taipei, Taiwan
jcchen@ym.edu.tw

Abstract. The term input function usually refers to the tracer plasma time activity curve (pTAC), which is necessary for quantitative positron emission tomography (PET) studies. The purpose of this study was to acquire the pTAC from the independent component analysis (ICA) estimated whole blood time activity curve (wTAC) using our proposed method: FDG blood-cell-two-compartment model (BCM). We also compared published models, which are linear haematocrit (HCT) correction, nonlinear HCT correction, and two-exponential correction. According to the results, the normalized root mean square error (NRMSE) and error of area under curve (EAUC) of BCM estimated pTAC were the smallest. Compartmental and graphic analyses were used to estimate metabolic rate of FDG (MR_{FDG}). The percentage error of MR_{FDG} (PE_{MRFDG}) estimated from BCM corrected pTAC was also the smallest. The BCM is a better choice to transfer wTAC to pTAC for quantification.

Keywords: input function, quantification, PET, tracer kinetic model.

1 Introduction

Positron emission tomography (PET) combined with tracer kinetic modeling is an excellent tool for quantification of interested parameters. For instance, after venous injection of FDG, the local metabolic rate of glucose can be accurately quantified. The arterial tracer plasma time activity curve (pTAC) is referred to as an input function because it delivers the tracer to all tissues. In addition, the arterial pTAC is necessary for rate constant calculations by serving as an input for tracer kinetic model. Accurate determination of the pTAC is important for kinetic modeling approach. The gold standard for the pTAC determination is arterial blood sampling [1, 2]. This technique relies on arterial cannulation and frequent blood sampling which is discomfort due to arterial puncture. Arterialized venous method [3] uses a heated limb to bate the invasion but still presents several drawbacks: repeated radiation exposure to the blood sampler, frequent sampling and spinning in the centrifuge affecting the accuracy of the pTAC due to gross error, and the relative

X. Gao et al. (Eds.): MIMI 2007, LNCS 4987, pp. 169–178, 2008.
© Springer-Verlag Berlin Heidelberg 2008

large amount of blood loss that affects the physiological parameters. These have led several groups to investigate alternative methods. For instance:

(1) A population-based pTAC were generated by averaging the pTACs from a sample population. After taking one or two individual's blood samples, the estimated pTAC can be obtained by scaling the population-based pTAC with the actual arterial plasma activity [4, 5]. The error of quantization may become larger due to different individual's physiological state and protocol.

(2) Positron-emitting nuclides emit positrons that traveling with finite range before undergoing annihilation. Thus it is possible to detect the positron before annihilation. Two β-sensitive probes are used to directly measure the whole blood time activity curve (wTAC) [6, 7]. One was inserted to the artery directly, and the other was inserted in the neighborhood of the artery to detect accumulated tracer in the surrounding tissue. After correct for sticking and dispersion of tracer to the probe by one compartment model, the wTAC was determined with subtracting the surrounding tissue signal to the arterial signal. There are several disadvantages in this method including invasive due to the surgically inserting the probe, and the large amount of annihilation photons to be counted.

(3) Catheters were inserted into the artery and vein. By the catheters, a fraction of whole blood flows outside through an arteriovenous shunt system [7, 8]. The wTAC was derived by the coincidence probe or β-sensitive probe, in the arteriovenous shunt system. Disadvantages of this method are: invasive due to the surgery of arteriovenous shunting, and the stick of tracer to the catheters affecting the accuracy.

(4) After correction for partial volume effect and spillover effect with dynamic images, the image based wTAC was determined with region of interest (ROI) within the blood pool [7, 9]. This method is noninvasive and simpler.

(5) Factor analysis (FA) and independent component analysis (ICA) are used to segment the blood pool from the dynamic images. The wTAC was derived from average of the segmented blood pool [7, 10, 11, 12]. This method is most attractive due to its noninvasive and simpler protocol than manual blood sampling, β-sensitive probe, and arteriovenous shunt system, showing higher precision than ROI method.

It is important to transfer the wTAC to pTAC accurately due to most of these methods described above only produce wTAC. The purpose of this study is to acquire the tracer pTAC from the ICA-estimated wTAC using our proposed method, FDG blood-cell-two-compartment model (BCM) and to compare with the published models: linear haematocrit (HCT) correction [12], nonlinear HCT correction [9], and two-exponential correction [1, 6, 8, 13].

2 Materials and Methods

2.1 Data Acquisition and Preprocessing

Imaging coverage from brain to heart apex was performed using the micro PET R4$^{®}$ (Concorde Microsystems, now Siemens). After a transmission scan using ^{68}Ge rod source for attenuation correction, dynamic PET image were acquired at rest for 3600 s that produced 31 time frames (6 images of 10 s, 6 images of 30 s, 6 images of 60 s, 5 images of 120 s, 8 images of 300 s) following the bolus injection of 18F-FDG. Transaxial images were reconstructed using the filtered backprojection (FBP) method for a 256×256×63×31 four dimensional matrix with pixel size of 0.423×0.423×1.121 mm. Arterial blood samples were taken at 0, 8, 15, 30, 45, 60, 120, 180, 300, 450, 600, 900, 1500, 2100, 2700 and 3600 s. After spinning for 5 min in a centrifuge, 40 μL plasma was counted in a gamma counter from each sample. HCT was obtained for linear HCT correction. Two groups of normal adult male Sprauge-Dawley rats (SD rats), weight: 350-450 g, were used in this study (group 1: n = 3 and group 2: n = 3).

2.2 ICA-Estimated wTAC by Su's Method

Su et al. proposed a method to extract image-derived wTAC from dynamic PET images using ICA [12]. Dynamic PET images can be treated as a mixed signal which is the spatial distribution of several tissues. ICA can estimate the tissues which are spatially statistically independent. After ICA estimation, the cardiac blood pool is segmented into dynamic component image. The mask of the cardiac blood pool ICA image is determined using the Gaussian fitting method and image dilation method. The wTAC is also corrected for partial volume and spillover effect.

2.3 WTAC and pTAC Processing

Both wTAC derived by an image and pTAC sampled manually are discrete points with different time intervals. When calculating the tracer kinetic model, the wTAC and pTAC need to have the same time intervals or available at any arbitrary time point due to convolution and numerical integration of differential equations. The wTAC and pTAC were linearly interpolated from post injection time to time of peak in the curve and fitted with three exponentials from time of peak to the end time [3, 5]. Equations are described as follows:

$$C(t) = m \times t \qquad 0 \le t < \text{time to peak} \tag{1}$$

$$C(t) = \sum_{i=1}^{3} A_i e^{-\lambda_i t} \qquad t >= \text{time to peak} \tag{2}$$

where C(t) is radiotracer concentration at time t and m is fitted parameter for linearly interpolation. A_i, and λ_i are fitted parameters for two-exponential correction.

2.4 Transferring wTAC to pTAC

Four methods of transferring wTAC to pTAC, our proposed method, FDG BCM, linear HCT correction proposed by Su et al. [12], nonlinear HCT correction proposed by Wahl et al. [9], and two-exponential correction proposed by Lammertsma et al. [1] were evaluated in this study.

FDG BCM. FDG two-tissue compartment model proposed by Phelps et al. [3] describes the kinetic of FDG between plasma and brain tissue. The rate constants between these compartments were estimated by the non-linear-lest-squares method using the pTAC as input and tissue time activity (tTAC) as output. After the parameter estimation, the metabolic rate of glucose can be calculated with these constants and lumped constant. FDG BCM was based on FDG two-tissue compartment model which is illustrated in Fig. 1. C_1 represents tracer in plasma, C_2 represents free and non-metabolized tracer in red blood cell etc, and C_3 represents metabolized tracer. K_1 is rate coefficient for transfer from C_1 to C_2, k_2 is rate coefficient for transfer from C_2 to C_1. k_3 is rate coefficient for transfer from C_2 to C_3, and k_4 is rate coefficient for transfer from C_3 to C_4. By mass balance, one obtains the following equations:

$$\frac{dC_2}{dt} = -(k_2 + k_3)C_2 + K_1C_1 + k_4C_3 \tag{3}$$

$$\frac{dC_3}{dt} = -k_4C_3 + k_3C_2 \tag{4}$$

By applying Laplace transforms on equations in (3) and (4), we have

$$\hat{C}_2 = \frac{K_1(s + k_4)}{s^2 + (k_2 + k_3 + k_4)s + k_2k_4}\hat{C}_1 \tag{5}$$

$$\hat{C}_3 = \frac{K_1k_3}{s^2 + (k_2 + k_3 + k_4) + k_2k_4}\hat{C}_1 \tag{6}$$

From equations (5) and (6), equations (7) can be derived as follows:

$$\hat{C}_1 = (\hat{C}_1 + \hat{C}_2 + \hat{C}_3)[1 + \frac{-K_1k_3 - K_1k_4}{\alpha_2 - \alpha_1}(\frac{1}{s + \alpha_1} - \frac{1}{s + \alpha_2}) + \frac{1}{\alpha_2 - \alpha_1}(\frac{K_1\alpha_1}{s + \alpha_1} - \frac{K_1\alpha_2}{s + \alpha_2})] \tag{7}$$

Applying inverse Laplace transform on equation (7), we have

$$C_1 = (C_1 + C_2 + C_3) + [\frac{K_1\alpha_1 - K_1k_3 - K_1k_4}{\alpha_2 - \alpha_1}e^{-\alpha_1 t} + \frac{-K_1\alpha_2 + K_1k_3 + K_1k_4}{\alpha_2 - \alpha_1}e^{-\alpha_2 t}] \otimes (C_1 + C_2 + C_3) \tag{8}$$

where

$$\alpha_1 = [(K_1 + k_2 + k_3 + k_4) - \sqrt{(K_1 + k_2 + k_3 + k_4)^2 - 4K_1k_3 - 4K_1k_4 - 4k_2k_4}\,)]/2 \qquad (9)$$

$$\alpha_2 = [(K_1 + k_2 + k_3 + k_4) + \sqrt{(K_1 + k_2 + k_3 + k_4)^2 - 4K_1k_3 - 4K_1k_4 - 4k_2k_4}\,)]/2 \qquad (10)$$

To transfer wTAC to pTAC, the following procedure was adopted: First, the wTACs from group 1 were corrected to $C_1 + C_2 + C_3$ with HCT of 0.45 for male SD rats using the following equation:

$$C_1 + C_2 + C_3 \cong C_1 + \frac{HCT}{1 - HCT}(C_2 + C_3) = \frac{wTAC}{1 - HCT} \qquad (11)$$

Second, BCM k values from Group 1 were estimated by the non-linear-lest-squares method. Standard BCM k values were calculated by averaging those k values. Second, the wTAC from group 2 was transferred to pTAC with standard BCM k values using equation (11) and (8).

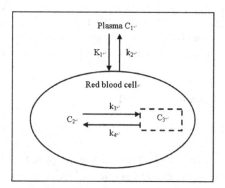

Fig. 1. FDG blood-cell-two-compartment model

Linear HCT correction. Su et al. [12] describes linear HCT correction which is defined as follows:

$$C_{p-lHCT}(t) = \frac{C_w(t)}{(1 - HCT)} \qquad (12)$$

Where $C_{p-lHCT}(t)$ is linear HCT corrected concentration of FDG in plasma at time t, $C_w(t)$ is concentration of FDG in whole blood at time t, and HCT is haematocrit. The wTAC from a rat was transferred to pTAC by equation (12) with the HCT itself.

Nonlinear HCT correction. Wahl et al. [9] describes a nonlinear HCT method which is defined as follows:

$$C_{p-nHCT}(t) = \frac{1 - HCT \ (1 - e^{-at})}{(1 - HCT \ )} C_w(t) \tag{13}$$

Where $C_{p-nHCT}(t)$ is nonlinear HCT corrected concentration of FDG in plasma at time t, HCT is 0.45 for male SD rat, and a is the equilibrium time constant. First, equilibrium time constants from group 1 were estimated. Second, the wTACs from group 2 were transferred to pTACs with mean equilibrium time constant by equation (13).

Two-exponential correction. Lammertsma et al. described multi-exponential method [1]. Optimum number of exponentials is two which was described by Weber et al. [8]. Two-exponential correction was defined as follows:

$$\frac{C_{p-exp}(t)}{C_w(t)} = A_1 e^{-\lambda_1 t} + A_2 e^{-\lambda_2 t} + C \tag{14}$$

Where $C_{p-exp}(t)$ is concentration of FDG in plasma at time t. $A_1, A_2, \lambda_1, \lambda_2$, and C are fitted parameters for two-exponential correction. The pooled time course of the ratio of FDG in plasma and whole blood from all rats were fitted by the equation (14). The wTACs from group 2 were transferred to pTACs with the fitted parameters from group 1.

2.5 Calculation of Metabolic Rate of FDG

Metabolic rate of FDG (MRFDG) in brain, which is directly proportional to the metabolic rate of glucose was estimated by FDG two-tissue compartment model proposed by Phelps et al. [3] and Patlak plot was proposed by Patlak et al. [15, 16]. The MRFDG derived from manually sampled pTAC was used as the reference for comparison with the MRFDG derived from estimated pTACs.

3   Results

Fig. 2 shows the PET image of cardiac section and the ICA segmented image. After segmentation, the cardiac blood pool image can be derived and the image-based wTAC also can be extracted. The manually sampled pTAC and estimated TAC of four methods are shown in Fig. 3. The normalized root mean square error (NRMSE) defined in equation (15), the error of area under curve (EAUC) defined in equation (16), and the percentage error of MR_{FDG} (PE_{MRFDG}) defined in equation (17) were showed in table 1.

$$\text{NRMSE} \quad = \quad \sqrt{\frac{\sum_{t=0}^{end} [C_{est}(t) - C_{ref}(t)]^2}{\sum_{t=0}^{end} [C_{ref}(t)]^2}} \tag{15}$$

where $C_{est}(t)$ is the estimated plasma concentration at time t, and $C_{ref}(t)$ is the manually sampled plasma concentration at time t.

$$\text{EAUC} \quad = \quad \left| \frac{AUC_{est} - AUC_{ref}}{AUC_{ref}} \right| \tag{16}$$

where AUC_{est} is the AUC of estimated pTAC, and AUC_{ref} is the AUC of manually sampled pTAC.

$$\text{PE}_{MRFDG} \quad = \quad \left| \frac{MRFDG_{est} - MRFDG_{ref}}{MRFDG_{ref}} \right| \times 100 \% \tag{17}$$

where $MRFDG_{est.}$ is the MR_{FDG} from estimated pTAC, and $MRFDG_{ref}$ is the MR_{FDG} from manually sampled pTAC.

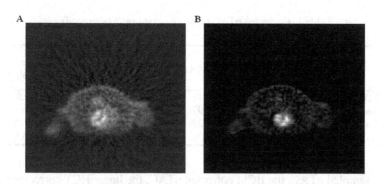

Fig. 2. (A) ^{18}F-FDG-PET image of cardiac section (B) ICA segmented cardiac blood pool image

4   Discussions

Image-based analysis with ICA segmented blood pool is the most attractive method in deriving input function for quantitative PET studies, because of its noninvasive, higher precision than the ROI method, and simplified protocol in comparison with manual blood sampling, β-sensitive probe, and arteriovenous shunt system. It is an important issue to transfer derived wTAC to pTAC accurately. Fig. 3 illustrates the

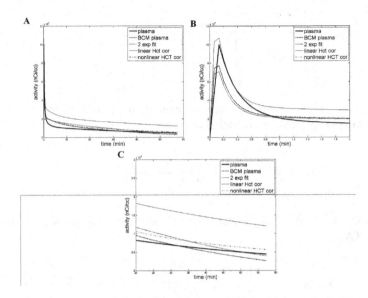

Fig. 3. (A) The manually sampled pTAC and estimated TAC of four methods. Plasma: manually sampling pTAC, BCM plasma: BCM corrected pTAC, 2 exp fit: two-exponential corrected pTAC, linear HCT cor: linear HCT corrected pTAC, and nonlinear HCT cor: nonlinear HCT corrected pTAC. (B) shows the same data that focused around the peak at earlier time. (C) shows the same data that focused on equilibrium area at later time.

Table 1. Corrected pTAC results from group 2 (averaged)

	NRMSE	EAUC	PE_{MRFDG} (%) (compartment model)	PE_{MRFDG} (%) (Patlak plot)
FDG BCM	0.33	0.17	9.44	6.67
Linear HCT cor.	0.85	0.93	55.47	56.51
Nonlinear HCT cor.	0.34	0.22	17.35	9.46
Two-exponential cor.	0.35	0.20	14.40	16.00

manually sampled pTAC, the BCM corrected pTAC, the linear HCT corrected pTAC, the nonlinear HCT corrected pTAC, and the two-exponential corrected pTAC of rats in group 2. At the earlier time around the peak that illustrated in Fig. 3 (B), the peak in all estimated pTACs shifted several seconds due to the blood sampling time difference from the frame time. The linear HCT corrected pTAC was estimated most accurate due to the metabolism of FDG in blood cell is not apparent in the short time course. The BCM corrected pTAC and the nonlinear HCT corrected pTAC that corrected for HCT also estimated more accuracy than the two-exponential corrected pTAC. The two-exponential corrected pTAC was under estimated due to simplicity. In the later time of equilibrium area that illustrated in Fig. 3 (C), the linear HCT corrected pTAC was over estimated due to ignorance of the blood uptake. The nonlinear HCT corrected pTAC was over estimated due to the one exponential was difficult to fit the detail of the pTAC. The two-exponential corrected pTAC was over estimated due to the two-exponential were not enough to fit the pTAC. The BCM corrected pTAC, which models the physiology of red blood cells, is the most accurate one.

Table 1 illustrates the corrected pTAC results. The NRMSE and EAUC can represent the differentiation between estimated pTAC and manually sampled pTAC. The NRMSEs and EAUCs of BCM pTAC are the smallest one in the four pTACs. It means that BCM estimated pTAC is very close to the one from manually sampled pTAC which is the gold standard. The MRFDG is an important parameter for quantitative PET studies using FDG. We used compartmental and graphic analysis to estimate the MRFDG. The PE_{MRFDG} estimated from BCM pTAC by compartmental and graphic analysis are also the smallest which is similar to the results of NRMSEs and EAUCs. It suggests that BCM can be used to transfer the wTAC to pTAC for use in quantification with compartmental or graphic analysis.

5 Conclusions

Linear HCT correction assumes that there is no FDG uptake in blood cell, but our results show that there is FDG uptake in blood cells. Nonlinear HCT and two exponentials correction are too simple to fit the detail of pTAC. Due to modeling the physiology of blood cell, the pTAC estimated by BCM is the most accurate one. Therefore, our proposed method, FDG BCM, can be widely used to transfer wTAC to pTAC for quantification of PET images.

Acknowledgments. The authors would like to thank Yueh-Ting Chou for arterial cannulating, and National Research Program for Genomic Medicine for imaging instrument support. This work was financially supported by National Science Council (NSC 95-2314-B-010-075 and NSC 95-3112-B-010-004).

References

1. Lammertsma, A.A., Bench, C.J., Price, G.W., Cremer, J.E., Luthra, S.K., Turton, D., Wood, N.D., Frackowiak, R.S.: Measurement of cerebral monoamine oxidase B activity using L-[11C]deprenyl and dynamic positron emission tomography. J. Cereb. Blood Flow Metab. 4, 545–556 (1991)
2. Sharp, T.L., Dence, C.S., Engelbach, J.A., Herrero, P., Gropler, R.J., Welch, M.J.: Techniques necessary for multiple tracer quantitative small-animal imaging studies. Nucl. Med. Biol. 32, 875 (2005)
3. Phelps, M.E., Huang, S.C., Hoffman, E.J., Selin, C., Sokoloff, L., Kuhl, D.E.: Tomographic measurement of local cerebral glucose metabolic rate in humans with (F-18)2-fluoro-2-deoxy-D-glucose: validation of method. Ann. Neurol. 5, 371–388 (1979)
4. Chen, K., Bandy, D., Reiman, E., Huang, S.C., Lawson, M., Feng, D., Yun, L.S., Palant, A.: Noninvasive quantification of the cerebral metabolic rate for glucose using positron emission tomography, 18F-fluoro-2-deoxyglucose, the Patlak method, and an image-derived input function. J. Cereb. Blood Flow Metab. 18(7), 716–723 (1998)

5. Eberl, S., Anayat, A.R., Fulton, R.R., Hooper, P.K., Fulham, M.J.: Evaluation of two population-based input functions for quantitative neurological FDG PET studies. Eur. J. Nucl. Med. 24(3), 299–304 (1997)
6. Pain, F., Laniece, P., Mastrippolito, R., Gervais, P., Hantraye, P., Besret, L.: Arterial input function measurement without blood sampling using a beta-microprobe in rats. J. Nucl. Med. 45(9), 1577–1582 (2004)
7. Laforest, R., Sharp, T.L., Engelbach, J.A., Fettig, N.M., Herrero, P., Kim, J., Lewis, J.S., Rowland, D.J., Tai, Y.-C., Welch, M.J.: Measurement of input functions in rodents challenges and solutions. Nucl. Med. Biol. 32(7), 679–685 (2005)
8. Weber, B., Burger, C., Biro, P., Buck, A.: A femoral arteriovenous shunt facilitates arterial whole blood sampling in animals. Eur. J. Nucl. Med. Mol. Imaging 2002 3, 319–323 (2002)
9. Wahl, L.M., Asselin, M.C., Nahmias, C.: Regions of interest in the venous sinuses as input functions for quantitative PET. J. Nucl. Med. 40(10), 1666–1675 (1999)
10. Lee, J.S., Lee, D.S., Ahn, J.Y., Cheon, G.J., Kim, S.K., Yeo, J.S., Seo, K., Park, K.S., Chung, J.K., Lee, M.C.: Blind separation of cardiac components and extraction of input function from H(2)(15)O dynamic myocardial PET using independent component analysis. J. Nucl. Med. 42(6), 938–943 (2001)
11. Ahn, J.Y., Lee, D.S., Lee, J.S., Kim, S.-K., Cheon, G.J., Yeo, J.S., Shin, S.-A., Chung, J.-K., Lee, M.C.: Quantification of regional myocardial blood flow using dynamic H 2 15 O PET and factor analysis. J. Nucl. Med. 42(5), 782–787 (2001)
12. Su, K.-H., Wu, L.-C., Liu, R.-S., Wang, S.-J., Chen, J.-C.: Quantification method in [F-18]fluorodeoxyglucose brain positron emission tomography using independent component analysis. Nuclear Medicine Communications 26, 995–1004 (2005)
13. Ashworth, S., Ranciar, A., Bloomfield, P.M.: Development of an on-line blood detector system for PET studies in small animals. In: Quantification of brain function using PET, pp. 62–66 (1996)
14. Takikawa, S., Dhawan, V., Spetsieris, P., Robeson, W., Chaly, T., Dahl, R., Margouleff, D., Eidelberg, D.: Noninvasive quantitative fluorodeoxyglucose PET studies with an estimated input function derived from a population-based arterial blood curve. Radiology 188(1), 131–136 (1993)
15. Patlak, C.S., Blasberg, R.G.: Graphical evaluation of blood-to-brain transfer constants from multiple-time uptake data. Generalizations. J. Cereb. Blood Flow Metab. 5(4), 584–590 (1985)
16. Patlak, C.S., Blasberg, R.G., Fenstermacher, J.D.: Graphical evaluation of blood-to-brain transfer constants from multiple-time uptake data. J. Cereb. Blood Flow Metab. 3(1), 1–7 (1983)

Prototype System for Semantic Retrieval
of Neurological PET Images

Stephen Batty[1], John Clark[2], Tim Fryer[2], and Xiaohong Gao[1]

[1] Middlsex University, The Burroughs, Hendon, London, UK
s.batty@prion.ucl.ac.uk
[2] WBIC, Addenbrookes Hospital, Cambridge University, UK

Abstract. Positron Emission Tomography (PET) is used within neurology to study the underlying biochemical basis of cognitive functioning. Due to the inherent lack of anatomical information its study in conjunction with image retrieval is limited. Content based image retrieval (CBIR) relies on visual features to quantify and classify images with a degree of domain specific saliency. Numerous CBIR systems have been developed semantic retrieval, has however not been performed. This paper gives a detailed account of the framework of visual features and semantic information utilized within a prototype image retrieval system, for PET neurological data. Images from patients diagnosed with different and known forms of Dementia are studied and compared to controls. Image characteristics with medical saliency are isolated in a top down manner, from the needs of the clinician - to the explicit visual content. These features are represented via Gabor wavelets and mean activity levels of specific anatomical regions. Preliminary results demonstrate that these representations are effective in reflecting image characteristics and subject diagnosis; consequently they are efficient indices within a semantic retrieval system.

Keywords: PET, neurological, content based image retrieval, dementia, semantic retrieval.

1 Introduction

Content based image retrieval (CBIR) is a widely researched field with a number of published reviews [1,2]. There is a developing emphasis towards the field of medical informatics [3,4] and also, to a degree, Positron Emission Tomography, or PET, images of the human brain [5,6]. Successful content based retrieval archives images using indices relevant to image's classification and enables semantic retrieval. Semantic retrieval pertains to the archiving and indexing of images based upon their real world classifications, and therefore in the case of medical imaging - the diagnosis. This is subtly different to CBIR which relates to the archiving and retrieval of images based on their visual content and characteristics - with no account, in the definition, for classification/diagnosis. Semantic retrieval is viewed as the benchmark for successful content based image retrieval, as retrieval results should have relevance and validity to the intended users (of the CBIR system). Indeed the difference between semantic and content based retrieval has previously been highlighted [2] with

X. Gao et al. (Eds.): MIMI 2007, LNCS 4987, pp. 179–188, 2008.
© Springer-Verlag Berlin Heidelberg 2008

the assertion that semantic has not been achieved using only visual characteristics [2]. This somewhat negates the large number of CBIR systems currently available [1, 2] and recently published [5], which perform content based retrieval using visual features alone, as they have no semantic significance. Semantic classification is fundamental to medical image retrieval and indeed information retrieval in general; if semantic classification of data cannot be achieved any developed system would offer little practical benefit.

Work presented in this paper outlines results from a prototype semantic retrieval system for PET neurological images. PET is a functional imaging technique utilized in the study of metabolic pathways; it is widely used in the treatment and diagnosis of neurodegenerative disorders, lesions and also in the drug discovery process. A key factor in PET imaging is the ability to label different metabolites, and thus analyze alternate pathways. PET images are intensity based visual representations of the concentration of a radioactive label, commonly ^{11}C, ^{18}F-FDG or FDG, ^{13}N or ^{15}O. This marker will have labeled, respectively, a specific metabolite such as raclopride, glucose, ammonia, or water. FDG-PET, for example, is an important tool for the diagnosis and treatment of Alzheimer's disease; this is due to functional differences in the glucose pathway can arise before any structural differences are apparent.

However, this process of radioactive labelling is prohibitively expensive (when compared to MRI), and coupled with the low resolution and inherent lack of anatomical information ensures that PET research is less widespread than alternate modalities. The role of PET is nevertheless assured due to the unique benefits metabolite marking provides; this and the large number of installed systems producing many volumes of data each day warrant research into PET image retrieval and archiving. Content based retrieval of dynamic PET images has previously been reported [6] in which the indexing data derives from time-activity-curves of dynamic PET images(possessing temporal information); the semantic classification of images is not explicit and time activity curves *do not pertain directly to visual content* [2].

The stimulus for PET CBIR research is provided by clinicians, cognitive psychologists, neuroscientists, and researchers in these or closely related fields who expend time collating, classifying and/or performing further processing of PET data. The storage strategy employed at the Wolfson Brain Imaging Centre (Cambridge University) reflects this requirement for retrieval research. Images are stored using Unix operating system in flat file form   with no provision for any indexing retrieval beyond that provided by in-built Unix commands (eg 'find' and 'grep'). Consequently there is a large number of disparate groups of data demarcated by folder name and file information, with very little cross-referencing. A second neurological research centre, the Institute of Cognitive Neuroscience (University College London) utilizes an identical methodology in the Microsoft Windows environment.   The development of a semantic retrieval system would therefore significantly increase the efficiency of data management and provide a means for further novel research, specifically that focusing on the meta-analysis of stored data.

Neurological image analysis and the process of mapping cognitive functioning to anatomical areas of the brain requires the fulfillment of two processing stages – spatial and intensity normalization. For a retrieval system to exhibit practical benefits and be scientifically valid these stages must be incorporated and/or accounted for. Inter-subject variability of size and shape of brain eliminates direct comparisons between image voxels without further spatial processing, (1) and (2); *AA* represents anatomical area, while *X*, *Y*, *Z* represents the Cartesian co-ordinates of voxels belonging to images *I* and *J*.

$$AA_I(X,Y,Z) \neq AA_J(X,Y,Z) \tag{1}$$

Where

$$(X_I, Y_I, Z_I) = (X_J, Y_J, Z_J) \tag{2}$$

The process of spatial normalization is therefore a fundamental stage in any neurological image archiving system to ensure the same anatomical areas are quantified, without which inter-subject comparison is redundant. In practice PET images are registered to a standardized template and anatomical atlas; when available functional PET data is also first registered to an anatomical MRI image from the same subject. Commonly utilized are the template image from the Montreal Neurological Institute [7] and the Talairach and Tournox anatomical atlas [8, 9]. The second factor to be accounted for is that of scanning protocol discrepancies that introduce variation in absolute metabolite activity levels and are directly derived from voxel intensity values.

Appropriate image processing techniques for feature extraction are limited by domain specific attributes. PET, and medical images in general, are intensity based grayscale images, evidently eliminating color based indexing. Attributes specific to PET are the high signal to noise ratio, lack of anatomical information and relatively smooth, when compared to alternate medical imaging domains, distribution of voxel intensity values. These factors and the narrow domain specificity ensure that feature extraction approaches utilized in well developed CBIR systems such as those outlined in [1,2], are not applicable in regard to PET. This is due to the fact that the systems listed in [1, 2] retain images from a variety of domains and commonly enlist color as the predominant feature group. These factors necessitate the design and development of novel feature extraction algorithms, which are applicable only to the PET domain and theoretically other neurological imaging formats.

2 Methodology

2.1 Anatomical Segmentation

In this research an analysis of the retrosplenial cortex (Brodmann's Area 29/30), Posterior Cingulate (Brodmann's Area 23/31/29/30), Parietal Lobes, Occipital Lobes and Hippocampus is presented and the results compared to those from an automated segmentation method employing spatial normalization, via SPM [10] and the MNI [7] template. This segmentation technique is again utilized in the measurement of texture using Gabor filters.

The process of segmentation requires spatial normalization of tested PET images to the MNI template [7] and subsequent mapping to the Talairach and Tournoux atlas [8-11]. Anatomical regions of interest are then isolated via the referenced Cartesian co-ordinates for that anatomical region, with no further image processing. This method of image segmentation is, clearly, only applicable to neurological data; furthermore the incorporation of this prior knowledge into segmentation algorithms for modalities such as MRI may not be advantageous. PET images contain a large amount of noise and are therefore difficult to segment. Low noise, high signal image modalities such as MRI may not produce better segmentation with the addition of prior knowledge in the manner outlined. Segmentation of anatomical regions of interest allows the further extraction of semantic visual features. A number of different measurements are obtained from the PET images utilizing the anatomical segmentation previously outlined.

2.2 Mean Intensity

The previously outlined anatomical segmentation method is utilized to calculate the mean intensity of specific anatomical regions in a completely autonomous manner. The measurements obtained are then compared to results from SPM analysis of hypometablism; this comparison ensures the validity of automated segmentation method.

SPM analysis required [12] co-registered images were spatially normalized to the T1-MRI template of SPM99, using MRI scan to define normalization parameters, and smoothed with a 16mm gaussian filter. Each patients scan was analysed individually, using a paired t-test, in comparison to the control group at a statistical threshold of $P_{uncorrected} < 0.001$. Scans showing no abnormality were also analysed at $P_{uncorrected} < 0.01$. The hypometabolic clusters for each subject were then projected back to onto subjects spatially normalized MRI scan (i.e. - FDG-PET and MRI were in same standardized space). Anatomical localization of hypometabolic clusters was assessed both by comparing the stereotaxic co-ordinates of cluster peaks to the co-planar sterotaxic atlas [8] and by visual comparison of the MRI projected sections with corresponding slices from the Duvernoy [13] brain atlas.

Mean intensity levels were measured via the previously outlined automated segmentation method. Specific anatomic regions that were quantified: Parietal Lobes; Occipital Lobes.; Posterior Cingulate (or Brodmann's areas 23/31/29/30); Hippocampus; Retrosplenial cortex (or Brodmann's Area's 29 and 30). These areas are traditionally associated with Alzheimers, Prodromal Alzheimers and PCA. The different diagnosis types were therefore accounted for by the anatomical regions specified and isolated.

2.3 Texture

The term texture refers to visual patterns or spatial arrangements of pixels that cannot be completely described using regional intensity alone. Quantification of texture is a fundamental technique within image processing and consequently is widely used within CBIR research. Gabor filters have been shown to quantify texture reliably and are theoretically based on the functioning of the human visual system [14]; they were therefore used in this research to characterize the texture of PET images and anatomical sub-regions. Six scales and four rotations of Gabor filter are applied [15]. Image represented as $I(X,Y)$ and Gabor Wavelet Transform is defined.

$$W_m(X,Y) = \int I(X_1 Y_1) g_m * (x - x_1, y - y_1) dx_1 dy_1 \tag{1}$$

Where

$$g_m(X,Y) = a^{-m} G(X'Y'), a > 1 \tag{2}$$

$$G(u,v) = \exp\left\{-\frac{1}{2}\left[\frac{(u-W)^2}{\sigma^2} + \frac{v^2}{\sigma_v^2}\right]\right\} \tag{3}$$

The filters are applied to the listed anatomical regions of interest and the whole brain. This results in a forty-eight element feature vector for each anatomical region i.

$$F^i = \left[\mu_{01}^i, \mu_{02}^i, ..., \mu_{24}^i, \sigma_{01}^i, \sigma_{02}^i, ..., \sigma_{24}^i\right] \tag{4}$$

2.4 Similarity Metric

The extracted texture data is then used, in conjunction with anatomical location and mean index ratio, as indices within a DBMS (Database Management System) for semantic retrieval. The similarity metric is represented in Eqs.(5-7), following on from Eqs.(1-4)

$$T = \sum_{i=1}^{n} F_i \tag{5}$$

Where, the different images are represented as J and K.

$$F = |\mu_{01}^J - \mu_{01}^K| + ... + |\mu_{24}^J - \mu_{24}^K| \, |\sigma_{01}^J - \sigma_{01}^K| + ... + |\sigma_{24}^{Ji} - \sigma_{24}^K| \tag{6}$$

The complete feature vector used in retrieval is therefore be expressed

$$T\left(|\frac{\overline{W_J}}{i_J} - \frac{\overline{W_K}}{i_K}|\right) \tag{7}$$

Where W refers to whole brain.
A schematic diagram of the complete prototype system is presented in Fig. 1.

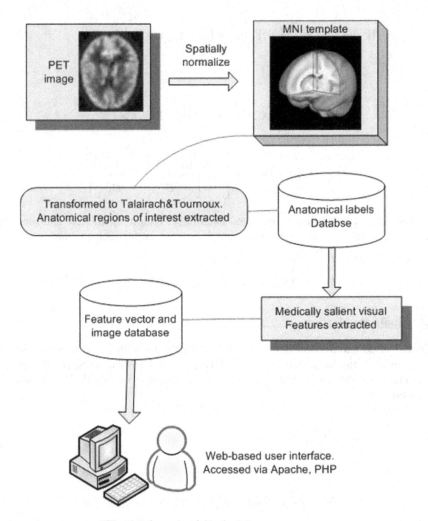

Fig. 1. Schematic of developed prototype system

3 Results

These results are as expected, when compared to the results from SPM analysis [12], the mean voxel intensities of tested experimental areas were found to be significantly less than controls (normal subjects, $p < 0.01$). The Parietal Lobes, Posterior Cingulate, Hippocampus, Brodmann's Area's 29 and 30, of patients diagnosed with Alzheimer's (prodromal form) were found to have a significantly reduced metabolism. Patients diagnosed with Posterior Cortical Atrophy exhibited hypometabolism in the Occipital Lobes, Parietal Lobes, Posterior Cingulate, Hippocampus, and Brodmann's Area 29 and 30.

Semantic retrieval of PET images has been performed; images from patients diagnosed with Dementia were retrieved in accordance to the expected results using a combination of mean index ratio and texture features. This procedure was evaluated iteratively and the product of texture and mean index ratio, of certain anatomical regions, was found to provide the best results. The anatomical structures conjoined are: the Occipital Lobe to assess Posterior Cortical Atrophy; Brodmann's Area 30, part of the Retrosplenial Cortex, and the Posterior Cingulate are included in relation to Alzheimer's. Improvements to this approach are suggested in Discussion (section IV).

Query by example produced results as predicted. Those images diagnostically closest to query are retrieved first, and vice versa, therefore semantic retrieval has been performed. Images are returned according to there respective diagnose, the order of retrieval possess medical saliency. Retrieval using dementia study was performed at the command line; no provision for user interface has yet been made; similarity metric utilized is nearest neighbor, the product of mean index ratio and the sum of squared differences of texture feature. The tuples for database indices are generated using *Matlab* algorithms, and retrieval is performed using LAMP (*Linux, Apache, MySQL, PHP*) architecture.

4   Discussion

Mean intensity levels from anatomical regions extracted using the automated method complement those from manual segmentation method; significant hypo-metabolism is found in the studied anatomical regions. However, absolute mean levels are not appropriate for indices within a retrieval system. Assuming differentiation based on tracer is part of pre-processing (due to DICOM header) it is still important to incorporate dosage disparities and inter-session/scanner noise variation [16, 17] to ensure practical robustness of semantic retrieval system. Utilization of mean index ratio provides this robustness by eliminating the variable of absolute intensity levels.

Semantic retrieval has been performed within the PET image domain utilizing a very specific feature set. This, when taken in the context of the DICOM standard and medical imaging in general, can viewed as a positive aspect. In medical informatics the DICOM standard instills a redundancy on inter-domain retrieval, based on visual content alone; this observation can also be levied at retrieval via anatomical areas (e.g. neurological opposed to cardiac) and imaging protocols. The DICOM standard contains this data in correctly implemented file headers[18] and consequently emphasizes the importance of classification based on diagnosis, and demarcation within specific image domains.

The small number of images in the dementia study group is an obvious limiting factor; however studies of dementia and cognition in general are prone to small experimental groups due the paucity of specific experimental data.

To create mean index ratio specific anatomical sub-regions are combined with whole brain measurements; an improvement, not implemented, would replace the whole brain value with that obtained from the cerebellum. This is due to the fact that the cerebellum is not considered to be a primary pathological focus in AD [19] and would provide a more robust distinction between diagnosis types.

Envisaged is a comprehensive PET archiving system for images from disparate sources, of which this prototype dementia study composes a constituent part. Figure 2

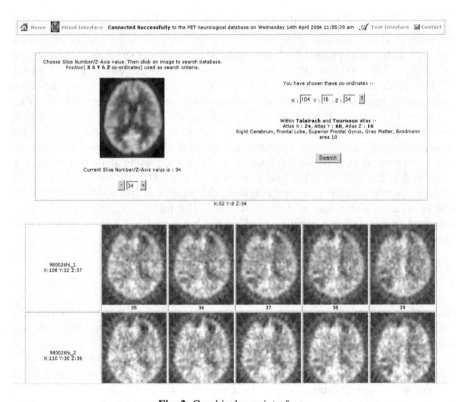

Fig. 2. Graphical user interface

shows web based UI for retrieval system managing images from patients with lesions [20-22]; the same database is utilized for Dementia retrieval and presented in this paper.

Further amalgamation will, in the future, provide functionality for retrieval and indexing of lesion, dementia and dynamic data simultaneously.

5 Conclusion

A prototype system for semantic retrieval of neurological PET images has been outlined and developed. This work accentuates the importance of domain specific knowledge to the problem of content based medical image retrieval; without which real-world benefits will remain limited. Of significance is the incorporation of a specific subset from within the PET image domain; the outlined system does not differentiate between an abstract collection of un-related images. The system provides a means to differentiate very closely related images based on medical saliency. Retrieval results have been presented for PET images based upon diagnosis, specifically classification of dementia.

Development of a practical and robust semantic retrieval system for PET neurological data would impact the research areas of *Decision Support* [2,3], *Computer Aided Diagnosis* [2,3] and also neurological/psychological research, specifically that which focuses on meta-analysis. Meta-analysis in these fields is composed by the combination of imaging data with cognitive, behavioral and diagnostic information across independent studies. The importance of CBIR research to the *Decision Support* and *Computer Aided Diagnosis* paradigms has previously been outlined and is well documented. The utilization of semantic retrieval within the fields of Psychology and Neuroscience research would be facilitated by providing a central database of diagnostically classified images – maintained by automated algorithms inherently reliable (compared to expert input); this would vastly increase the efficiency of meta-analysis and enable novel studies. Efficiency is improved by decreasing the time consuming aspects of administering imaging data and enabling rapid access to stored images, of specified diagnoses , to all users (with appropriate privileges). Novel inquires that cross reference individual imaging studies separated by scan date, scanning investigator; and imaging protocol would be enabled with the development of a semantic retrieval system; this is applicable to all neurological imaging modalities and not only PET.

It is therefore important to closely incorporate these paradigms into the research and development process of content based, and semantic, image retrieval. Greater knowledge transfer between the fields of CBIR and, in the case of PET imaging, the fields of Neurology and Psychology facilitates the evolution of content based image retrieval to semantic retrieval, which is the previously stated target of CBIR: *"Semantic retrieval based on images that are segmented automatically into objects and where diagnoses can be derived easily from the objects visual features."* [2].

Acknowledgments

This work was funded by the EPSRC (Engineering and Physical Sciences Research Council) in the UK.

References

1. Smeulders, A.W.M., Worring, M., Santini, S., Gupta, A., Jain, R.: Content-based image retrieval at the end of the early years. IEEE Trans. Pattern Anal. Machine Intel. 22(12), 1349–1380 (2000)
2. Muller, H., Michoux, N., Bandon, D., Geissbuhler, A.: A review of content-based image retrieval systems in medical applications-clinical benefits and future directions. Int. J. Med. Inform. 73(1), 1–23 (2004)
3. Shyu, C.R., Brodley, C.E., Kak, A.C., Kosaka, A., Aisen, A.M., Broderick, L.S.: ASSERT: A physician-in-the-loop content-based retrieval system for HRCT image databases. Comput. Vis. Image Understand 75(1–2), 111–132 (1999)
4. Liu, Y., Dellaert, F.: Classification-driven medical image retrieval. In: Proceedings of the ARPA Image Understanding Workshop (1997)

5. Rahman, M.M., Bhattacharya, P., Desai, B.C.: A Framework for Medical Image Retrieval Using Machine Learning and Statistical Similarity Matching Techniques With Relevance Feedback. IEEE transactions on Information Technology in Biomedicine 11(1), 58–69 (2007)
6. Cai, W., Feng, D.D., Fulton, R.: Content-based retrieval of dynamic PET functional images. IEEE Trans. Information Technol. Biomed. 4(2), 152–158 (2000)
7. Montreal Neurological Institute, http://www.bic.mni.mcgill.ca
8. Talairarch, J., Tournoux, P.: Co-planar stereotaxic atlas of the human brain. Thieme. New York (1988)
9. Lancaster, J.L., Woldorff, M.G., Parsons, L.M., Liotti, M., Freitas, C.S., Rainey, L., Kochunov, P.V., Nickerson, D., Mikiten, S.A., Fox, P.T.: Automated Talairach Atlas labels for functional brain mapping. HBM 10, 120–131 (2000)
10. Friston, K.J., Ashburner, J., Poline, J.B., Frith, C.D., Heather, J.D., Frackowiak, R.S.J.: Spatial Registration and Normalization of Images. Human Brain Mapping 2, 165–189 (1995)
11. Brett, M.: Cambridge University, MRC, http://www.mrc-cbu.cam.ac.uk/matthew/abstracts/MNITal/mnital.html
12. Nestor, P.J., Fryer, T.D., Ikeda, M., Hodges, J.R.: Retrosplenial cortex (BA 29/30) hypometabolism in mild cognitive impairment (prodromal Alzheimer's disease). European Journal of Neuroscience 18(9), 2663 (2003)
13. Duvernoy, H.M.: The Human Brain: Surface, three dimensional sectional anatomy with MRI, and blood supply. Springer, New York
14. Smith, J.R., Chang, S.: Automated Image Retrieval Using Color and Texture, Columbia, University Technical Report TR# 414-95-20 (July 1995)
15. Ma, W.Y., Manjunath, B.S.: Texture Features for Browsing and Retrieval of Image Data. IEEE transactions on Pattern Analysis and Machine Intelligence 18(8) (1996)
16. Friston, K.J., Frith, C.D., Liddle, P.F., Dolan, R.J., Lammertsma, A.A., Frackowiak, R.S.: The relationship between global and local changes in PET scans. J. Cereb. Blood Flow Metab. 10(4), 458–466 (1990)
17. Scarmeas, N., Habeck, C.G., Zarahn, E., Anderson, K.E., Park, A., Hilton, J., Pelton, G.H., Tabert, M.H., Honig, L.S., Moeller, J.R., Devanand, D.P., Sterna, Y.: Covariance PET patterns in early Alzheimer's disease and subjects with cognitive impairment but no dementia: utility in group discrimination and correlations with functional performance. NeuroImage 23, 35–45 (2004)
18. Güld, M.O., Kohnen, M., Keysers, D., Schubert, H., Wein, B.B., Bredno, J., Lehmann, T.M.: Quality of DICOM header information for image categorization. In: Proceedings of the International Symposium on Medical Imaging, vol. 4685, pp. 280–287 (2002)
19. Rapoport, M., Reekum, R., Mayberg, H.: A Selective Review: The Role of the Cerebellum in Cognition and Behavior. J. Neuropsychiatry Clin Neurosci. 12, 193–198 (2000)
20. Batty, S., Gao, X.W., Clark, J., Fryer, T.: Content-based Retrieval of PET images via Localised Anatomical texture measurements and mean activity levels. In: Proceedings of International Conference on Medical Imaging and Telemedicine, pp. 70–74 (2005) ISBN:1-85924-252-9
21. Burns, M., Leung, K., Rowland, A., Vickers, J., Hajnal, J.V., Rueckert, D., Hill, D.L.G.: Information eXtraction from Images (IXI) - Grid Services for Medical Imaging. In: DiDaMIC 2004, Rennes, France (2004)
22. US patent number 7,158,961; Methods and apparatus for estimating similarity. Assigned to Google Inc. (2007)

Evaluation of Reference Tissue Model for Serotonin Transporters Using [123I] ADAM Tracer

Bang-Hung Yang[1,2], Shyh-Jen Wang[1], Yuan-Hwa Chou[3,4], Tung-Ping Su[3,4], Shih-Pei Chen[1], Jih-Shian Lee[2], and Jyh-Cheng Chen[2,5,*]

[1] Department of Nuclear Medicine, Taipei Veterans General Hospital, Taiwan, R.O.C
[2] Department of Biomedical Imaging and Radiological Sciences, National Yang-Ming University, Taipei, Taiwan, R.O.C
[3] National Yang-Ming University Medical School, Taipei, Taiwan, R.O.C
[4] Department of Psychiatry, Taipei Veterans General Hospital, Taipei, Taiwan, R.O.C
[5] Department of Education and Research, Taipei City Hospital, Taipei, Taiwan, R.O.C
jcchen@ym.edu.tw
Tel.: 886-2-28267282
Fax: 886-2-28201095

Abstract. The serotonin transporters are target-sites for commonly used antidepressants. [123I] ADAM is a novel radiotracer that selectively binds the serotonin transporters (SERTs) of the central nervous system. The aim for this study was to evaluate a non-invasive reference tissue model for SERTs quantification using the cerebellum as the indirect input function. The four-parameter model (FPM) was compared with the three-parameter model (TPM) using [123I] ADAM dynamic brain SPECT images. The binding potential values derived from both models were the same, but the ratio of delivery (R_1) in TPM had a smaller standard deviation than the FPM model. In conclusion, the simplified reference tissue model (TPM) was the better choice because of its stability (small standard deviation) and convenient implementation for non-invasive quantification of brain SPECT studies.

Keywords: serotonin transporters, reference tissue model, [123I] ADAM, binding potential.

1 Introduction

Depression has become an important disease in this century. Thus, its diagnostic methods have drawn much attention recently among e tmedical community. [123I] ADAM (2-((2-((dimethylamino)methyl)phenyl) thio)-5-iodophenylamine) is a novel radiopharmaceutical that selectively binds the serotonin transporters (SERTs) of the central nervous system (CNS) as midbrain, pons etc. [1,2]. The SERTs are target-sites for commonly used antidepressants, such as fluoxetine, paroxetine, sertraline, and so on. Imaging of these sites in the living human brain may provide an important tool to

---

* Corresponding author.

X. Gao et al. (Eds.): MIMI 2007, LNCS 4987, pp. 189–196, 2008.
© Springer-Verlag Berlin Heidelberg 2008

evaluate the mechanisms of action as well as to monitor the treatment of depressed patients [3-5].

Tracer kinetic modeling of receptor studies provides not only its delivery to the tissue (input function), but also an estimation of the uptake and biodistribution of the tracer in tissue as a function of time. The conventional method of obtaining input function required arterial blood sampling that was time-consuming and invasive. Recently, a reference tissue model has been proposed to eliminate the need to suffer an arterial catheter [6-8]. However, there were choices between a four-parameter model [6,7] and a three-parameter model [8,9] used to estimate neuroreceptor binding potential (BP) [10]. There are a great many studies on quantification of brain dopamine system but few on SERT discussions. The purpose in this study was to evaluate a reference tissue model for BP of SERTs, which correlates well with SERT densities [4, 5], and was obtained from the reference tissue compartment model using the cerebellum as indirect input function.

2   Materials and Methods

2.1   Subjects

Seven healthy volunteers who gave written informed consent were included. The healthy subjects included 4 men (age range 26.8 ± 6.4) and 3 women (age range 22.87 ± 3.1). No subject had any current psychiatric disorder according to DSM-IV (Diagnostic and Statistical Manual of Mental Disorders, American Psychiatric Association). The subjects were given 400 mg potassium perchlorate 30 minutes before injection in order to reduce [^{123}I] uptake in the thyroid and salivary glands.

2.2   SPECT Imaging Acquisition

Dynamic imaging data were collected for a total period of 6.6 hours and resulted in 12 frames (17.5min, 35min, 52.5min, 74.5min, 96.5min, 118.5min, 154.5min, 190.5min, 232min, 274min, 334min, 393min per frame) after injection of 185 MBq [^{123}I]ADAM using a SPECT scanner in TPE-VGH. Images were acquired using a SIEMENS e.soft dual-head SPECT scanner equipped with a low energy fan-beam collimator. Data were collected in step and shoot mode at 3^0 intervals over 180^0, and sixty 30-sec projection views were obtained per camera head. The radius of rotation was fixed at 14 cm. The image matrix size was 128×128 and pixel size was 3.9 mm. All images were obtained through a filtered back-projection (FBP) reconstruction algorithm with a Metz filter, using a Nyquist frequency cutoff at 0.55 and order of 30. Attenuation correction was performed by Chang's correction (μ=0.12 cm^{-1}) [11] and no scatter correction was employed.

2.3   Magnetic Resonance Imaging Acquisition

Images of the seven healthy volunteers had also been collected by MRI with T1-weighting in order to confirm there was no dysfunction or atrophic cortex. MR images were obtained using a 1.5T GE scanner Excite-II system in TPE-VGH.

(TR/TE =8.54 ms / 1.836; FOV =260 * 260 * 1.5; Matrix = 256 * 256 * 124; NEX = 1; TI = 400 ms; Filp angle = 15; BW = 15.63)

2.4 Image Co-registration and ROI Definition

Each subject's MRI scan was co-registered to the [^{123}I] ADAM SPECT images using a normalized mutual information algorithm provided by the SPM2 software [12,13]. Region of interest (ROI) as midbrain and cerebellum defined on co-registered MR images were used to sample the dynamic SPECT data to obtain regional time–activity radioactivity concentrations (Fig.1). Regional radioactivity was determined for each frame, corrected for decay, and plotted versus time.

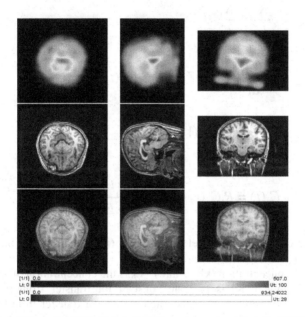

Fig. 1. ROI Definition was performed on MRI-based images using the PMODE version 2.7 software package .The first row presents [^{123}I] ADAM static image. The second row is presents individual MRI-T1 image. The third row is overlay images between MRI and SPECT image.

2.5 Reference Tissue Model

Using the reference tissue model for dynamic PET or SPECT kinetic modeling analysis is a non-invasive method without arterial blood sampling and has been widely demonstrated in many literatures of neuroreceptor quantification. The pixel-wise modeling tool (PMOD) is aimed at the processing of quantitative PET or SPECT studies. All dynamic SPECT images in our study were analyzed by a commercial kinetic modeling tool (PKIN) from the PMOD version 2.7 software package.

The reference tissue compartment model (Fig 2) is based on the following differential equations extracted from Lammertsma and Hume's paper [6-8]:

$$\frac{dC_r(t)}{dt} = K_1' C_p(t) - k_2'(t)Cr(t) \tag{1}$$

$$\frac{dC_f(t)}{dt} = K_1 C_p(t) - k_2 C_f(t) - k_3 C_f(t) + k_4 C_b(t) \tag{2}$$

$$\frac{dC_b(t)}{dt} = k_3 C_f(t) - k_4 C_b(t) \tag{3}$$

$$\frac{K_1'}{k_2'} = \frac{K_1}{k_2} \tag{4}$$

$$\frac{dC_t(t)}{dt} = K_1 C_p(t) - k_{2a} C_t(t) \tag{5}$$

$$\frac{K_1}{k_{2a}} = (\frac{K_1}{k_2}) * (1 + BP) \tag{6}$$

$$C_t(t) = R_1 C_r(t) + \left\{ k_2 - \frac{R_1 k_2}{(1+BP)} \right\} C_r(t) * e^{\left\{ \frac{-k_2 t}{(1+BP)} \right\}} \tag{7}$$

where C_r is the concentration in reference tissue (kBq $\cdot$ml^{-1}) in the brain, C_f is the concentration of non-specific bound radioligand (kBq $\cdot$ml^{-1}), C_p is the metabolite corrected plasma concentration (kBq $\cdot$ ml^{-1}) , C_b is the concentration of specific bound radioligand (kBq $\cdot$ml^{-1}), K_1 is the rate constant for transfer from plasma to free compartment (ml $\cdot$ml^{-1} $\cdot$min^{-1}), k_2 is the rate constant for transfer from free to plasma compartment (min^{-1}), k_3 is the rate constant for transfer from free to bound compartment (min^{-1}), k_4 is the rate constant for transfer from bound to free compartment (min^{-1}), K_1' is the rate constant for transfer from plasma to reference compartment (ml $\cdot$ml^{-1} $\cdot$min^{-1}), k_2' is the rate constant for transfer from reference to plasma compartment (min^{-1}), k_{2a} (min^{-1}) is the overall rate constant for transfer from specific compartment to plasma, and t is time (min). Because C_f and C_b cannot be measured, the total concentration in tissue was presented C_t (=C_f +C_b).

Equation (1) describes the exchange between plasma and reference tissue, while Eqs. (2) and (3) relate to the free and bound compartments of the ROI, respectively. According to Eqs (1) to (3) relationship, we could get six parameters (K_1, k_2, k_3, k_4, K_1', and k_2'). $R_1 = \frac{K_1}{K_1'}$ is defined as the ratio of tracer delivery, and the binding potential as $BP=k_3/k_4$. From Eqs (4) we can further simplify the computation by assuming that the distribution volume is the same for the tissue of interest and the reference tissue. Therefore, k_2' can be replaced by k_2/R_1 and k_4 by k_3/BP, then an operational equation with four parameters (R_1, k_2, k_3, and BP) is obtained [6, 7].

Although BP is robust in the four-parameter model, convergence rates are slow and other parameters can have large standard deviation. In order to overcome these problems, a simplified reference tissue containing only three parameters (R_1, k_2, and BP) was developed [8, 9]. Because in the target region of SPECT images it is difficult to distinguish between free and specific compartments, the reference tissue model can be simplified to a three-parameter model (Eq. (7)) which was derived from Eq. (1), (4), (5), and (6).

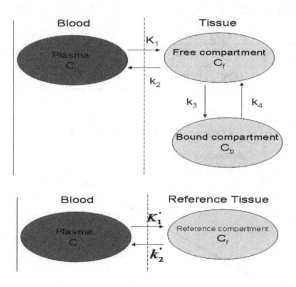

Fig. 2. Two-tissue compartment model sketch

3   Results

The results of reference tissue kinetic analysis for the midbrain are listed in Table1. Linear regression statistical analysis was used in the relationships between midbrain BP and R_1 estimates obtained with three- and four-parameter models for [123I] ADAM tracer study. The two methods gave similar BP results and a high coefficient regression slope (BP, $r^2=0.9682$; R_1, $r^2=1$) (Fig3, Fig4). The results of ratio of tracer delivery (R_1) were 0.595 ± 0.379 in the three-parameter model and 0.545 ± 0.349 in the four-parameter model. In addition, the three-parameter model was further simplified and produced stable results for other parameters because of the small standard deviation (SD) (Table1).

Table 1. Rate constant of the midbrain region for different parameter models

	4-parameter model			3-parameter model		
	BP	R_1	k_2	BP	R_1	k_2
Subject 01	2.169	0.389	0.046	2.169	0.364	0.038
Subject 02	1.016	0.417	0.029	1.013	0.384	0.025
Subject 03	1.996	1.084	0.061	1.999	0.875	0.031
Subject 04	1.395	0.479	0.067	1.396	0.448	0.055
Subject 05	1.273	0.158	0.024	1.271	0.152	0.022
Subject 06	2.473	1.168	0.014	2.472	1.166	0.014
Subject 07	1.075	0.467	0.042	1.072	0.425	0.035
Average	1.628	0.595	0.040	1.627	0.545	0.031
SD	0.578	0.379	0.019	0.579	0.349	0.013

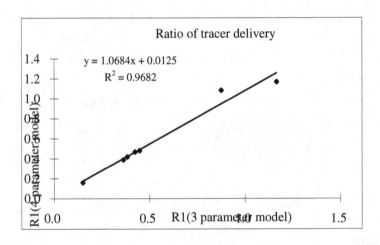

Fig. 3. Correlation coefficient of rate constant R_1 (ratio of tracer delivery) derived with different parameter model analysis.

4   Discussion and Conclusion

Our results have demonstrated that a simplified reference tissue model can be adopted for dynamic SPECT imaging as well as some PET non-invasive studies of SERTs quantification [6-8, 14-16]. Using either a three-parameter model or four-parameter model to derive BP or R_1 gave nearly identical results for each outcome measure across the cerebellum as indirect input function. However, another possible cause for

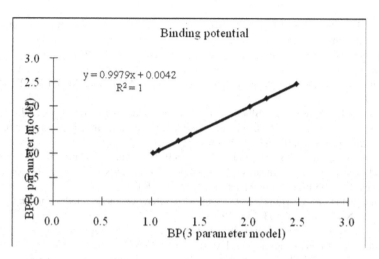

Fig. 4. Correlation coefficient of rate constant BP (binding potential) derived with different parameter model analysis

the differences in BP and R_1 might be associated with different reference tissue such as occipital cortex [17] or the imaging registration algorithm. Although further studies are required, it is important to evaluate a suitable and non-invasive compartment model for quantitative SPECT studies. Our study was to provide simplified reference tissue approach derived from the images alone as the input function to the mathematic modeling of tracer distribution. In conclusion, for the [^{123}I] ADAM quantification, the three-parameter model is a better choice with increased stability.

Acknowledgments. This study was supported by the National Science Council under grants NSC 94-2623-7-075-001, 95-2314-B-075-077-MY2, and 96-NU-7-075-001.The preparation of [^{123}I] ADAM was in INER. The authors would like to thank Ms. Chi Tai-Hua from the Department of Psychiatry at Taipei Veterans General Hospital for the collection of healthy subjects.

References

1. Goodman, M.M., Chen, P., Plisson, C., Martarello, L., Galt, J., et al.: Synthesis and characterization of iodine-123 labeled 2-beta- carbomethoxy-3-beta-(4'-((Z)-2-iodoethenyl) Phenyl)nortropane. A ligand for in vivo imaging of serotonin transporters by single-photon-emission tomography. J. Med. Chem. 46, 925–935 (2003)
2. Oya, S., Kung, M.P., Acton, P.D., Hou, C., Mu, M., Kung, H.: A new SPECT imaging agent for serotonin transporters, [123I]IDAM: 5-iodo-2-[[2-2-[(dimethylamino) methyl]phenyl]thio]benzyl alcohol. J. Med. Chem. 42, 333–335 (1999)
3. Newberg, A.B., Plossl, K., Mozley, P.D., Stubbs, J.B., Kung, H.F., et al.: Biodistribution and imaging with (123)I-ADAM: a serotonin transporter imaging agent. J. Nucl. Med. 45, 834–841 (2004)

4. Oya, S., Choi, S.R., Hou, C., Mu, M., Kung, M.P., Kung, H.F., et al.: 2-((2-((dimethylamino)methyl)phenyl)thio)-5-   iodophenylamine   (ADAM):   an improvedserotonin transporter ligand. Nucl. Med. Biol. 27, 249–254 (2000)
5. Zhuang, Z.P., Choi, S.R., Hou, C., et al.: A novel serotonin transporter ligand: 5-iodo-2-(2-dimethylaminomethylphenoxy)-benzyl alcohol (ODAM). Nucl. Med. Biol. 27, 169–175 (2000)
6. Hume, S.P., Myers, R., Bloomfield, P.M., Opacka-Juffry, J., Cremer, J.E., et al.: Quantitation of carbon-11-labeled raclopride in rat striatum using positron emission tomography. Synapse 12, 47–54 (1992)
7. Lammertsma, A.A., Bench, C.J., Hume, S.P., Osman, S., Gunn, K., Brooks, D.J., Frackowiak, R.S.J.: Comparison of methods for analysis of clinical [11C]raclopride studies. J. Cereb.Blood Flow Metab. 16, 42–52 (1996)
8. Lammertsma, A.A., Hume, S.P.: Simplified reference tissue model for PET receptor studies. NeuroImage 4, 153–158 (1996)
9. Wu, Y., Carson, R.E.: Noise reduction in the simplified reference tissue model for neuroreceptor functional imaging. J. Cereb. Blood Flow Metab. 22, 1440–1452 (2002)
10. Mintun, M.A., Raichle, M.E., Kilbourn, M.R., et al.: A quantitative model for the in vivo assessment of drug binding sites with positron emission tomography Ann. Neurol. 15, 217–222 (1984)
11. Chang, L.-T., et al.: A method for attenuation correction in radionucleide computed tomography. IEEE Trans. Nucl. Sci. 25, 638–643 (1978)
12. Ashburner, J., Friston, K.J.: Nonlinear spatial normalization using basis functions. Human Brain Mapping 7, 254–266 (1999)
13. Friston, K.J., Ashburner, J., Frith, C.D., et al.: Spatial registration and normalization of images. Human Brain Mapping 2, 165–189 (1995)
14. Frankle, W.G., Slifstein, M., Gunn, R.N., Huang, Y., Hwang, D.-R., et al.: Estimation of Serotonin Transporter Parameters with 11C-DASB in Healthy Humans:Reproducibility and Comparison of Methods. J. Nucl. Med. 47, 815–826 (2006)
15. Lundberg, J., Odano, I., Olsson, H., Halldin, C., Farde, L.: Quantification of 11C-MADAM Binding to the Serotonin Transporter in the Human Brain. J. Nucl. Med. 46, 1505–1515 (2005)
16. Kim, J.S., Ichise, M., Sangare, J., Innis, R.B.: Innis: PET Imaging of Serotonin Transporters with [11C]DASB: Test–Retest Reproducibility Using a Multilinear Reference Tissue Parametric Imaging Method. J. Nucl. Med. 47, 208–214 (2006)
17. Turkheimer, F.E., Edison, P., Pavese, N., Roncaroli, F., Anderson, A.N., et al.: Reference and Target Region Modeling of [11C]-(R)-PK11195 Brain Studies. J. Nucl. Med. 48, 158–167 (2007)

A Fast Approach to Segmentation of PET Brain Images for Extraction of Features

Xiaohong Gao[1] and John Clark[2]

[1] School of Computeing Science, Middlesex University, London, NW4 4BT,
United Kingdom
x.gao@mdx.ac.uk
[2] Wolfson Brain Imaging Centre, University of Cambridge, Cambridge, CB2 2QQ,
United Kingdom
jcc24@wbic.cam.ac.uk

Abstract. Position Emission Tomography (PET) is increasingly applied in the diagnosis and surgery in patients thanks to its ability of showing nearly all types of lesions including tumour and head injury. However, due to its natures of low resolution and different appearances as a result of different tracers, segmentation of lesions presents great challenges. In this study, a simple and robust algorithm is proposed via additive colour mixture approach. Comparison with the other two methods including Bayesian classified and geodesic active contour is also performed, demonstrating the proposed colouring approach has many advantages in terms of speed, robustness, and user intervention. This research has many medical applications including pharmaceutical trials, decision making for drug treatment or surgery and patients follow-up and shows potential to the development of content-based image databases when coming to characterise PET images using lesion features.

Keywords: PET imaging, segmentation, additive colour mixture, Lesion detection.

1 Introduction

Positron emission tomography (PET) is an important tool for enabling quantification of human brain function in three dimensions [1]. Through the use of a diverse range of tracers, PET can provide quantitative information on, for example, blood flow, glucose metabolism and neurotransmitter receptor binding potential. However, due to the nature of PET imaging with high noise to signal ratios and its inability of showing anatomic structure, segmentation of lesions, such as head injury and tumour poses great challenge. Due to its many medical applications including pharmaceutical trials, decision making for drug treatment or surgery and patients follow-up, lesion segmentation have been studied extensively by many researchers proposing many promising methods. One group of researchers [2] study the tissue transformation and expansion or contraction effects in order to analysis Multiple Sclerosis (MS) on brain MR images. Mathematical morphological operations have been applied in their study which

X. Gao et al. (Eds.): MIMI 2007, LNCS 4987, pp. 197–206, 2008.

are also utilised to delineate lesion regions [3]. Active contour is another popular technique in region detection and boundary delineation, which develops geometric and probabilistic models for shapes and their dynamics in real time. However it suffers the problem of false attraction on noisy images and computational cost [4]. Intelligent mesh algorithm is hence developed by researchers [5] to detect lesion/tumour on CT and Mammography images. Other well known methods for region detection and segmentation include multi-resolution segmentation [6], wavelet based detection [7], texture segmentation [8], and neural network [9]. Multi-resolution scheme has been studied by [10] on the detection of speculated lesions in mammograms, which specifically addresses the difficulty on predetermining the neighbourhood size for feature extraction and fundamentally bases on a linear phase non-separable 2-D wavelet transform.

Conventionally, each method only works well for one particular group of images and performs worse on the other images. At most cases, the methods mentioned above only work well for images with high contrast and low noise. For the images with high noise to signal ratios, such as PET images, most of lesion detection methods do not work well without considerable enhancements.

Statistical methods, for example, Bayes theorem, hence were introduced into this field [11]. Although very promising, Bayesian classified requires large sample data or called training data sets, which sometimes may not be obtained easily. This is due to the fact that different tracer will generate different PET appearance of images for the same subject, resulting different training sets have to be provided.

In this study, a new approach is studied which applies additive colour mixture approach, or called colouring approach, and is under the assumption that a human brain bears similarity with reference of middle plane or middle line in a 2D image form. This approach not only segments lesion robustly but also visualises the lesion in colour, showing an advantage over the other approaches.

2   Methodology

Although most radiological images are in grey scale, colour has been widely introduced in them primarily for the purpose of visualization to increase the contrast between different regions [12]. The most common method is colour map, or a lookup table, by which each colour corresponds to each intensity value in an image. After replacing each pixel with its corresponding colour, the image becomes colourful, generating a pseudo colour image with high contrast.

In some cases, colouring image becomes necessary, especially for fusing multi-modality images, e.g., MR with PET, or CT with PET, to increase high contrast of composite image while maintaining the property of each individual modality. The common method is to colour interleaved pixels using independent colour scales for each modality [13], showing the results of both visually pleasing and easy to interpret.

A colour normally is represented by three independent values, hue, chroma or saturation, and brightness/lightness. Hue is mostly applied in colouring and contains three primary colours, red, green, and blue. The other hues, i.e., yellow, orange, purple, can be generated by proper mixing of any of these three primary hues (either by mixing coloured lights, e.g, in a computer monitor, or by mixing ink as applied in a ink-jet printer). The mixing procedure can be additive, whereby red, green, and blue are the primary colours (i.e., in a colour monitor), producing white when all three hues of equal part being mixed together. The opposite mixture is subtractive where cyan, magenta and yellow are the primary colours, which is mostly applied in printers in a CMYK colour system (K represents black), producing black colour when mixing all these three primary pigments with equal amounts. Additive colour mixture has been widely applied to viewing medical images and implemented in some open source imaging software including ImageJ(http://rsb.info.nih.gov/ij/), which is a convenient way increasing colour contrast. In this study, additive colour mixture technique is investigated to segment lesions of brain PET images.

2.1   Image Colouring

When an image displayed on a computer monitor, one pixel (or voxel in 3D form) can be represented using Red (R), Green (G), Blue (B) colours. For example, in an 8-bits monitor, the intensity range for each colour is 0-255. If all of R, G, and B values are the same for a pixel, this pixel is presented in grey colour, arriving at the intensity value being the average of the sum of these three colour values. As such, other colours can be achieved by the proper mixture of these three primary colours. For example, a yellow pixel can be achieved by the mixture of R, G, and B where B=0, R>0 and G>0, whilst the combination of B>0, R>0 and G=0 will produce a purple colour.

If a 2D brain image with a lesion is represented as I and its reflected image with reference of its middle line as I_R (a flip over image), I and I_R can then be expressed as

$$I = I_L + I_O \tag{1}$$

$$I_R = I_{R_L} + I_{R_O} \tag{2}$$

where L represents lesions in the image, whilst O the rest (other) part of the image. If I is coloured as red as $R(I)$, and I_R green and blue and are represented as $G(I_R)$ and $B(I_R)$ respectively, then

$$R(I) + G(I_R) + B(I_R)$$

$$\Rightarrow R(I_L + I_O) + G(I_{R_L} + I_{R_O}) + B(I_{R_L} + I_{R_O})$$
$$\Rightarrow R(I_L) + R(I_O) + G(I_{R_L}) + G(I_{R_O}) + B(I_{R_L}) + B(I_{R_O})$$
$$\Rightarrow R(I_L) + Cyan(I_{R_L}) + Grey(I_O) \tag{3}$$

Since a brain image is symmetrical with reference to the middle line (to be discussed below), apart from the lesion part, the rest of brain is more or less the same as its reflected counterparts, resulting $I_O = I_{RO}$. Therefore the mixture of red, green and blue for the non-lesion pixel would produce grey colour. Similarly

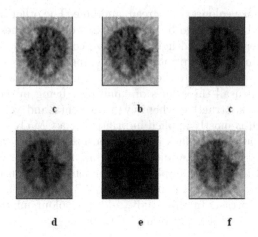

a

b

c

d

e

f

Fig. 1. The procedure of additive colour mixture. From left to right: a). original image, b). reflection of (a), c). (a) in red, d). (b) in green, e). (b) in blue, f). (c) + (d) + (e).

the adding of green and blue colour for the reflected lesion region would produce a region with cyan colour. Fig. 1 illustrates the procedure of Eq. (3). The final colour image only contains two colours of red and cyan with one colour associated to the reflected lesion region, i.e., a false region. It is therefore helpful to get rid of that colour first before delineation of lesion boundary. In Fig. 1, the false lesion region is in cyan colour. In order to use meaningful colour attributes instead of RGB space, HSI space is applied in this study to calculate hue, saturation, and intensity values of each pixel. As there are only two hues in the image, it is the saturation attribute that contributes more in processing the image, which is calculated as Eq.(4) [14].

$$H = arccos \frac{\frac{(R-G)+(R-B)}{2}}{\sqrt{(R-G)^2 + (R-B)(G-B)}} \tag{4}$$

where H=360°-H. If (B/I)>(G/I)

$$S = 1 - \frac{3min(R,G,B)}{R+G+B} \tag{5}$$

$$I = \frac{R+G+B}{3} \tag{6}$$

The elimination of cyan colour can then be performed using hue attribute alone. In order to get rid of some red colour that is very close to grey colour, i.e., the background, saturation can be added to the process in addition to hue. For example, the images in Fig. 1 apply 10% saturation as threshold, i.e., any pixel with less than 10% saturation will be classified as grey colour. It should be noted that the threshold varies according to the tracers applied administrated to the subject, which giving rise to different appearances of PET images and resulting in different thresholds of saturation.

Once an image has only one colour left, a simplified k-mean clustering method is utilised to cluster the lesion region. First, the image is divided into four equal sub-regions (more sub-regions can be generated according to the need). Then the centre of the red colours will be worked out, from which, colour clustering is performed. Then the boundary is delineated using a circular cylinder co-ordinate system with origin located at the centre of the lesion region. When the angle coordinate rotates from 0° to 360°, the radius reached to the edge of the lesion region.

2.2 Locating Middle Line

The success of the above approach depends in some ways on the correctly located symmetrical line of the brain , so that the reflection image with reference to this symmetrical line is similar to the original image apart from the lesion regions.

There are two coordination systems when defining a 3D brain. The *ideal head co-ordinate system* is defined as centred in the brain with positive X_0, Y_0, Z_0 axes pointing in the right, anterior and superior direction respectively [15]. With respect to this co-ordinate system, the bilateral symmetry plane of the brain is defined as the plane $X_0 = 0$, passing through the nose. This plane is often referred to as the mid-sagittal plane of the brain. It is expected that a set of axial (coronal) slices is cut perpendicular to the Z_0 (Y_0) axis, and the intersection of each slice with the bilateral symmetry plane appears as a vertical line on the slice [16]. In clinical practice however, a *working co-ordinate system* XYZ is applied. X and Y are oriented along the rows and columns of each image slice, and Z is the actual axis of the scan. The orientation of the working co-ordinate system differs from the ideal co-ordinate system by three rotation angles, *pitch, roll* and *yaw*, and three translation differences, ∇X_0, ∇Y_0, and ∇Z_0, respectively.

For each sagittal slice of brain PET image, its left pattern is symmetrical or similar to its right pattern around middle symmetrical line. Hence, its reflection image is similar to the original one. The cross-correction between the original one and the reflected (and rotated) one can then be calculated. The biggest cross-correction (CC) value should be achieved when the corrected rotation angle (θ_j) and translation (c_k) distance are located using Eq. (7).

$$CC(c_k, \theta_j) = max(max(XCorr(S_i, rot(2\theta, ref(S_i, c_k))))) \qquad (7)$$

where CC is the cross-correlation value, θ_j the yaw angle, and c_k the symmetrical line on the 2D slice S_i. Whlist $ref(S_i, c_k)$ refers to the reflected image of S_i with reference of line at c_k, and rot represents rotation. When an image rotates θ degrees, its reflected image rotates 2θ with reference to the original image.

3 Results

Table 1 lists the images studied in this research. One hundred and one slices of 2D images with head injuries and tumors from 9 subjects are collected to evaluate

Table 1. The images used in this study with visible lesions (Ls) head injury (HI) and tumour (T)

ID	Diagnisis	No slices	L'ed slices	Multi-Ls	No detected Ls
1	HI	35	10		10
2	HI	35	5		5
3	HI	70	19		17
4	HI	35	7		7
5	HI	70	24	yes	22
6	HI	70	8		8
7	HI	70	8		8
8	T	69	5	yes	5
9	T	69	15		15
Total		**523**	**101**		**97**

this approach. Although subject number 7 in Table 1 has images with 5 tracers i.e., FDG2D, FDG3D, O15CO2D, O15CO3D, O15water3D, only images with tracer of O15water3D have visible lesions and are included in the study. Similar cases applied to the other subjects. The tumor data are with ^{18}F-FLT (3_-Deoxy-3_-18F-fluorothymidine) tracer and are used to study cell proliferation, during which ten subjects are recruited in the ^{18}F-FLT study with two normal subjects as control. Again, only two sets of data are visible and used in our study. Experimental results show that all the lesions are correctly delineated using colouring approach. Figure 2 shows the delineation results for some images with different tracers in-take, showing the appearance of images appears differently. These images have been aligned correctly, i.e., the symmetrical line is in the middle with 0° rotation. Due to the movement of subject, some images are not aligned around the central line. Finding the symmetrical line is then to be performed first as shown in Fig. 3.

Since the edges are delineated using cylinder co-ordinate systems with the scanning line starting from the lesion centre and going from 0° to 360°, some edges may look zigzagged, which is however can be overcome using a smoothing algorithm. After the lesion has been delineated on the rotated and translated image, the delineation of lesions from the original images can then be performed by adding cropping distance and then rotating back the rotated degrees $(-\theta)$ obtained during middle line finding.

4   Comparisons

Comparison with two other popular algorithms are made. The first one is Bayesian algorithm and the other is geodesic active contour approach. The Bayesians classifier applied in this research is illustrated in Eq.(8).

$$d_i(\bar{x}) = lnP(C_i) - \frac{1}{2}((\bar{x} - \bar{m}_i)^T C_i^{-1}(\bar{x} - \bar{m}_i)) \tag{8}$$

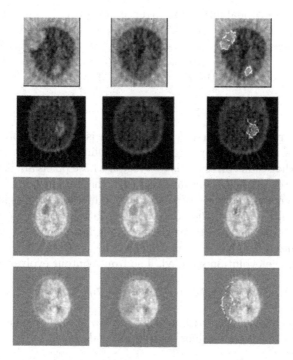

Fig. 2. Delineation results for images. The left column shows the original images, the middle column the images with lesions in red colour, and the right column the lesions with delineated boundary.

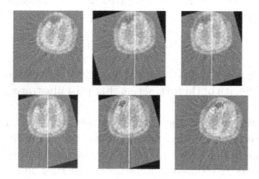

Fig. 3. The steps to from finding symmetrical line to delineating lesion boundary. Top row: (left) original image, (middle) its rotated image with middle line, (right) cropped image from middle. Bottom row: (left) images with coloured lesion region, (middle) edge delineation of lesion region, (right) edge delineation on the original image based on the middle image.

where $P(C_i)$ is the probability of occurrence of class C_i, i = 1, 2, ..., N, $\bar{x}$ the sample pattern, $\bar{m}_i$ the mean of $\bar{x}$ from C_i, and d_i the decision function. For example, if a pixel is represented as $\bar{x}$, and $d_i(\bar{x}) > d_j(\bar{x})$, then $\bar{x}$ belongs to class C_i class (e.g., background) rather than C_j (lesions). Sometimes, a error threshold ϵ is introduced to the Eq. (8) so that if $\bar{x} \in C_i$, then

$$d_i(\bar{x}) > d_j(\bar{x}) + \epsilon \tag{9}$$

The second approach studied in this research is geodesic active contour [4], an expansion of snake contour algorithm. To delineate a lesion from 2D PET images, where the lesion corresponds to a region whose pixels are of different grey level intensity, the geodesic contour evolves to the desired boundary according to intrinsic geometry measures of the image. When a user provided an initial guess of the contour (seed), the contour propagates inward or outward in the normal direction driven toward the desired boundaries by image-driven forces. The initial contour should be placed inside the lesions. The final contour is extracted when the evolution stopped. The front contour evolves according to

$$C_t = g(I)((1 - \varepsilon k)\bar{N}) - (\nabla g \cdot \bar{N})\bar{N} \tag{10}$$

where level set equation takes form of Eq.(10) to detect boundaries with high differences in their gradient values, as well as small gaps.

$$\phi_t + g_I(1 - \varepsilon k)|\nabla \phi| - \beta \nabla P \cdot \nabla \phi = 0 \tag{11}$$

where

$$g_I(x, y) = \frac{1}{1 + |\nabla(G_\sigma * I(x, y)|} \tag{12}$$

which shows that the image I(x,y) convolves with a Gaussian smoothing filter G_σ whose characteristic width is σ. And

$$P(x, y) = -|\nabla(G_\sigma * I(x, y)| \tag{13}$$

which attracts the surface to the edges in the image. Whlist coefficient β in Eq. (11) controls the strength of this attraction. Figure 4 illustrates some comparison results.

On the surface, Fig. 4 shows the delineation results are very much comparable between these three methods. However, for Bayesian approach, the training sets of data will be needed in order to get accurate results, which is not always easy. Different tracers give different appearances of PET images, leading to the requirement of different sets of training data. User intervention will therefore be needed. In Fig. 4, 3rd row, the black dots in the right image represents edges of the lesion detected using Bayesian classifier, whilst the white dots the smoothed edge combining the edges of both lesion and the brain. For the data in Table 1, 96% lesions have been delineated accurately using Bayesian classifier, the remaining 4% being the cases with very confuing boundary between lesions and the image background.

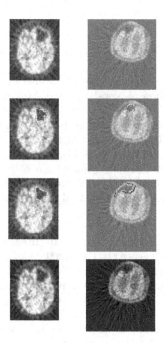

Fig. 4. Comparison results of delineation of lesion using 3 approaches. From top to bottom: original image, the method proposed in the paper, Bayesian classifier, and geodesic active contour.

As for geodesic active contour approach, seed point is needed from users. Due to the heavy calculation involved, this approach takes much longer than the other two methods (up to a few minutes sometimes). in Fig. 4. Although 100% successful rate has been achieved for delineation of the data given in Table 1, sometimes, the arrived contour is not always the desired boundary.

5   Conclusion and Discussion

In this study, three methods have been studied and compared for lesion delineation, including additive colour mixture, Bayesian classifier, and geodesic contour approaches. Each method has its own pros and cons. Overall, additive colour mixture, or colouring, approach appears to be better in terms of robust, speed, and automation. However, the colouring method has its own limitations. It only applies to the images with symmetry, by which colour adding can then be applied. For any other images without symmetry, the colour additive mixture can also utilised as long as there is a template available where the image of interest is registered to spatially.

Acknowledgments. This work is part of TIME (Tele-imaging in Medicine) project funded by European Commission under Asia ICT programme.

References

1. Bendriem, B., Townsend, D.W. (eds.): The Theory and Practice of 3D PET. Kluwer Academic Publishers, London (1998)
2. Thirion, J., Calmon, G.: Measuring Lesion Grouwth from 3D Medical Images. In: IEEE Workshop on Motion of Non-Rigid and Articulated Objects (NAM 1997), pp. 112–119 (1997)
3. He, R., Narayana, P.A.: Detection and Delineation of Multiple Sclerosis Lesions in Gadolinium-Enhanced 3D T1-Weighted MRI Data. In: 13th IEEE Symposium on Computer-Based Medical Systems (CBMS), pp. 201–205 (2000)
4. Gao, X.W., Birhane, D., Clark, J.: Application of Geodesic Active Contours to the Segmentation of Lesions of PET (Positron Emission Tomography) Images. In: Gao, X., Lin, C., Müller, H. (eds.) Medical Imaging and Telemedicine, pp. 45–50 (2005)
5. Yin, L., Deshpande, S., Chang, J.K.: Automatic Lesion/Tumour Detection Using Intelligent Mesh-Based Active Contour. In: IEEE International Conference on Tools with Artificial Intelligence (ICTAI) (2003)
6. Cai, W., Feng, D.D., Fulton, R.: Content-Based Retrieval of Dynamic PET Functional Images. IEEE Trans. on Info. Tech. in Biome. 4, 152–158 (2000)
7. Sawle, G.V., Playford, E.D., Brooks, D.J., Quinn, N., Frackowiak, R.S.J.: Asymmetrical Pre-synaptic and Post-synaptic Changes in the Striatal Dopamine Projection in Dopa Nave Parkinsonism: Diagnostic Implications of the D2 Receptor Status. Brain 116, 853–867 (1993)
8. Ullmann, J.R.: Pattern Recogntion Techniques. Crane Russak, New York (1973)
9. Lammertsma, A.A., Brench, C.J., Hume, S.P., Osman, S., Gunn, K., Brooks, D.J., Frackowiak, R.S.: Comparison of Methods for Analysis of Clinical [^{11}C]raclopride Studies. J. Cereb. Blood Flow Metab. 16, 42–52 (1996)
10. Liu, S., Babbs, C., Delp, E.: Multiresolution Detection of Spiculated Lesions in Digital Mammpgrams. IEEE Trans. on Image Processing 10, 874–884 (2001)
11. Huang, C.C., Yu, X., Bading, J., Conti, P.S.: Computer-Aided Lesion Detection with Statistical Model-Based Features in PET Images. IEEE Trans. on Nucl. Science 44, 2509–2521 (1997)
12. Ogata, Y., Naito, H., et al.: Novel Display Technique for Reference Images for Visibility of Temporal Change on Radiographs. Radiation Med. 24, 28–34 (2006)
13. Rehm, K.R.: Display of Merged Multimodality Brain Images Using Interleaved Pixels with Independent Color Scales. J. Nucl. Med. 35, 1815–1821 (1994)
14. Zhao, B.: Colour Space. Computer Vision Laboratory Stony Brook University, New York (2002)
15. Talairach, J., Tournoux, P.: Co-Planar Steriotaxic Atlas of the Human Brain. Theme Medical Publishers (1988)
16. Gao, X.W., Batty, S., Clark, J., Fryer, T., Blandford, A.: Extraction of Sagittal Symmetry Planes from PET Images. In: Visualization, Imaging, and Image Processing (VIIP), pp. 428–433 (2001)

New Doppler-Based Imaging Method in Echocardiography with Applications in Blood/Tissue Segmentation

Sigve Hovda, Håvard Rue, and Bjørn Olstad

Norwegian University of Science and Technology, Trondheim, Norway
sigveh@idi.ntnu.no
http://idi.ntnu.no/~sigveh

Abstract. Knowledge Based Imaging is suggested as a method to distinguish blood from tissue signal in transthoracial echocardiography. Parametric model for the autocorrelation functions for turbulent blood flow and slowly moving tissue are augmented for in this paper. The model also includes the presence of stationary clutter noise and system white noise. Knowledge Based Imaging utilizes the maximum likelihood function to classify blood and tissue signal. In amplitude imaging blood and tissue are separated by their difference in signal powers. This effect is also present in Knowledge Based Imaging. In addition, this method utilizes the fact that blood flow is turbulent and moves faster than tissue. Some images of Knowledge Based Imaging with different parameter settings are visually compared with Second-Harmonic Imaging, Fundamental Imaging and Bandwidth Imaging [1].

1 Introduction

The state of art echocardiographic modes for defining endocardium of left ventricle of the human heart are; Fundamental Imaging, Second-Harmonic Imaging and Left Ventricle Opacification. These methods distinguish blood signal from tissue signal by their differences in power [2].

Alternatively, Doppler signal from blood flow differs from tissue motion, since it is less coherent with depth. In Power Doppler, blood is distinguished from tissue signal by the power of the highpass filtered Doppler signal. Here a packetsize of above 6 is required to achieve the desired filter characteristics [3].

In paper [1], Bandwidth Imaging was introduced and the experiment indicated that tissue and blood could be distinguished with a packetsize as small as 3. The small packetsize enables a resolution that is interesting for endocardial border definition. In this paper, we seek to discuss the potential of Knowledge Based Imaging, where the pulse strategy of the optimized Bandwidth Imaging method is taken as a starting point.

In section2 a parametric models for signal from blood and tissue are outlined and Knowledge Based Imaging is defined. In section 3, some premature Knowlege based Images with different parameter settings are compared with a Fundamental Image, a Bandwidth Imaging and a Second-Harmonic Image.

X. Gao et al. (Eds.): MIMI 2007, LNCS 4987, pp. 207–215, 2008.

2   Signal Model and Definition of Knowledge Based Imaging

Torp et. al. [4] introduced a parametric model for the autocorrelation functions in regions with rectilinear flow, under the assumption that signal is a complex Gaussian process. In this section, this model is expanded to yield turbulent flow as well. The signal model is also further expanded to include additive white noise and clutter noise in a similar manner as in Heimdal et. al. [5]. This is the theoretical framework for defining, instrumenting and discussing Knowledge Based Imaging and Bandwidth Imaging.

2.1   Parametric Model for the Autocorrelation Function of Signal from Blood and Tissue

As mentioned above the signal model of [4] is used. Here the authors assume a random continuum model for blood scattering [6]. The spatial fluctuation in mass density and compressibility, which determine the incoherent part of the scattering, is assumed proportional to the fluctuation of blood cell concentration $n_b(\mathbf{r}, t)$, where $\mathbf{r}$ is position and t is time. Here, $n_b(\mathbf{r}, t)$ is a zero mean random process. For a short correlation in space, for a fixed time and neglecting diffusion, the autocorrelation function of $n_b(\mathbf{r}, t)$ is approximated in [6] by

$$< n_b(\mathbf{r}, t), n_b(\mathbf{r} + \xi, t + \tau) > = \mathbf{\Upsilon}(\mathbf{r}, t)\, \delta(\xi - \zeta(\mathbf{r}, t, \tau))$$

$$\mathbf{\Upsilon}(\mathbf{r}, t) = \frac{var(n_b(\mathbf{r})) \cdot \Delta V}{\Delta V} \tag{1}$$

where $\zeta(\mathbf{r}, t, \tau)$ is the displacement of the fluid element in position $\mathbf{r}$ during the time interval t to $t + \tau$. The function $\mathbf{\Upsilon}(\mathbf{r}, t)$ is the variance per unit volume in numbers of blood cells inside a small volume ΔV, and this quantity is proportional to the backscattering coefficient in blood.

Assuming a Gaussian shaped beam profile and a rectangular shaped receiver filter impulse response, the authors outline an expression for the expected value of the two dimensional autocorrelation function for any time and radial lag. In general it is necessary to assume rectilinear flow, but in the case of no radial lag, this assumption has to be valid inside only one range cell. The expected value of the autocorrelation function with only time lag for an electronically steered probe is

$$r(m) = r(0)\beta(m)e^{i\,2\,m\,k\,v_1\,T}$$

$$\beta(m) = e^{-\frac{3}{2}m^2\left[\left(\frac{v_1 T}{L}\right)^2 + \left(\frac{v_2 T}{\Theta_1}\right)^2 + \left(\frac{v_3 T}{\Theta_2}\right)^2\right]} \tag{2}$$

according to [4]. Here the respective velocity components are v_1, v_2, v_3. Further, L is pulse length, and Θ_1 and Θ_2 are the lateral and elevation resolutions corresponding to -3.25 dB opening angle. The repetition time is T and k is the wave number, which is equal to 2π divided by the wavelength. This model yields for laminar flow. Moreover, flow in left ventricle is turbulent [7], and in the next subsection this model is expanded to yield for turbulent flow as well.

2.2   Model for Turbulent Blood Flow

For turbulent flow we assume that the autocorrelation function for $n_b(\mathbf{r}, t)$ is

$$<n_b(\mathbf{r},t), n_b(\mathbf{r}+\xi, t+\tau)> = \Upsilon(\mathbf{r}, t) \frac{1}{(2\pi)^{\frac{3}{2}}\sigma_1\sigma_2\sigma_3} e^{-\frac{1}{2}\left(\frac{(\xi_1-\zeta_1)^2}{\sigma_1^2}+\frac{(\xi_2-\zeta_2)^2}{\sigma_2^2}+\frac{(\xi_3-\zeta_3)^2}{\sigma_3^2}\right)}$$

(3)

where ζ_1, ζ_2 and ζ_3 are mean displacements and σ_1, σ_2 and σ_3 are standard deviations of displacements. Here we assume a Gaussian shaped velocity profile to describe turbulent flow. With this extra assumption, the development of the expected value of the autocorrelation function $r(m)$ can follow the same path as in paper [4]. The difference is to multiply $r(m)$ with the Gaussian probability density function of velocities and integrate over all velocities.

$$r(m) = r(0) \int_{-inf}^{inf} \partial v_x, \partial v_y \, \partial v_z \beta(m) \, e^{i \, 2 \, m \, k \, v_1 T} e^{-\frac{1}{2}\left(\frac{(v_x-v_1)^2}{\sigma_1^2}+\frac{(v_y-v_2)^2}{\sigma_2^2}+\frac{(v_z-v_3)^2}{\sigma_3^2}\right)}$$

(4)

Here σ_1, σ_2 and σ_3 are redefined as the standard deviations of the velocity components. Further, v_1, v_2 and v_3 refer to the means of the velocity components. Integrating this gives

$$r(m) = r(0)\hat{\beta}(m)\hat{\alpha}(m) \, e^{i \frac{2 \, m \, k \, v_1 T}{a_1}} \qquad \text{where}$$

$$\hat{\alpha}(m) = e^{-\frac{2 \, m^2 \, k^2 \, T^2 \, \sigma_1^2}{a_1^2}}, \qquad \hat{\beta}(m) = \frac{1}{a_1 \, a_2 \, a_3} e^{-\frac{3}{2}m^2\left[\left(\frac{v_1 T}{L \, a_1}\right)^2+\left(\frac{v_2 T}{\Theta_1 \, a_2}\right)^2+\left(\frac{v_3 T}{\Theta_2 \, a_3}\right)^2\right]},$$

$$a_1 = \sqrt{3m^2\frac{\sigma_1^2 T^2}{L^2}+1}, \quad a_2 = \sqrt{3m^2\frac{\sigma_2^2 T^2}{\Theta_1^2}+1} \quad \text{and} \quad a_3 = \sqrt{3m^2\frac{\sigma_3^2 T^2}{\Theta_2^2}+1}$$

(5)

The coefficients a_1, a_2 and a_3 are close to one when $\sigma_1 T$ is small compared to L, $\sigma_2 T$ is small compared to θ_1 and $\sigma_3 T$ is small compared to θ_2. Therefore $\beta(\hat{m})$ is close to $\beta(m)$. A simplified model for turbulent flow is therefore

$$r(m) = r(0)\beta(m)\alpha(m) \, e^{i \, 2 \, m \, k \, v_1 T} \quad \text{where} \quad \alpha(m) = e^{-2 \, m^2 \, k^2 \, T^2 \, \sigma_1^2} \qquad (6)$$

The effect of turbulence is covered in the $\alpha(m)$ parameter, which is a function of the radial velocity distribution alone.

2.3   Model Including White Noise and Clutter Noise

Signal is assumed to be described by three components in Heimdal's model [5]. These three components are the signal from the range cell, additive white noise with power σ_n^2 and DC clutter noise from stationary echo with power σ_c^2. We assume the same, and the autocorrelation estimate for blood $r_b(m)$ and for tissue $r_t(m)$ is modeled as:

$$
\begin{aligned}
r_b(0) &= \sigma_b^2 + \sigma_c^2 + \sigma_n^2 & r_t(0) &= \sigma_t^2 + \sigma_c^2 + \sigma_n^2 \\
r_b(1) &= \sigma_b^2\,\beta(1)\alpha(1)\,e^{\mathrm{i}\,2\,k\,v_1\,T} + \sigma_c^2 & r_t(1) &= \sigma_t^2\,\beta(1)\,e^{\mathrm{i}\,2\,k\,v_1\,T} + \sigma_c^2 \\
r_b(2) &= \sigma_b^2\,\beta(2)\alpha(2)\,e^{\mathrm{i}\,8\,k\,v_1\,T} + \sigma_c^2 & r_t(2) &= \sigma_t^2\,\beta(2)\,e^{\mathrm{i}\,8\,k\,v_1\,T} + \sigma_c^2
\end{aligned}
\tag{7}
$$

Notice that the power terms of white noise are zero for $r_b(1)$, $r_t(1)$, $r_b(2)$ and $r_t(2)$. This is because white noise from different shots are uncorrelated. Transversing velocities are neglected in the tissue model and taken into account by the turbulent parameter in the blood model.

The probability density function for a signal $\mathbf{z}$ in blood is P_b and the probability density function for a signal $\mathbf{z}$ in tissue P_t is

$$
\begin{aligned}
P_b(\mathbf{z}|\sigma_b, \sigma_c, \sigma_n, v_b, \sigma_{v_b}) &= \frac{1}{\pi^N\,|\mathbf{C_b}|}\,e^{\bar{\mathbf{z}}\,\mathbf{C_b}^{-1}\,\mathbf{z}} \\[4pt]
P_t(\mathbf{z}|\sigma_t, \sigma_c, \sigma_n, v_t) &= \frac{1}{\pi^N\,|\mathbf{C_t}|}\,e^{\bar{\mathbf{z}}\,\mathbf{C_t}^{-1}\,\mathbf{z}}
\end{aligned}
\tag{8}
$$

where v_b and v_t are the radial velocity components in blood and tissue and σ_{v_b} is the standard deviation of the velocity profile inside one range cell in blood. Here $\mathbf{C_b}$ and $\mathbf{C_t}$ are:

$$
\mathbf{C_b} = \begin{bmatrix} r_b(0)\ \overline{r_b(1)}\ \overline{r_b(2)} \\ r_b(1)\ r_b(0)\ \overline{r_b(1)} \\ r_b(2)\ r_b(1)\ r_b(0) \end{bmatrix} \qquad \mathbf{C_t} = \begin{bmatrix} r_t(0)\ \overline{r_t(1)}\ \overline{r_t(2)} \\ r_t(1)\ r_t(0)\ \overline{r_t(1)} \\ r_t(2)\ r_t(1)\ r_t(0) \end{bmatrix}
\tag{9}
$$

In general the parameters defining P_b and P_t are not known. If their distributions are known then

$$
\begin{aligned}
P_b(\mathbf{z}) &= \int_{-\inf}^{\inf} d\sigma_b, d\sigma_c, d\sigma_n, dv_b, d\sigma_{v_b}\, P_b(\mathbf{z}|\sigma_b, \sigma_c, \sigma_n, v_b, \sigma_{v_b})\, P_{\sigma_b}\, P_{\sigma_c}\, P_{\sigma_n}\, P_{v_b}\, P_{\sigma_{v_b}} \\
P_t(\mathbf{z}) &= \int_{-\inf}^{\inf} d\sigma_t, d\sigma_c, d\sigma_n, dv_t, P_t(\mathbf{z}|\sigma_t, \sigma_c, \sigma_n, v_t)\, P_{\sigma_t}\, P_{\sigma_c}\, P_{\sigma_n}\, P_{v_t}
\end{aligned}
\tag{10}
$$

where $P_{\sigma_b}\, P_{\sigma_c}\, P_{\sigma_n}\, P_{v_b}\, P_{\sigma_{v_b}}\, P_{\sigma_t}$ and P_{v_t} are the probability density functions for the σ_b, σ_c, σ_n, v_b, σ_{v_b}, σ_t and v_t. In practice, these probability density functions can potentially be found from a priory knowledge, estimation or experimental trial and error.

2.4   Knowledge Based Imaging

The echocardiographic mode Knowledge Based Imaging index is proposed as

$$
\text{Knowledge Based Imaging index} = 20\cdot\log_{10}\left[\ln\left(\frac{P_t(\mathbf{z}) + P_b(\mathbf{z})}{P_b(\mathbf{z})}\right)\right]
\tag{11}
$$

Here $\mathbf{z}$ is the measured complex signal vector with length equal to packet size. Knowledge Based Imaging is basically a histogram manipulated version of the maximum likelihood ratio of a signal sample. The maximum likelihood ratio is $P_t(\mathbf{z})/P_b(\mathbf{z})$, and this is described in Van Trees [8].

The histogram manipulation can be argued for in the following way: The expression $(P_t(\mathbf{z}) + P_b(\mathbf{z}))/P_t(\mathbf{z})$ is close to 1 when $P_t(\mathbf{z})$ is dominating, equal to 2 when $P_t(\mathbf{z}) = P_b(\mathbf{z})$ and approaches infinity when $P_b(\mathbf{z})$ is dominating. The natural logarithm of this becomes a number between zero and infinity. Notice that this number is dominated by the difference of the exponents in equation (8). These exponents are dominated by the power of the signal, and this motivates for the final log compression. This histogram becomes reasonably uniform.

Another interesting method is the generalized likelihood ratio test that is also described in Van Trees. In the case of Knowledge Based Imaging, this is the same as calculating Knowledge Based Imaging from equation (11), where $P_t(\mathbf{z})$ and $P_b(\mathbf{z})$ are substituted with $\hat{P}_t(\mathbf{z})$ and $\hat{P}_b(\mathbf{z})$;

$$\hat{P}_b(\mathbf{z}) = \max_{R_b}(P_b(\mathbf{z}|\sigma_b, \sigma_c, \sigma_n, v_b, \sigma_{v_b})) \quad \text{where} \quad (\sigma_b, \sigma_c, \sigma_n, v_b, \sigma_{v_b}) \in R_b$$

$$\hat{P}_t(\mathbf{z}) = \max_{R_t}(P_t(\mathbf{z}|\sigma_t, \sigma_c, \sigma_n, v_t)) \quad \text{where} \quad (\sigma_t, \sigma_c, \sigma_n, v_t) \in R_t \tag{12}$$

Obviously, Knowledge Based Imaging requires definition of parameter space in tissue R_t and blood R_b. In this manuscript, this is done by defining the upper and lower limits of the parameters. This is hereby referred to as Knowledge Based Imaging with box constraints.

2.5 Fundamental Imaging

In the computer simulation, Fundamental Imaging index is defined as

$$\text{Fundamental Imaging index} = 20 \log_{10}(r(0)) where \quad r(m) = \frac{1}{3-m} \sum_{n=0}^{3-m-1} \overline{z_n} z_{n+m} \tag{13}$$

Note that no highpass filter is used prior to Fundamental Imaging calculation.

2.6 Bandwidth Imaging

In paper [1] Bandwidth Imaging index is defined as

$$\text{Bandwidth Imaging index} = \frac{|r(1)|}{r(0)} \tag{14}$$

and prior to the autocorrelation estimate the signal is filtered with this 2-tap Finite Impulse Response filter

$$x_1 = z_2 - \left(1 - 10^{-\frac{\text{AF}}{20}}\right) z_1$$

$$x_2 = z_3 - \left(1 - 10^{-\frac{\text{AF}}{20}}\right) z_2 \tag{15}$$

where AF is the attenuation factor at zero frequency.

Table 1. Parameters related to the transducer for Fundamental Imaging, Bandwidth Imaging, Knowledge Based Imaging and Second-Harmonic Imaging

Parameter	Fundamental Imaging Bandwidth Imaging Knowledge Based Imaging	Second-Harmonic Imaging
Center frequency trans./rec.	2.5/2.5 MHz	1.7/3.4 MHz
Pulse repetition frequency	3.75 kHz	4.25 kHz
Multi-Line Acquisition	4	2
Packetsize	3	1
Radial resolution	$6.67 \cdot 10^{-4}$ m	$4.6 \cdot 10^{-4}$ m
Aperture	$1.8 \times 2.0 \cdot 10^{-4}\,\mathrm{m}^2$	$2.2 \times 2.0 \cdot 10^{-4}\,\mathrm{m}^2$
Depth	0.15 m	0.15 m
Focal point (single)	0.15 m	0.09 m
Framerate	44	44
Number of beams	127	193

2.7 Pulse Strategy

The pulse strategy of Bandwidth Imaging, Knowledge Based Imaging and Fundamental Imaging is given in Table 1. The center frequency for Bandwidth Imaging, Knowledge Based Imaging and Fundamental Imaging is a trade off between resolution and penetration and is set to 2.5 MHz. The pulse length (0.7 mm) is chosen as a trade off between radial resolution and sensitivity. The pulse repetition frequency is set to 3750, as a trade off between reverberation noise from earlier shots and transit time effects in tissue. The transit time effect is the effect of decorrelation of signal due to movement of scatterers in the range cell. The packet size is 3, which is the lowest possible for calculating Bandwidth Imaging with the filter given by equation (15).

3   Discussion of Instrumentation of Knowledge Based Imaging

The strategy for implementation of Knowledge Based Imaging is to use the pulse strategy of Table 1 on a scanner (Vivid 7, GE Vingmed Ultrasound AS (Horten)). If we use the generalized maximum likelihood definition of Knowledge Based Imaging with box constraints, there are 14 parameters to adjust. These are the upper and lower limits of $\sigma_t, \sigma_b, \sigma_c, \sigma_n, v_t, v_b$ and σ_{v_b}. This section contains some examples of instrumentation of Knowledge Based Imaging with box constraints. In this case, the box constraints can be tuned so Knowledge Based Imaging can look similar to both Bandwidth Imaging and Fundamental Imaging.

Knowledge Based Imaging at one range cell is calculated in this way: A five dimensional array of values of $\sigma_b, \sigma_c, \sigma_n, v_b$ and σ_{v_b} is created and limited by the box constraints. Next, all $P_b(\mathbf{z})$ are calculated and the maximum value determined. A similar path is followed to calculate maximum of $P_t(\mathbf{z})$. Finally, Knowledge Based Imaging is calculated by equation (11).

Fig. 1 shows six four-chamber view images of a healthy mature male with different echocardiographic modes. Fig. 1(a), 1(b) and 1(c) show Second-Harmonic Imaging, Fundamental Imaging and Bandwidth Imaging, respectively.

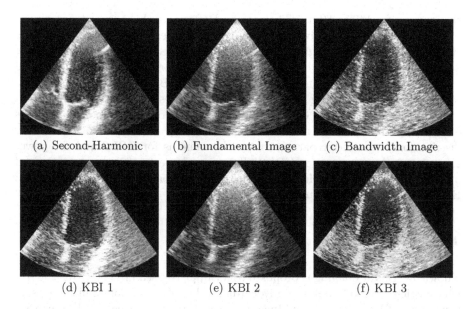

(a) Second-Harmonic   (b) Fundamental Image   (c) Bandwidth Image

(d) KBI 1   (e) KBI 2   (f) KBI 3

Fig. 1. Four-chamber views of a healthy heart with different imaging modes. Fig. 1(a), 1(b) and 1(c) show Second-Harmonic Image, Fundamental Image and Bandwidth Image, respectively. In Fig. 1(e) Knowledge Based Imaging is adjusted so that blood and tissue signal are separated by their differences in power. This image (KBI 2) is therefore similar to Fig. 1(b). In Fig. 1(f) (KBI 3) parameters are adjusted so that blood and tissue signal are separated by their differences in velocities and turbulence parameters. This image is therefore similar to Fig. 1(c). Fig. 1(d) (KBI 1) shows a Knowledge Based Image, which is a combination of the parameter settings of KBI 2 and KBI 3.

Fig. 1(d), 1(e) and 1(f) show three variants of Knowledge Based Imaging. In these images, σ_n is set to increase from 10 dB to 20 dB downward in the image. In Fig. 1(e) KBI 2 is shown. Here, v_b and v_t are set at 7 steps between - 1 to 1 m/s. Here, σ_{v_b} and σ_c are both set to zero. The only parameters separating $\hat{P}_t(\mathbf{z})$ and $\hat{P}_b(\mathbf{z})$, are σ_b and σ_t. These are given at 3 equally spaced steps from 50 to 100 dB in blood and 120 to 150 dB in tissue. We see that the KBI 2 is similar to Fundamental Imaging. They are related in the way that they both separate blood from tissue signal by their difference in power.

KBI 3 is shown in Fig. 1(f). Here there is no separation by power at all and σ_b and σ_t are set in three steps between 40 to 140 dB. The separation between blood and tissue signal is by velocity and velocity distribution. Here, v_b is set at seven steps between - 1 to 1 m/s. Further, the magnitude of velocity in tissue v_t is limited by 0.013 m/s in the apical region, and this magnitude is increased linearly to 0.13 m/s at 15 cm depth. This is because the radial velocities in myocardium are higher in the atrial ventricular plane region, than closer to apex. Moreover, the turbulence parameter σ_{v_b} is set to 0.12 m/s. It is important to mention that the image is enhanced by setting this parameter. Also the clutter parameter is set. The clutter parameter is set to decrease linearly downward in the image from 140 to 80 dB. The net effect of setting this parameter is similar to clutter filtering in Bandwidth Imaging. It is interesting that KBI 3 becomes similar to Bandwidth Imaging. The fact that Knowledge Based Imaging can be adjusted between the two extremes that look similar to Fundamental Imaging and Bandwidth Imaging, indicates that Knowledge Based Imaging can be used to find an optimal imaging method that compromises these two extremes.

KBI 1 is shown in Fig. 1(d). KBI 1 is a mixture of these two extreme ways of setting parameters of Knowledge Based Imaging. Here the velocity, velocity distributions and clutter parameter are the same as for KBI 3 and the power settings are the same as for KBI 2. This gives hope for finding an optimized imaging setup of Knowledge Based Imaging that balances the advantages of Bandwidth Imaging and Fundamental Imaging.

4   Conclusion

Knowledge Based Imaging is proposed as a Doppler-based method to distinguish left-ventricular blood pool from myocardial wall in echocardiographic images. A few images of Knowledge Based Imaging are supplied in this paper, showing that Knowledge Based Imaging can be adjusted to look similar to both Fundamental Imaging and Bandwidth Imaging.

Finally, we acknowledge that more optimization and research are needed for a clinical valuable implementation of Knowledge Based Imaging. First, the implementation should be real time, and the challenges here are the maximizations in equation (12) or integrations in equation (10). In the case of maximisations in equation (12), the maximizations could be done by a Preconditioned Conjugate Gradient Method.

Second, the box constraints of Knowledge Based Imaging have to be set everywhere in the image. To some degree they could be found. The level of white noise could be measured, while the transmitter is turned off. The velocity and turbulence parameters in tissue and blood could be found from a priory knowledge. Further, the signal characteristic could potentially be estimated by for instance a Levenberg-Marquardt method with box constraints [9]. Also, the potential of manual adjustment of parameters may also be investigated.

References

1. Hovda, S., Rue, H., Olstad, B.: Bandwidth of the ultrasound doppler signal to distinguish blood from tissue signal in the left ventricle. In: Proceedings of Medical Imaging and Informatics (MIMI) (2007)
2. Angelsen, B.A.: 7.4,9,3, 10.4. In: Ultrasound Imaging Wawes, Signals and Signal Processing, Emantec, Trondheim, Norway (2000)
3. Torp, H.: Clutter rejection filters in color flow imaging a theoretical approach. IEEE Transactions on Ultrasonics, Ferroelectriscs. and Frequency Control 44, 417–424 (1997)

4. Torp, H., Kristoffersen, K., Angelsen, B.A.J.: Autocorrelation techniques in color flow imaging: Signal model and statistical properties of the autocorrelation estimates. IEEE Transactions on Ultrasonics, Ferroelectriscs. and Frequency Control (1994)
5. Heimdal, A., Torp, H.: Detecting small blood vessels in colorflow ultrasound imaging: a statistical approach. IEEE Transactions on Ultrasonics, Ferroelectriscs. and Frequency Control (1999)
6. Angelsen, B.A.J.: A theoretical study of the scattering of ultrasound from blood. IEEE Trans. Biomed. Eng. 27(2), 61–67 (1980)
7. Schoephoerster, C., Chandran, K.B.: Velocity and turbulence measurements past mitral valve prostheses in a model left ventricle. Journal of Biomechanics 24(7), 549–562 (1991)
8. Trees, H.L.V.: Detection, Estimation, and Modulation Theory, vol. 1. John Wiley and Sons, Inc., Chichester (1968)
9. An, L.T.H., Tao, P.D.: A branch and bound method via d.c. optimization algorithms and ellipsoidal technique for box constrained nonconvex quadratic problems. Journal of Global Optimization 13(2), 171–206 (1998)

Comparison of Chang's with Sorenson's Attenuation Correction Method by Varying Linear Attenuation Coefficient Values in Tc-99m SPECT Imaging

Inayatullah Shah Sayed[1,*], Ahmed Zakaria[2], and Norhafiza Nik[1]

[1] School of Health Sciences, Universiti Sains Malaysia, Health Campus
16150 Kubang Kerian, Kota Bharu, Kelantan, Malaysia
s_ishah@hotmail.com
[2] Department of Nuclear Medicine, Oncology and Radiotherapy,
School of Medical Sciences, Universiti Sains Malaysia, Health Campus,
16150 Kubang Kerian, Kota Bharu, Kelantan, Malaysia

Abstract. Attenuation (scattering and absorption) of gamma photons in the patient's body is one of the major limitations among the others in single photon emission computed tomography (SPECT). It reduces quantitative accuracy of measured radioactivity concentration and causes hot rim artifacts in reconstructed images if not corrected for. A variety of approximate attenuation correction methods has been developed or proposed by various groups to date, but all methods have some limitations. In this paper two attenuation correction methods have been investigated and compared. Data are acquired with both the collimators either LEGP or LEHR by scanning R. A. Carlson cylindrical phantom over 360^{0} with an acrylic block of holes simulating hot regions of various sizes at different locations with respect to the walls of the phantom, which was filled with water and Tc-99m solution was uniformly distributed. Results show that the Chang's attenuation correction method works better as compared to the Sorenson's method in terms of the linearity in measured counts in hot regions. However, Chang's method is sensitive with linear attenuation coefficient values and also gives higher standard deviation values particularly in smaller hot regions count density – with LEHR collimator data - compared to the Sorenson's method.

Keywords: Attenuation correction, SPECT, Nuclear medicine.

1 Introduction

Accurate quantitative analysis of SPECT images is desired for a number of clinical studies. This can be accomplished to some extent by correcting the data for attenuation (absorption and scattering) of gamma photons within the patient's body [1 – 4]. There exists a number of such approximate attenuation correction techniques which are categorized into pre-processing, iterative techniques and post-processing.

---

* Present address: Institute of Physics, University of Sindh, Jamshoro, Pakistan.

X. Gao et al. (Eds.): MIMI 2007, LNCS 4987, pp. 216–222, 2008.
© Springer-Verlag Berlin Heidelberg 2008

Pre-processing techniques are based on the simple assumption that linear attenuation coefficient is uniform within the object boundaries (considered known) and can be easily implemented with filtered back projection reconstruction [5]. These techniques can reduce image distortion (hot rim artifacts) but does not give accurate quantification of radioactivity uptake, particularly for non-uniform absorbing media [6]. These procedures make correction to raw projection data before reconstruction. This is the preferred approach because correcting the data before formation of the image allows errors in the subsequent image to be reduced. These attenuation correction approaches consider a constant attenuation coefficient throughout the material within the object contour. Therefore they can be used for head and abdomen regions, where most body constituents are soft tissue types with similar attenuation coefficients [7].

Iterative processing techniques compensate for attenuation during reconstruction. These procedures require an extra term in the reconstruction algorithm in order to implement the compensation for gamma photon attenuation. They have been incorporated in both filtered back projection reconstruction algorithms [8] and iterative algorithms [6]. In the case of filtered back projection implementation, a constant linear attenuation coefficient is assumed, while with iterative algorithms a variable attenuation coefficient can be employed provided that the mapping of the linear attenuation coefficient within the object is known. One approach is via a modified version of ART algorithm, in which an additional factor representing the attenuation is incorporated into the calculations of the projections. The distribution of linear attenuation coefficient can be either assumed to be constant, or if an accurate linear attenuation map of the object is available from a transmission scan, for example, then spatially varying linear attenuation coefficient can be accommodated [9-13]. In these, a separate transmission image of the object is acquired before an emission scan. The limitations of measurements are that the imaging time is increased and that there is a possibility of miss-registration between transmission and emission scans due to patient movement [12]. These techniques provide more satisfactorily quantitative results. However, generally, iterative techniques have the disadvantage of longer computational times.

Post-processing attenuation correction techniques have been proposed by [14-16]. Chang's [14] approach considers a constant attenuation coefficient and requires prior knowledge of the edge of the object. For this attenuation compensation method, an image is first reconstructed without attenuation correction by using filtered back projection image reconstruction algorithm and a correction matrix is generated by the formula

$$C(x, y) = \frac{1}{\frac{1}{M} \sum_{i=1}^{M} \exp(-\mu l \theta_i)} \tag{1}$$

Where M is the number of projections, $l\theta_i$ is the attenuation distance between point (x,y) and the boundary of the object for θ_i.

To achieve a first order attenuation corrected image, the uncorrected image is (point) divided by the correction matrix. For better results, new projection data are calculated from the first order attenuation corrected image including an attenuation term, i.e.

$$p_c = \sum_{i=1}^{N} c_i \exp(-\mu l_{ij}) \qquad (2)$$

Where N is the number of pixels that contributes to the projection and l_{ij} is the length of intersection of the ray-sum with the attenuating medium. The error projections are then obtained by subtracting the new reprojected data from the original projections.

$$P_{error} = P_{original} - P_{corrected} \qquad (3)$$

The second order correction is achieved by adding the corrected error image to the first order corrected image and can be repeated if necessary.

The first order Chang's attenuation correction in most of SPECT scanning situations provides satisfactory results, if the edges of the object are obtained accurately; scattered gamma photons are reduced / rejected. However, this method has some drawbacks, e.g. its high noise sensitivity, the number of iterations until more accurate results are met and the generation of artifacts during processing [17, 18].

The Sorenson's attenuation correction method employs modified projection values, which are based upon the geometric mean of two opposing ray-sums and hyperbolic sine corrector [19, 20]. This method considers a region of uniform activity distribution within a larger absorbing medium of constant attenuation.

$$P_{new} = x.e^x \sqrt{P_a.P_b} / \sinh(x) \qquad (4)$$

Where $x = \mu L/2$, P_{new} is the modified projection, μ the attenuation coefficient for correction, L the path length through the attenuating medium, P_a and P_b is one and the opposite projection bin values, respectively.

In this study Chang's [14] and Sorenson's [21] techniques are evaluated and compared which are commercially available and installed in the system used in this study. These attenuation compensation techniques are relatively easy to implement and take low computational time.

2 Methodology

The data were collected with a Toshiba Gamma camera GCA901A/HG. Both the collimators either LEGP or LEHR were used and images were produced by using the reconstruction software available with the gamma camera. An acrylic (R A Carlson) walled cylindrical phantom was used. The dimensions of the phantom are 21.6 cm inner diameter and 17.00 cm in length, and it was filled uniformly with Tc-99m solution. Phantom was placed on the patient coach, with axis parallel to the face of collimator and in the centre of field of view (FOV) of the gamma camera. An acrylic block simulating hot regions in cold back ground with various sizes of hot regions was placed in the phantom. Eight pairs of circular holes (in a V shape) are drilled through the block, each pair separated by distance equal to the hole diameter (4.7, 5.9, 7.3, 9.2, 11.4, 14.3, 17.9 and 22.4 mm). In addition a pair of holes 30 mm diameter near the edges of the insert (opposite to each other at $180°$ from the centre of insert) is also drilled.

A filtered back projection algorithm has been applied with a ramp filter of second order Butterworth window having 0.30/cm cut-off frequency. Results were processed using commercially available software (Toshiba GCM5500UI). All necessary corrections, such as, uniformity and centre of rotation corrections are performed before sending the data for image reconstruction.

3 Results

3.1 Relative Count Ratio (RCR) in Count Densities of Hot Regions

An approximate procedure to calculate the relative count ratios (RCR) of hot regions of various sizes (30, 22.4, 17.9 and 14.3 mm diameter) located at different positions in the phantom was carried out. For the measurement of hot region relative count ratios, region of interest (ROI) were drawn within each of hot region and maximum pixel counts (relative) were noted (maximum count pixels were averaged for a pair of regions of the same diameter). In Tables 1 and 2 results are presented for the comparison of relative count ratios. The deeper hot regions relative count ratios were compared to the relative count ratios of hot regions located nearer the boundary of the phantom insert. The closer the calculated relative count ratio for deeper and more superficial hot regions are to their ideal values, the more accurate attenuation correction procedure is assumed to be.

Two attenuation correction methods [14, 21] are evaluated and compared in terms of various values of linear attenuation coefficients (0.121, 0.131, 0.141 and 0.151/cm). Attenuation correction techniques are applied to those data that were obtained by using material filter which reduces the influence of scattered gamma photons from SPECT projection data [22 – 23].

Table 1. Relative count ratio (RCR) in the count densities of hot regions with LEGP collimator

Hot region diameter mm	LEGP Collimator							
	Linear attenuation coefficient cm^{-1}							
	0.121		0.131		0.141		0.151	
	RCR Chang's Method	RCR Sorenson's Method	RCR Chang's Method	RCR Sorenson's Method	RCR Chang's Method	RCR Sorenson's Method	RCR Chang's Method	RCR Sorenson's Method
22.4/30	0.755	0.761	0.762	0.762	0.775	0.765	0.781	0.767
17.9/30	0.512	0.511	0.511	0.512	0.590	0.513	0.611	0.512
14.3/30	0.305	0.295	0.309	0.295	0.335	0.295	0.350	0.290

Table 2. Relative count ratio (RCR) in the count densities of hot regions with LEHR collimator

Hot region diameter mm	LEHR Collimator							
	Linear attenuation coefficient cm^{-1}							
	0.121		0.131		0.141		0.151	
	RCR Chang's Method	RCR Sorenson's Method	RCR Chang's Method	RCR Sorenson's Method	RCR Chang's Method	RCR Sorenson's Method	RCR Chang's Method	RCR Sorenson's Method
22.4/30	0.825	0.817	0.827	0.818	0.835	0.817	0.841	0.816
17.9/30	0.621	0.561	0.639	0.562	0.650	0.562	0.680	0.562
14.3/30	0.351	0.311	0.352	0.311	0.352	0.312	0.353	0.312

3.2   Standard Deviation (SD) in Count Densities of Hot Regions

Tables 3 and 4 shows standard deviation in relative count densities in hot regions (30, 22.4, 17.9 and 14.3 mm diameter) of reconstructed images located at different positions in the phantom, respectively. It was measured from noting the average count density within the hot regions by drawing regions of interest (ROI) in each pairs of hot region. The standard deviation is calculated by the following formula

$$SD = \sqrt{\frac{\sum_{i=1}^{N}(Z_i - D_{mean})^2}{(N-1)}} \qquad (5)$$

D_{mean} is the mean count density / pixel, and measured by using the following equation:

$$D_{mean} = \sum_{i=1}^{N}(1/N)Z_i \qquad (6)$$

Where N represents the number of pixels within a region of interest (ROI) and Z_i is the number of counts in the ith pixel.

Table 3. Standard deviation in the count densities of hot regions with LEGP collimator

Hot region diameter mm	LEGP Collimator							
	Linear attenuation coefficient cm^{-1}							
	0.121		0.131		0.141		0.151	
	SD Chang's Method	SD Sorenson's Method	SD Chang's Method	SD Sorenson's Method	SD Chang's Method	SD Sorenson's Method	SD Chang's Method	SD Sorenson's Method
30	280	300	285	320	315	315	292	290
22.4	150	145	180	150	175	160	175	180
17.9	110	80	115	90	120	92	130	195
14.3	25	19	26	21	28	21	29	22

Table 4. Standard deviation in the count densities of hot regions with LEHR collimator

Hot region diameter mm	LEHR Collimator							
	Linear attenuation coefficient cm^{-1}							
	0.121		0.131		0.141		0.151	
	SD Chang's Method	SD Sorenson's Method	SD Chang's Method	SD Sorenson's Method	SD Chang's Method	SD Sorenson's Method	SD Chang's Method	SD Sorenson's Method
30	140	165	150	175	175	210	190	190
22.4	65	90	66	105	90	110	110	150
17.9	56	55	58	50	65	50	75	52
14.3	23	20	26	18	30	20	29	16

4   Discussion

Geometric mean based attenuation correction techniques are largely dependent on the body thickness, weakly dependent on the source thickness, and independent of source depth. These methods tend to give connecting count density between separated radioactive sources in the reconstructed image [7, 24].

It is clear in Tables 1 and 2 that, 17.9/30mm relative count ratio is improved by the Chang's method in all cases. At 0.121 and 0.131/cm linear attenuation coefficients there is no relative improvement for 22.4/30mm diameter hot region but at 0.141 and 0.151/cm values improvement is noticed with the Chang's method – LEGP collimator. The trend of results shows that with all linear attenuation coefficient values, Sorenson's method gives stable relative count ratio results. Moreover, these results indicate the depth dependence of the Chang's method is reduced. Overall with both the collimators improvement in relative count ratio with the Chang's method is achieved.

It is noted that Chang's method has higher standard deviation values than Sorenson's method (Tables 3 and 4). With increasing linear attenuation coefficient values the standard deviation increases rapidly. This suggests that Chang's method is sensitive to the linear attenuation coefficient values. Sorenson's method also gives higher standard values although much lower than Chang's method (not in all cases), but it isn't sensitive to varying linear attenuation coefficient values.

5 Conclusion

For two different types of collimators, relative count ratio is higher for low energy high resolution collimator than low energy general purpose collimator. For the standard deviation calculations low energy high resolution collimator shows smaller standard deviation compared to low energy general purpose collimator.

Chang's method provides relatively more quantitatively accurate results compared to Sorenson's method at the cost of high level standard deviation particularly at higher linear attenuation coefficient values. This indicates that Chang's method is sensitive to the choice of this parameter that must be chosen carefully in clinical studies.

Acknowledgements. Authors are grateful to the Department of Nuclear Medicine, Oncology and Radiotherapy, School of Medical Sciences, Universiti Sains Malaysia, Health Campus, 16150 Kubang Kerian, Kota Bharu, Kelantan, Malaysia for allowing conducting experiments and the staff for cooperation and some technical help in this regard.

References

1. Hayashi, M., Deguchi, J., Utsunomiya, K., Yamada, M., Komori, T., Takuchi, M., Kana, K., Narabayashi, I.: Comparison of Methods of Attenuation and Scatter Correction in Brain Perfusion SPECT. Journal of Nuclear Medicine Technology 33, 224–229 (2005)
2. El Fakhri, G., Kijewski, M.F., Albert, M.S., Johnson, K.A., Moore, S.C.: Quantitative SPECT Leads to Improved Performance in Discrimination Tasks Related to Prodromal Alzheimer's Disease. J. Nucl. Med. 45, 2026–2031 (2004)
3. Kim, K.M., Varrone, H., Watabe, H., Shidahara, M., Fujita, M., Innis, R.B., Iida, H.: Contribution of Scatter and Attenuation Compensation to SPECT Images of Nonuniformly Distributed Brain Activities. J. Nucl. Med. 44, 512–519 (2003)
4. Zaidi, H., Hasegawa, B.: Determination of the Attenuation Map in Emission Tomography. J. Nucl. Med. 44, 291–315 (2003)
5. Budinger, T.F., Gulberg, G.T., Huesman, R.H.: Emission Computed Tomography. In: Herman, G.T. (ed.) Image reconstruction from projections: implementation and applications, pp. 147–246. Springer, New York (1979)

6. Gullberg, G.T., Huesman, R.H., Malko, G.A., Plec, N.J., Budinger, T.F.: An attenuated projector-backprojector for iterative SPECT reconstruction. Phy. Med. Bio. 30, 799–816 (1985)
7. Rosenthal, M.S., Cullom, J., Hawkins, W., Moore, S.C., Tsui, B.M.W., Yester, M.: Quantitative SPECT imaging: A review and recommendations by the Focus Committee of the Society of Nuclear Medicine Computer and Instrumentation Council. J. Nucl. Med. 36, 1489–1513 (1995)
8. Tanaka, E., Toyama, H., Murayama, H.: Convolutional image reconstruction for quantitative single photon emission computed tomography. Phy. Med. Bio. 29, 1489–1500 (1984)
9. Glick, S.J., Penney, B.J., King, M.A.: Filtering of SPECT reconstruction made using Bellini's attenuation correction method: a comparison of three pre-reconstruction and a post reconstruction Wiener filter. IEEE Trans. Nucl. Sci. NS-38, 663–669 (1991)
10. Liang, Z., Turkington, T.G., Gilland. Jaszczak, R.J., Coleman, R.E.: Simultaneous compensation for attenuation, scatter, and detector response for SPECT reconstruction in three dimensions. Phys. Med. Bio. 37, 587–603 (1992)
11. Galt, J.R., Cullom, S.J., Garcia, E.V.: SPECT quantification: a simplified method of attenuation correction method for cardiac imaging. J. Nucl. Med. 33, 2232–2237 (1992)
12. Tung, C.H., Gullberg, G.T., Zeng, G.L., Christian, P.E., Datz, F.L., Morgan, H.T.: Nonuniform attenuation correction using simultaneous transmission and emission converging tomography. IEEE Trans. Nucl. Sci. NS-39, 1134–1143 (1992)
13. Maze, A., Le Cloirec, J., Collorec, R., Bizais, Y., Braindet, P., Bourguet, P.: Iterative Reconstruction Methods for Nonuniform Attenuation Distribution in SPECT. J. Nucl. Med. 34, 1204–1209 (1993)
14. Chang, L.T.: A method for attenuation correction in radionuclide computed tomography. IEEE Trans. Nucl. Sci. NS-35, 638–643 (1978)
15. Walters, T.E., Simon, W., Chesler, D.A., Correia, J.A.: Attenuation correction in gamma emission computed tomography. J. Comp. Asst. Tomogr. 1, 89–94 (1981)
16. Moore, S.C., Brunelle, J.A., Kirsch, C.: An iterative attenuation correction for a single photon scanning multidetector tomography system. J. Nucl. Med. 22, 65 (1981)
17. Mas, J., Ben Younes, R., Bidet, R.: Improvement of quantification in SPECT studies by scatter and attenuation compensation. Eur. J. Nucl. Med. 15, 351–356 (1989)
18. Jaszczak, R.J., Coleman, R.E., Lim, C.B.: Single photon emission computed tomography. IEEE Trans. Nucl. Sci. NS- 27, 1137–1152 (1980)
19. Faber, T.L., Lewis, M.H., Corbett, J.R., Stokely, E.M.: Attenuation correction for SPECT: An evaluation of Hybrid approaches. IEEE Trans. Medical Imaging MI-3, 101–107 (1984)
20. Murase, K., Itoh, H., Mogami, H., Ishine, M., Kawamura, M., Iio, A., Hamamoto, K.: A comparative study of attenuation correction algorithms in single photon emission computed tomography (SPECT). Eur. J. Nucl. Med. 13, 55–62 (1987)
21. Sorenson, J.A.: Methods for quantitative measurement of radioactivity in vivo by whole-body counting. In: Hine, G.J., Sorenson, J.A. (eds.) Instrumentation in Nuclear Medicine, vol. 2, pp. 311–348. Academic Press, New York (1974)
22. Spinks, T.J., Sayed, I.S.: Effect of lead filters on the performance of a Neuro-PET tomography operated without septa. IEEE Trans. Nucl. Sci. NS-40, 1087–1091 (1993)
23. Sayed, I.S.: Reduction of Scattered gammas and Attenuation Correction in SPET. Ph D Thesis, King's College London, University of London (1996)
24. Tsui, B.M.W., Zhao, X., Frey, E.C., McCartney, W.H.: Quantitative single photon emission computed tomography: basics and clinical considerations. Seminars in Nucl. Med. 24, 38–65 (1994)

An Improved Median Filtering System and Its Application of Calcified Lesions' Detection in Digital Mammograms

Kun Wang, Yuejian Xie, Sanli Li, and Yunpeng Chai

Department of Computer Science and Technology, Tsinghua University, Beijing, 100084, China
wangkun00@mails.tsinghua.edu.cn

Abstract. Median filtering is an important approach in digital image processing for noise elimination or extraction. The time cost and detection quality of the filtering system are two convention measures, depending on the sliding window size. In this paper, an improved median filter, Adaptive Sliding Window – Simultaneous Deleting and Inserting (ASW-SDI) system, is proposed for calcified lesions' detection in digital mammograms, increasing the quality of detection and also reducing the time cost. It changes the size of sliding windows adaptively and uses the same pixels in two neighboring windows, deleting and inserting a line of pixels in a single array traverse. It is especially appropriate for images with a small quantity of large noises and a mass of salt & pepper noises. In the breast cancer computer-aided diagnosis experiments, ASW-SDI works efficiently in calcified lesion extraction.

Keywords: median filtering; complexity; adaptive; calcified lesion.

1 Introduction

Image processing is an aspect of digital mammography which offers benefits to clinicians to aid in both the detection of abnormal features and the diagnosis of cancer. Among those abnormal features, calcified lesion detection is of clinical significance [1], as the detection rate of calcified lesions in malignant group is much higher than that in the benign breast mass group. Most of the calcified lesions belong to the micro-calcified type, represented in the breast X-Ray images as a mass of salt & pepper noises. In the computer-assisted detection[2,3] process, median filtering, wavelet transform, and artificial neural networks are used to pick out these noises[4]. Median filtering is mainly used for noise elimination or extraction [6, 7] and is of great importance in digital image processing. Time cost and quality[8] are two convention measures of it. The traditional algorithm is based on full sorting of pixels in the sliding window. At worst, the computational complexity is $O(m^2n^2)$, where m and n are the sliding window's length and width. The computational complexity grows rapidly with the square of sliding window area. With the large image size, computational cost is even higher[9]. To improve the quality of noise detection, the

X. Gao et al. (Eds.): MIMI 2007, LNCS 4987, pp. 223–232, 2008.
© Springer-Verlag Berlin Heidelberg 2008

sliding window size should be appropriately chosen: if the sliding window area is n = $2k^2+1$, noises of area k^2+1 or larger are kept, while those of k^2 or smaller are erased [10].The ASW-SDI system pays attention to both aspects: time cost and quality of noise detection. An adaptive sliding window size strategy is used for different noises' extraction, and in the median filtering process an improved full sorting algorithm is devised for time diminishment.

The rest of this paper is organized as follow: section 2 introduces some related works; section 3 describes the architecture of ASW-SDI system; section 4 puts forward the Sorting Unit and its simultaneous deleting and inserting algorithm; section 5 introduces the Judgment Unit and its adaptive sliding window strategy; section 6 introduces the experiment results of breast X-Ray images' calcified lesions extraction as well as the comparison with other techniques; conclusion and future works are given in section 7.

2 Related Work

Methods for calcified lesion detection[11] and types classification[3] as well as the serial analysis of gene expression[12] are paid much attention by researches from both computer science and medicine areas. As a classical method for calcified lesion detection[4], median filter can be applied to both gray-scale images and color images [13]. This paper just focuses on the gray-scale image processing, since each pixel in a RGB color image is composed of three components (red, green and blue). Some improved algorithms derived from the classical algorithm are categorized into full sorting algorithms and non-full sorting algorithms. A full sorting algorithm is designed and applied to a Doppler radar information processing system [9]. At worst, $2m\log_2 mn$ comparisons are needed. An improved non-full sorting method is put forward by [8], its complexity is $O(mn)$. Adaptive methods are designed by [14], which both work on reducing the loss of valid information, and [15] gives out a solution on adjusting the sliding window size. Some other parallel solutions suggest allocating the computation to distributed computational nodes, such as [6]. Hardware implementation is also made, for instance [16].

The ASW-SDI system guarantees the complexity of $O(mn)$ as the non-full sorting algorithm while it completes a full sort and reduces the number of comparisons to $2\log_2 m+2\log_2(m-1)+2mn-m$ in the worst case. In the process of adaptively adjusting the size of its sliding window, sorted array information is also used to reduce the time cost and improve the quality.

3 ASW-SDI System

ASW-SDI system deals with mammograms, in DICOM[17] or JPEG format, producing detection results of calcified lesions. The architecture of ASW-SDI is shown in Fig.1, including a Sorting Unit and a Judgment Unit.

When sorting pixels in the current sliding window by the Sorting Unit, a simultaneous deleting and inserting algorithm based on the former sorted information

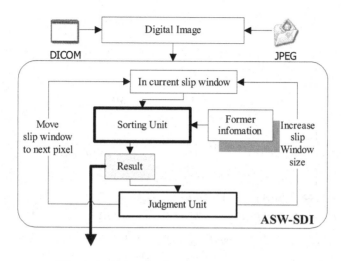

Fig. 1. Architecture of the ASW-SDI system

is used. Results are sent to the Judgment Unit for noise-probability calculation, according to which, the sliding window is increased in size or moved to the next pixel. For the previous occasion, the simultaneous deleting and inserting algorithm is used again to reduce the time cost. This mechanism is especially efficient in the case of images with large amount of salt & pepper noises and a sprinkle of larger noises.

4   The Sorting Unit

When a sliding window is specified, the Sorting Unit uses the simultaneous deleting and inserting algorithm to get the median filtering results, aiming at reducing the time cost of sorting.

4.1   Median Filtering Problem

The process of median filtering can be represented as follows: a matrix $A_{H,B} =$

$\begin{bmatrix} a_{0,0} & a_{0,1} & \cdots & a_{0,B-1} \\ a_{1,0} & a_{1,1} & \cdots & a_{1,B-1} \\ \vdots & \vdots & \vdots & \vdots \\ a_{H-1,0} & a_{H-1,1} & \cdots & a_{H-1,B-1} \end{bmatrix}$ is used to represent the gray scale values of all the pixels

in a digital image with the size of H×B.

For description convenience, the following definitions are given:

Definition 1: The operation of making median filtering for matrix $A_{H,B}$ is defined as $MF(A_{H,B}, W_{n,m})$. The operation of sorting elements in matrix $A_{H,B}$ by a sliding window with the size of n×m is defined as Sort($A_{H,B}$). The operation of getting the median value of array V_n with the length of n is defined as mid(V_n).

If $n < H \wedge m < B$,

$$MF\,(A_{H,B}, W_{n,m}) = \begin{bmatrix} MF(A'_{(0,0),(n-1,m-1)}, W_{n,m}) & \cdots & MF(A'_{(0,B-m),(n-1,B-1)}, W_{n,m}) \\ MF(A'_{(1,0),(n,m-1)}, W_{n,m}) & \cdots & MF(A'_{(1,B-m),(n,B-1)}, W_{n,m}) \\ \vdots & \vdots & \vdots \\ MF(A'_{(H-n,0),(H-1,m-1)}, W_{n,m}) & \cdots & MF(A'_{(H-n,B-m),(H-1,B-1)}, W_{n,m}) \end{bmatrix} \tag{1}$$

$A'_{(i,j),(i',j')} = \begin{bmatrix} a_{i,j} & a_{i,j+1} & \cdots & a_{i,j'} \\ a_{i+1,j} & a_{i+1,j+1} & \cdots & a_{i+1,j'} \\ \vdots & \vdots & \vdots & \vdots \\ a_{i',j} & a_{i',j+1} & \cdots & a_{i',j'} \end{bmatrix}$. Let $V_{(i,j)(i',j')} = \{a_{i,j}, a_{i,j+1}, ..., a_{i,j'}, \ a_{i+1,j}, ..., a_{i',j}$

$, a_{i',j+1}, ..., a_{i',j'}\} \implies Sort(A'_{(i,j),(i',j')}) = Sort(V'_{(i,j),(i',j')})$;

If $n = H \wedge m = B$, $MF(A'_{(i,j),(i',j')}, W_{i'-i+1,j'-j+1}) = mid(V_{(i,j)(i',j')})$, $MF\ (A_{H,B}, W_{n,m}) =$

$$\begin{bmatrix} mid(V_{(0,0),(n-1,m-1)}) & \cdots & mid(V_{(0,B-m),(n-1,B-1)}) \\ mid(V_{(1,0),(n,m-1)}) & \cdots & mid(V_{(1,B-m),(n,B-1)}) \\ \vdots & \vdots \vdots & \vdots \\ mid(V_{(H-n,0),(H-1,m-1)}) & \cdots & mid(V_{(H-n,B-m),(H-1,B-1)}) \end{bmatrix} \tag{2}$$

Definition 2: For operation C, its computation complexity is defined as $Comp(C)$. When use traditional algorithms to sort $V_{(i,j)(i+n-1,j+m-1)}$, for example quick-sort algorithm, the number of comparison is $Comp(QuickSort(V_{(i,j)(i+n-1,j+m-1)}))$, $nm\log_2 nm \leq Comp(Quick\ Sort(V_{(i,j)(i+n-1,j+m-1)})) \leq n^2 m^2$. Next section will introduce the simultaneously deleting and inserting algorithm.

4.2 Simultaneous Deleting and Inserting Algorithm

According to formula(1), redundant information exists in neighboring sliding windows. Take $A'_{(i,j),(i+n-1,j+m-1)}$, $A'_{(i-1,j),(i+n-2,j+m-1)}$ and $A'_{(i,j-1),(i+n-1,j+m-2)}$ for

example. $A'_{(i,j),(i+n-1,j+m-1)} = \begin{bmatrix} A'_{(i,j),(i+n-2,j+m-1)} \\ a_{i+n-1,j}, ..., a_{i+n-1,j+m-1} \end{bmatrix} = \begin{bmatrix} A'_{(i,j),(i+n-1,j+m-2)} & \begin{matrix} a_{i,j+m-1} \\ \vdots \\ a_{i+n-1,j+m-1} \end{matrix} \end{bmatrix} \tag{3}$

$A'_{(i-1,j),(i+n-2,j+m-1)} = \begin{bmatrix} a_{i-1,j}, ..., a_{i-1,j+m-1} \\ A'_{(i,j),(i+n-2,j+m-1)} \end{bmatrix} \tag{4}$

$A'_{(i,j-1),(i+n-1,j+m-2)} = \begin{bmatrix} a_{i,j-1} \\ \vdots & A'_{(i,j),(i+n-1,j+m-2)} \\ a_{i+n-1,j-1} \end{bmatrix} \tag{5}$

$Sort(V_{(i-1,j),(i+n-2,j+m-1)})$ has been done when $Sort(A'_{(i-1,j),(i+n-2,j+m-1)})$ is accomplished. Operation $Sort(A'_{(i,j),(i+n-1,j+m-1)})$ equals to deleting $\{a_{i-1,j}, ..., a_{i-1,j+m-1}\}$ from the result of $Sort(A'_{(i-1,j),(i+n-2,j+m-1)})$ and inserting $\{a_{i+n-1,j}, ..., a_{i+n-1,j+m-1}\}$ to it. If deleting $\{a_{i-1,j}, ..., a_{i-1,j+m-1}\}$ and inserting $\{a_{i+n-1,j}, ..., a_{i+n-1,j+m-1}\}$ is implemented to result of $Sort(A'_{(i-1,j),(i+n-2,j+m-1)})$, even when the fastest quick-sort algorithm is used, the number of comparison is $m\log_2 mn$ and number of movements is $\frac{(2mn-1-n)*n}{2}$ for

the   worst   case.   That   means
$\max(Comp(Sort(A'_{(i,j),(i+n-1,j+m-1)}))) = m\log_2 mn + m\log_2(mn-m) + (2mn-1-n)*n$.

This paper describes an algorithm which makes the operation of deleting and inserting finished in a single traverse of the array, as shown in Fig.2.

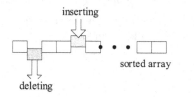
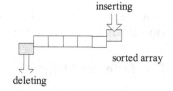

Fig. 2. Deleting and inserting arrays   **Fig. 3.** Deleting and inserting elements

1) Sort array $\{a_{i-1,j},...,a_{i-1,j+m-1}\}$ (named del-array) and array $\{a_{i+n-1,j},..., a_{i+n-1,j+m-1}\}$ (named insert-array); *del-array* and *insert-array* can be got from array $\{a_{i-1,j-1},...,a_{i-1,j+m-2}\}$ and array $\{a_{i+n-1,j-1},...,a_{i+n-1,j+m-2}\}$ when operation $Sort(A'_{(i,j-1),(i+n-1,j+m-2)})$ is accomplished.

$\{a_{i-1,j},...,a_{i-1,j+m-1}\} = \{a_{i-1,j-1},...,a_{i-1,j+m-2}\} - \{a_{i-1,j-1}\} + \{a_{i-1,j+m-1}\}$; $\{a_{i+n-1,j},...,a_{i+n-1,j+m-1}\} = \{a_{i+n-1,j-1},...,a_{i+n-1,j+m-2}\} - \{a_{i+n-1,j-1}\} + \{a_{i+n-1,j+m-1}\}$, as shown in Fig.3.

2) Let array $\{\alpha_0,\alpha_1,...,\alpha_{nm-1}\}$ be the result of $Sort(A'_{(i-1,j),(i+n-2,j+m-1)})$. *index_del* and *index_insert* are used to indicate the to-be-operated element in array $\{a_{i-1,j},...,a_{i-1,j+m-1}\}$ and array $\{a_{i+n-1,j},...,a_{i+n-1,j+m-1}\}$, *index_a'* indicates the element to be operated in array $\{\alpha_0,\alpha_1,...,\alpha_{nm-1}\}$. β_i stands for the ith element in the result array of $Sort(A'_{(i-1,j),(i+n-2,j+m-1)})$. The algorithm is shown as follow:

```
Delete_and_Insert(del, insert, α )
index_del = 0; index_add = 0; index_a' = 0;
for i=0 to nm, do
if  α_index_a' > add[index_add] then
β_i = add[index_add] ; index_insert++; i++;
else if  α_index_a' = del[index_del] then index_del++;
else  β_i = α_index_a' ; index_a'++; i++;
```

This algorithm uses historical information to simplify the current sort. Complexity analysis is given as below:

1) Sort *del_array* and *insert_array*. Take *del_array* for example: as array $\{a_{i-1,j-1},...,a_{i-1,j+m-2}\}$ has been sorted, the number of comparison for deleting element $\{a_{i-1,j-1}\}$ is log_2m for the worst case, and for inserting element $\{a_{i-1,j+m-1}\}$ is $log_2(m-1)$ Similarly, when *insert_array* is being sorted, deleting element $\{a_{i+n-1,j-1}\}$ from array

$\{a_{i+n-1,j-1},...,a_{i+n-1,j+m-2}\}$ and inserting element $\{a_{i+n-1,j+m-1}\}$ need log_2m and $log_2(m-1)$ comparisons.

2) Delete the sorted *del_array* from array $\{\alpha_0,\alpha_1,...,\alpha_{nm-1}\}$, and at the same time insert the sorted *insert_array*. This process needs $2mn-m$ comparisons for the greatest quantity.

The sum of the above two parts is the number of comparison needed for this algorithm, meaning $\max(Comp(Sort(A'_{(i,j),(i+n-1,j+m-1)}))) = 2log_2m+2log_2(m-1)+2mn-m$. In the above analysis, the sliding window size is set as $n\times m$. The next section will introduce the Judgment Unit, which uses the adaptive sliding window.

5   The Judgment Unit

The Judgment Unit is the kernel component of ASW-SDI system, which adaptively changes the size of sliding window, and thus guarantees the effect of noises extraction.

5.1   Sliding Window Size

The sliding window size affects the results of median filtering. As shown in Fig. 4(a), size of the noises are 2×3, 1×1 and 1×1, the median filtering results are as shown in Fig. 4(b) and Fig. 4(c).

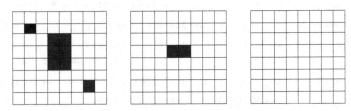

Fig. 4. (a). Image with noises.   **(b).** Window size 3*3.   **(c).** Window size 5*5.

When sliding window size is 3x3, noise is kept partially, while with 5x5 window, noise is removed completely.

5.2   Workflow of the Judgment Unit

At the initial stage of the Judgment Unit, the size of the sliding window is set to a minimal value. The filtering result of the Sorting Unit is sent to the Judgment Unit. The principle of the Judgment Unit is: if the number of pixels in the current sliding window is larger than a gray-scale value threshold, increase the sliding window size; if it is smaller than the threshold, current sliding window's calculation is ended and the sliding window should be moved to the next pixel. The algorithm is shown as below:

```
(1) m = Window_min; n = Window_min;
```
(2) $MF(A'_{(i-(n-1)/2,j-(m-1)/2,i+(n-1)/2,j+(m-1)/2)},W_{n,m})$
```
(3) if Noise_count(
```
$A'_{(i-(n-1)/2,j-(m-1)/2,i+(n-1)/2,j+(m-1)/2)}$) > 0.5×

```
pixel_count( A'_(i-(n-1)/2,j-(m-1)/2,i+(n-1)/2,j+(m-1)/2) ) and m<Window_max,
n<Window_max  then m = m+•; n=n+•; Goto (2)
end if
```

Windows_max can be set according to the largest noise's size to prevent m and n from increasing illimitably, Δ and Ω, which are the increasing step for m and n, can be chosen as steady values or increasing values, determined by the idiographic character of different images. When the size of large noises is far greater than those salt-pepper noises, the growth pattern of Δ and Ω could be arithmetic growth or exponential; while if the discrepancy is not so great, the pattern could be constant or arithmetic growth. In the processing of adjusting sliding window size, former sorted information can be used to make further decrease of time cost:

$$MF(A'_{(i-(n-1)/2,j-(m-1)/2,i+(n-1)/2,j+(m-1)/2)},W_{n,m}) = mid(V_{(i-(n-1)/2,j-(m-1)/2,i+(n-1)/2,j+(m-1)/2)})$$

$$m' = m - \Delta , n' = n - \Omega$$

$$Sort(V_{(i-(n-1)/2,j-(m-1)/2,i+(n-1)/2,j+(m-1)/2)}) = Sort(V_{(i-(n'-1)/2,j-(m'-1)/2,i+(n'-1)/2,j+(m'-1)/2)})$$

$$+V_{(i-(n-1)/2,j-(m-1)/2,i-(n'-1)/2-1,j+(m-1)/2)} + V_{(i+(n'-1)/2+1,j-(m-1)/2,i+(n-1)/2,j+(m-1)/2)}$$

$$+V_{(i-(n'-1)/2,j-(m-1)/2,i+(n'-1)/2,j-(m'-1)/2-1)} +V_{(i-(n'-1)/2,j+(m'-1)/2+1,i+(n'-1)/2,j+(m-1)/2)})$$

temp1=Delete_and_Insert $(\quad V_{(i-(n-1)/2,j-(m-1)/2,i-(n'-1)/2-1,j+(m-1)/2)} \quad , \quad$ null,

$V_{(i-(n-1)/2,j-(m-1)/2,i+(n-1)/2,j+(m-1)/2)})$

temp2= Delete_and_Insert $(V_{(i+(n'-1)/2+1,j-(m-1)/2,i+(n-1)/2,j+(m-1)/2)},$ null, temp1)

temp3= Delete_and_Insert $(V_{(i-(n'-1)/2,j-(m-1)/2,i+(n'-1)/2,j-(m'-1)/2-1)},$ null, temp2)

result= Delete_and_Insert $(V_{(i-(n'-1)/2,j+(m'-1)/2+1,i+(n'-1)/2,j+(m-1)/2)},$ null, temp3)

For most of the pixels in current sliding window, the size is of minimal value.

6 Application in Breast Images' Calcified Lesions Extraction

The ASW-SDI is deployed on a breast cancer grid environment and uses medical breast X-Ray images to validate its performance. The experiment uses 4 computational nodes of the breast cancer grid. The tumor hospital attached to the Shanghai Fudan University provides the breast X-Ray images. Calcified lesions can be got by the original image minus the result image of the ASW-SDI., as shown in Fig.5.

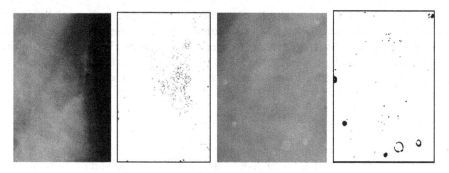

Fig. 5. Original images and their calcified lesions' character

The validating experiment is organized in two stages: first, it compares the improved simultaneous deleting and inserting algorithm with the other two algorithms. At the second stage, for a given image, it compares the adaptive sliding window strategy with algorithms of different sliding window size.

6.1 The First Stage

In the first stage three sorting algorithms are used: classical full sorting algorithm (quick-sort), classical non-full sorting algorithm and the simultaneous deleting and inserting algorithm. Fig.6-Fig.9 shows their time cost(s) with different sliding window size ($m=n$).

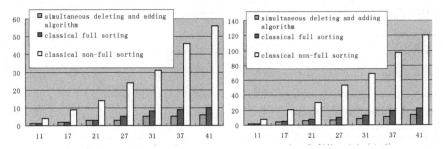

Fig. 6. Image of 400×400 pixels   **Fig. 7.** Image of 600×600 pixels

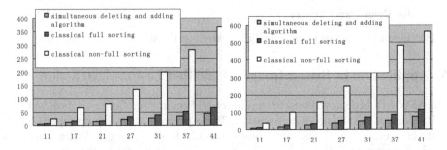

Fig. 8. Image of 800×800 pixels   **Fig. 9.** Image of 1000×1000 pixels

The time cost of the classical full sorting algorithm increases exponentially as the accretion of sliding window area, which means it is almost unavailable when image area or sliding window area increase to a certain tolerance. From the experiment, conclusions can also be made that the Sorting Unit, using the simultaneous inserting and deleting method is superior to the other two algorithms as the sliding window size grows larger.

6.2 The Second Stage

In the second stage, the same image is used to validate the filtering effect: Fig.10(a). shows an enlargement of a breast X-Ray image, the adaptive sliding window and sliding window with size 31×31, and 21×21(using simultaneous inserting and deleting algorithm). The median filtering results are shown in Fig.10(b)., Fig.10(c). and Fig. 10(d).. Window_min is 11 and Window_max is 41, according to the image character. Table 1 compares the time cost of these three methods.

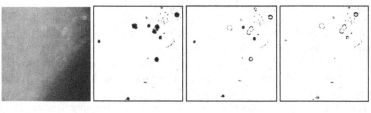

Fig. 10.   **(b).**Adaptive window.   **(c).** 31×31 .   **(d).** 21×21.

Table 1. Time cost comparison

Sliding window size	Calcified lesions Distortion	Time cost(s)
Adaptive	0	46
31×31	6	78
21×21	9	51

A sliding window of size 21×21 distorts 9 calcified lesions, and 31×31 distorts 6 calcified lesions. The adaptive sliding window strategy gets the best extraction effect of 0 distortions and the least time cost.

7   Conclusion and Future Work

Median filtering problem has always been a hotspot in the digital image processing field, aiming at spending the least time on getting the best effect. For images with a large amount of salt & pepper noises and a sprinkling of larger noises, the ASW-SDI system, which synthesizes the adaptive sliding window strategy and the simultaneous deleting and inserting algorithm, has been proved to be able to get better filtering effect with less time cost, both on the theory analysis stage and mammograms' processing validation stage. The ASW-SDI system's kernel idea is: do not increase the sliding window size unless it is necessary, and use as much as former sorted information as possible.

References

1. Xiao, Y., Wu, Y., Luo, H.: Clinical Significance of Calcified Lesion Detection in Breast Mass with Ultrasonography. Journal of Clinical Research 21(3), 233–239 (2004)
2. Jorg, S., Raymond, T.N., Monica, C.S., et al.: A methodology for analyzing SAGE libraries for cancer profiling. ACM Transactions on Information Systems 23(1), 35–60 (2005)
3. Seral, Ş., Kemal, P., Halife, K.: A new hybrid method based on fuzzy-artificial immune system and k-nn algorithm for breast cancer diagnosis. Computers in Biology and Medicine 37(3), 415–423 (2007)

4. Wan, B.K., Wang, R.P., Zhu, X.: A novel technique to detect the microcalcifications in digital mammograms based on a synthetic processing method. Chinese Journal of Biomedical Engineering 21(6), 536–542 (2002)
5. Wang, J.H., Lin, L.D.: Improved median filter using minmax algorithm for image processing. Electronics Letters 33(16), 1362–1363 (1997)
6. Amir, R.F., Babak, N.A.: Iterative Median Filtering for Restoration of Images with Impulsive Noise. In: Electronics, Circuits and Systems, Proceedings of the 2003 10th IEEE International Conference on, vol. 1, pp. 232–235 (2003)
7. Lu, R., Shen, Y., Wang, Q.: Edge Detection Based on Early Vision Model Incorporating Improved Directional Median Filtering. In: Instrumentation and Measurement Technology Conference, 2004. Proceedings of the 21st IEEE, vol. 1, pp. 441–443 (2004)
8. Li, G., Fan, R.X.: A New Median Filter Algorithm in Image Tracking Systems. Journal of Beijing Institute of Technology, 116–118 (2002)
9. Cui, Z.H., Cheng, M.H., Wu, Q.L.: A Technique of Fast Median Filtering and Its Application to Data Quality Control of Doppler Radar. Plateau Meteorology, 727-733 (2005)
10. Li, G., Fan, R.X.: A New Median Filter Algorithm in Image Tracking Systems. Journal of Beijing Institute of Technology, 116–118 (2002)
11. Qian, W., Mao, F., Sun, X.J., et al.: An improved method of region grouping for microcalc-ification detection in digital mammograms. Computerized Medical Imaging and Graphics 26(6), 361–368 (2002)
12. Thomadaki, H., Talieri, M., Scorilas, A.: Prognostic value of the apoptosis related genes BCL2 and BCL2L12 in breast cancer. Cancer Letters 247(1), 48–55 (2007)
13. Carlo, S.R., Andrea, T.: A New Approach to Vector Median Filtering Based on Space Filling Curves. Image Processing, IEEE Transactions 6(7), 1025–1037 (1997)
14. Nallaperumal, K., Saudia, S., Vinsley, S.S.: Selective Switching Median Filter for the Removal of Salt & Pepper Impulse Noise. In: Wireless and Optical Communications Networks, 2006 IFIP International Conference, p. 5 (2006)
15. Hwang, H., Haddad, R.A.: Adaptive Median Filters: New Algorithms and Results. IEEE Transactions on image processing 4(4), 499–502 (1995)
16. Alejandro, D.S., Jaime, R.A., Antonio, L.M., et al.: A Fully Parallel CMOS Analog Median Filter. Circuits and Systems II: Express Briefs. IEEE Transactions on [see also Circuits and Systems II: Analog and Digital Signal Processing, IEEE Transactions on] 51(3), 116–123 (2004)
17. David, P., Eugenia, P., Mark, S., et al.: A relational approach to the capture of DICOM files for Grid-enabled medical imaging databases. In: Proceedings of the 2004 ACM symposium on applied computing, pp. 272–279 (2004)

Bandwidth of the Ultrasound Doppler Signal with Applications in Blood/Tissue Segmentation in the Left Ventricle

Sigve Hovda, Håvard Rue, and Bjørn Olstad

Norwegian University of Science and Technology, Trondheim, Norway
sigveh@idi.ntnu.no
http://idi.ntnu.no/~sigveh

Abstract. A new estimator, Bandwidth Imaging, related to the bandwidth of the ultrasound Doppler signal is proposed as a classification function of blood and tissue signal in transthoracial echocardiography of the left ventricle. An in vivo experiment is presented, where the apparent error rate of Bandwidth Imaging is compared with the apparent error rate of Second-Harmonic Imaging on 15 healthy men. The apparent error rates are calculated from the 16 myocardial wall segments defined in [1]. A hypothesis test of Bandwidth Imaging having lower apparent error rate than Second-Harmonic Imaging is proved for a p-value of 0.94 in 3 segments in end diastole and in 1 segment in end systole. When data was averaged by a structural element of 5 radial, 3 lateral and 4 temporal samples the numbers of segments increased to 9 in end diastole and to 6 in end systole. This experiment indicates that Bandwidth Imaging can supply additional information for automatic border detection routines on endocardium.

1 Introduction

The ejection fraction is one of the most commonly measured parameters in diagnosis and follow up of coronary heart disease, valve decease and heart failure. The ejection fraction is the ejected volume divided by the maximum volume of the left ventricle, and measuring ejection fraction involves defining the endocardial border, either automatically or by manual tracing.

Many approaches have been suggested to solve the endocardium tracking problem. We mention here briefly; active contour models (snakes) [2] and [3], active shape models [4] and [5], region-growing scheme [6] and Hough transform [7]. Common for all these approaches is that they are all applied on Second-Harmonic Imaging data.

It is an important point, that Bandwidth Imaging is not the same as the Variance-mode, available on most conventional Color Flow Imaging systems. The variance estimates are calculated from the bandwidth of the highpass filtered Doppler signal [8] (page 10.20) and these measurements are related to the accuracy of blood flow measurements.

X. Gao et al. (Eds.): MIMI 2007, LNCS 4987, pp. 233–242, 2008.
© Springer-Verlag Berlin Heidelberg 2008

In Bandwidth Imaging contradictory, the Doppler signal is only partially attenuated before the bandwidth estimate. The signal from tissue has therefore a narrow bandwidth, while signal from blood has broader bandwidth, since this signal is a mixture of blood signal and clutter noise. Bandwidth Imaging is therefore used as a classification function.

In Power Doppler the packetsize has to be at least 6 to achieve a useful stopband in the highpass filter [9]. However in Bandwidth Imaging, a 2-tap Finite Impulse Response highpass filter is sufficient and this filter is available with a packetsize of 3. The temporal resolution is proportional to the packetsize and this gives an important resolution gain compared to Power Doppler. Further, spatial resolution and frame rate are increased by using Multi-Line acquisition. Multi-Line acquisition is reconstruction of multiple scan lines from sparsely transmitted scan lines. This means that Bandwidth Imaging is available at a temporal and spatial resolution that is interesting in endocardial border detection. In table 1 in section 2.1 we see that Bandwidth Imaging is available at a frame rate of 44 with 127 beams available per frame.

In order to discuss the usefulness of Bandwidth Imaging, an in vivo experiment on 15 healthy male is introduced. A similar experiment is suggested by Spencer et. al. in [10]. Here, the visualization of Second-Harmonic Imaging and Fundamental Imaging were rated by expert cardiologists in all myocardial segments outlined in [1]. However, the visual differences between Bandwidth Imaging and Second-Harmonic Imaging are more radical than the visual differences between Fundamental Imaging and Second-Harmonic Imaging. Therefore, a test which is less dependent on visual perception is introduced in this paper.

2   Bandwidth Imaging

The bandwidth estimator is found to be

$$B^2 = 2 - 2\frac{|r(1)|}{r(0)} \quad \text{where} \quad r(m) = \frac{1}{N-m} \sum_{n=0}^{N-m-1} \overline{z_n} z_{n+m} \quad \text{for} \quad 0 \le m \le N-1 \tag{1}$$

in [8] and [11]. Here $r(m)$ is the autocorrelation function z_n is the signal. In Bandwidth Imaging the packet size N is set to 3. Notice that the signal dependent part of B^2, is dependent on the absolute value of the normalized autocorrelation function with lag one. For simplicity, the Bandwidth Imaging index is defined as:

$$\text{Bandwidth Imaging index} = \frac{|r(1)|}{r(0)} \tag{2}$$

Bandwidth Imaging index is therefore high when bandwidth is small and visa verse. This is because Bandwidth Images should be white in tissue and black in blood, similar to Second-Harmonic Images.

The appearance of white noise biases the estimate downward, while clutter noise biases the estimate upward. To compensate for the effect of clutter noise, a 2-tap Finite Impulse Response highpass filter prior to autocorrelation calculation is introduced

$$
\begin{aligned}
x_1 &= z_2 - (1 - 10^{-\frac{AF}{20}}) z_1 \\
x_2 &= z_3 - (1 - 10^{-\frac{AF}{20}}) z_2
\end{aligned}
\tag{3}
$$

where AF is the attenuation factor at zero frequency in dB. When AF is high the filter can be regarded as a stationary canceling filter and the transfer function is given in [11] (page 209). In apical views, the clutter noise level is high in the near field and the white noise level increases by depth due to depth gain compensation. We have therefore found it reasonable to let AF decrease linearly from 40 dB to 15 dB in images from apical views with depth 15 cm.

2.1 Instrumentation of Bandwidth Imaging

The strategy for implementation of Bandwidth Imaging is by trial and error of various pulse strategies on a scanner (Vivid 7, GE Vingmed Ultrasound AS (Horten)) . A reasonable pulse strategy for Bandwidth Imaging is given in Table 1. The pulse strategy for Second-Harmonic Imaging, which is used in section 3, is shown for comparison.

The center frequency for Bandwidth Imaging is a trade off between lateral resolution and penetration and is set to 2.5 MHz. The pulse length of 0.7 mm is chosen as a trade off between radial resolution and sensitivity. The pulse repetition frequency is set to 3750, as a trade of between reverberation noise from earlier shots and transit time effects in tissue. The transit time effect is the effect of decorrelation of signal due to movement of scatterer inside the range cell. The packet size is 3, which is the lowest possible for calculating Bandwidth Imaging with the filter given by equation (3).

Note that the pulse length is about 50 % longer in Bandwidth Imaging than in Second-Harmonic Imaging. Also, Bandwidth Imaging contains approximately 33 % less beams per frame than Second-Harmonic Imaging. This is because the frame rate of Bandwidth Imaging is equal to the frame rate of Second-Harmonic Imaging, the packet size is three times higher, the Multi-Line acquisition parameter is doubled and pulse repetition frequency is about the same.

The In Quadrature (signal after complex demodulation in the signal chain) data is recorded and saved to a file for further post-processing in Matlab (The MathWorks Inc.). In Bandwidth Imaging, signal is highpass filtered by equation (3) and then calculated by equation (2). Second-Harmonic Imaging is calculated by log compressing the square root of $r(0)$. The images are then scan converted to get physical scale and histogram equalized to get comparable contrast.

Table 1. Parameters related to the transducer for Bandwidth Imaging and Second-Harmonic Imaging

Parameter	Bandwidth Imaging	Second-Harmonic Imaging
Center frequency trans./rec.	2.5/2.5 MHz	1.7/3.4 MHz
Pulse Repetition frequency	3.75 kHz	4.25 kHz
Multi-Line Aqusition	4	2
Packetsize	3	1
Radial resolution	$6.67 \cdot 10^{-4}$ m	$4.6 \cdot 10^{-4}$ m
Aperture	$1.8 \times 2.0 \cdot 10^{-4}\,\mathrm{m}^2$	$2.2 \times 2.0 \cdot 10^{-4}\,\mathrm{m}^2$
Depth	0.15 m	0.15 m
Focal point (single)	0.15 m	0.09 m
Frame Rate	44	44
Number of beams	127	193

3   Experiment for Comparing Bandwidth Imaging with Second-Harmonic Imaging

3.1   Methods

The test included 15 healthy male persons aged 24 to 32. The image qualities were acceptable, which means that substantial agreement with Magnetic Resonance Images [12] were expected. The three standard apical views, four-chamber, two-chamber and long-axis view were recorded in one loop each. The pulse strategy and the instrumentation details were the same as given in section 2.

The depth was set to 15 cm and a single transmit focus was chosen in both Second-Harmonic Imaging and Bandwidth Imaging to get better resolution. In this study all depth gain compensations were equalized for all depths to eliminate for this variability.

The subjects were asked to hold their breath and keep still during recording. This enabled the examiner to compare Second-Harmonic Imaging and Bandwidth Imaging from the same positions. The examiner traced the endocardium in the Second-Harmonic Images in both end systole and end diastole in all three views. Immediately after tracing in the Second-Harmonic Images, the same traces were shown in the corresponding Bandwidth Images. In cases where the subject moved under the examination, the examiner retraced on the Bandwidth Images.

In article [1], recommendations for nomenclature and standardized segmentation of myocardium are given. The sixteen segmentation model for eckocardiaography is shown in the bulls-eye diagram in Fig. 1(d).

From the manual traces of the endocardium, the shape and position of myocardial segments were calculated according to the procedure explained in [1]. These segments are seen in figure 1(a), 1(b) and 1(c). Here corresponding blood segments are shown on the inside of endocardium. The number labels are denoted in the blood segments, corresponding to the myocardial segments.

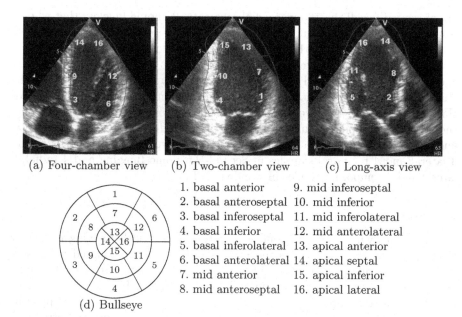

(a) Four-chamber view   (b) Two-chamber view   (c) Long-axis view

1. basal anterior	9. mid inferoseptal
2. basal anteroseptal	10. mid inferior
3. basal inferoseptal	11. mid inferolateral
4. basal inferior	12. mid anterolateral
5. basal inferolateral	13. apical anterior
6. basal anterolateral	14. apical septal
7. mid anterior	15. apical inferior
8. mid anteroseptal	16. apical lateral

(d) Bullseye

Fig. 1. Display, on circumferential polar plot, of the 16 myocardial segments and recommended nomenclature recommended for echocardiography

All recorded data inside each myocardial segment and each blood segment were stored in an array, with labels of subject number, segment name, segment type (blood or tissue), method (Second-Harmonic Imaging of Bandwidth Imaging) and time instance (end diastole or end systole).

Evaluation Criteria for Classification Functions. A comprehensive discussion of classification theory can be found in [13]. The quantity apparent error rate is chosen to evaluate the performance of the classification functions Bandwidth Imaging and Second-Harmonic Imaging. Advantages of apparent error rate are that it is easy to implement and not dependent of the form of the parent populations. We suggest this definition of apparent error rate:

$$\text{Apparent error rate} = \min_{T} \left(\frac{m_{tT} + m_{bT}}{a_t + a_b} \right) \tag{4}$$

Here, a_t is the total area of one particular tissue segment. Correspondingly, a_b is the total area of the neighboring blood segment. An image of both the blood and the tissue segment is thresholded at T, making this image binary. The value m_{tT} is the total area of the black pixels in the tissue segment. This value is therefore the area in the tissue segment, where the classification by thresholding at T failed. Correspondingly, the value m_{bT} is the area of white pixels in the blood segment. The apparent error rate is therefore the proportion of misclassified area, given the best possible threshold. In this paper, results of apparent error rates are presented for all the 16 myocardial segments. It should be clear that when a result of for instance the mid anterior segment is presented, the apparent error rate calculation uses both the myocardial and the blood segment.

Prior to apparent error rate calculation the images have either been non averaged, moderately averaged or strongly averaged. In moderate averaging, the structural element is 3 radial, 2 lateral and 3 temporal samples in Second-Harmonic Imaging. To account for the resolution loss in Bandwidth Imaging, the structural element in moderate averaging is reduced to 2 radial, 2 lateral and 2 temporal samples. In strong averaging, the structural element is 5 radial, 3 lateral and 4 temporal samples in Second-Harmonic Imaging and 4 radial, 2 lateral and 4 temporal samples in Bandwidth Imaging.

3.2   Results

The occasions where the apparent error rate of Bandwidth Imaging is smaller than apparent error rate of Second-Harmonic Imaging are counted in all segments. This number ranges from 0 to 15, since 15 subjects attended the study. The result is shown in column one and three in Fig. 2. If numbers are 11 or above, the p-values are higher than 0.94 on the hypothesis test; true apparent error rate of Bandwidth Imaging is equal or lower than true apparent error rate of Second-Harmonic Imaging.

This indicates that Bandwidth Imaging classifies better than Second-Harmonic Imaging in these segments, and these segments are therefore marked green. Segments with numbers four and below are marked red, where the test is favoring Second-Harmonic Imaging. In segments with black numbers, the experiment can not indicate which method works best.

The first column shows results of end diastole and the third column shows results of end systole. In apical septal and in apical lateral segments a super-index and a sub-index are given. The super-index tells us which view has the lowest mean apparent error rate taken over subjects in Bandwidth Imaging. Correspondingly, the sub-index shows the best view of Second-Harmonic Imaging. Here 4 means four-chamber view and L means long-axis view. In these segments, the test compares the apparent error rate of Second-Harmonic Imaging and the apparent error rate of Bandwidth Imaging from their respective best views.

In the top, mid and bottom row of Fig. 2 the test is performed on non, moderately and strongly averaged data, respectively. The effect of averaging is therefore that the number of green segments is increased from 3 to 7 to 9 in end diastole and from 1 to 2 to 6 in end systole. Also, the number of red segments is reduced from 6 to 5 to 3 in end diastole and from 9 to 5 to 4 end systole. Note that the apparent error rate decreases with averaging in every segment at any time instance (end diastole or end systole).

In column two and four in Fig. 2, we see that the apparent error rate is very different in various segments. On non averaged data, the apparent error rate of Bandwidth Imaging, varies from 0.21 to 0.37 in end diastole and 0.27 to 0.38 in end systole, while apparent error rate of Second-Harmonic Imaging, varies from 0.11 to 0.38 in end diastole and 0.16 to 0.40 in end systole. The smallest numbers

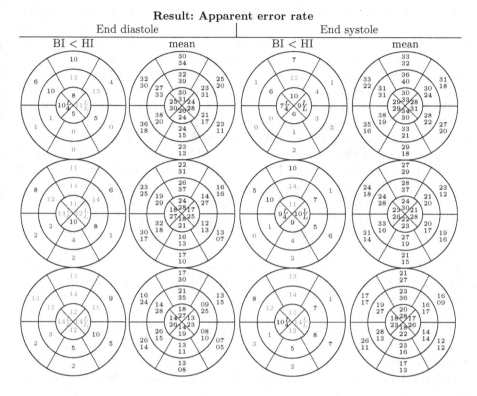

Fig. 2. Column one and three show numbers where apparent error rate is lower in Bandwidth Imaging BI than in Second-Harmonic Imaging HI in end diastole and end systole, respectively. Numbers of 11 and above are marked green indicating that BI is best there. Numbers of 4 and below are marked red indicating HI is best there. In column two and four, the mean values of apperant error rate in percent are shown in end diastole and end systole. The top values are for Bandwidth Imaging and the bottom values are for Second-Harmonic Imaging. The top, mid and bottom row shows result when images are not, moderate and strongly averaged.

of the apparent error rate are found in segments where Second-Harmonic Imaging works best, and the largest numbers of apparent error rate are found in segments where Bandwidth Imaging works best.

3.3   Discussion of the Comparison Experiment

In comparing Second-Harmonic Imaging and Bandwidth Imaging, the ground truth of the endocardial borders are found by manual traces on Second-Harmonic Images. It can be objected that there is a flaw in comparing two methods, when the ground truth is determined by one of them. On the other side, manual traces of endocardium on images of reasonable image quality as basis for ejection fraction measurements are reported to have reasonable agreement with ejection fraction measurements of Magnetic Resonance Imaging [12]. In this study the subjects had reasonable image qualities, and this suggests that more thrust can be placed on the manual traces as ground truth of endocardium. Moreover, if the manual traces are biased, it can be argued that they are biased in favor of Second-Harmonic Imaging, since they are drawn on Second-Harmonic Images. This would therefore only strengthen the results in favor of Bandwidth Imaging.

We have selected apparent error rates as the quantitative evaluation criteria of Bandwidth Imaging and Second-Harmonic Imaging. This measure is intuitive because it calculates the proportion of misclassified area, given the best threshold. In a practical clinical setting this threshold level is not known. However, automatic border detection routines are in general more dependent on a good tissue to blood contrast, rather than evenly distributed intensity levels in an image. We therefore postulate that the apparent error rate is related to the potential of an automatic detection routine of endocardium.

In the experiment we found the lowest values of apparent error rate in segments where Second-Harmonic Imaging worked best, and the largest values of apparent error in segments where Bandwidth Imaging worked best. This indicates that the great regional differences seen in Fig. 2 are more a matter of regional differences in Second-Harmonic Imaging, rather than regional differences in Bandwidth Imaging.

Since the traces of endocardium in end diastole and end systole are needed for ejection fraction calculation, only these time instances are considered in this experiment. Notice also the difference between end diastole and end systole in Fig.2. These differences are greater in Bandwidth Imaging than in Second-Harmonic Imaging.

Many automatic detection routines involve using several or all frames in a heart beat. Therefore averaged images have been considered in this study. It is important to notice from Fig. 2 that apparent error rate decreases with averaging in every segment at any time instance (end diastole or end systole). If this was not the case, it would not be fair to compare averaged data of Second-Harmonic Imaging with averaged data of Bandwidth Imaging. The result that averaging seems to favor Bandwidth Imaging can be taken as an argument for employing Bandwidth Imaging data in detection routines that use many frames.

3.4   Discussion of Instrumentation of Bandwidth Imaging

In the process of instrumenting Bandwidth Imaging, we tried a variety of pulse repetition frequencies, pulse lengths, center frequencies and beam sizes. Also a great number of AF were tested. There is not room for a comprehensive discussion of parameter tuning in this paper. Fig. 3(b) shows Bandwidth Imaging from two-chamber view at six equally sparsed time steps in the heart cycle. Image 1 indicates end diastole and image 4 indicates end systole. In Fig. 3(a) the corresponding Second-Harmonic Images are shown. These effects are important in Bandwidth Imaging:

Tissue surrounding the cardiac muscle is more similar to tissue in the cardiac muscle in Bandwidth Imaging than in Second-Harmonic Imaging. This is

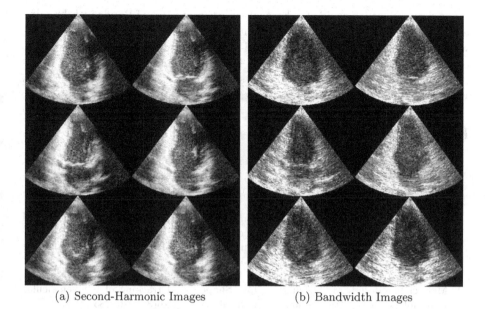

(a) Second-Harmonic Images   (b) Bandwidth Images

Fig. 3. In Fig. 3(a) Second-Harmonic Images from two-chamber view are shown at six equally spaced time steps in the cardiac cycle. The end diastole is shown in the first image and the end systole is shown in the fourth image. In Fig. 3(b) the corresponding Bandwidth Images are shown.

because Bandwidth Imaging is more dependent on the motion of the scatterers, while Second-Harmonic Imaging is dependent on the reflection coefficient of the scatterers.

Next, the mitral valve and apparatus are not visible in Fig. 3(b). Signal from mitral valve and apparatus is a mixture of blood and tissue signal and has therefore a broader bandwidth. Moreover, signal from vibrating muscles such as in mitral apparatus is known to have broader bandwidth [14].

Further, Bandwidth Imaging is dependent of the movement of the scatterers and the image quality is therefore dependent on the acquisition time in the cardiac cycle. This can be seen as image four is much brighter than image one. This can also explain the differences between end diastole and end systole seen in Fig. 2.

4   Conclusion

A new echocardiographic mode has been proposed, where the difference in Doppler signal from blood flow and tissue motion is utilized. A reasonable instrumentation setup of Bandwidth Imaging is outlined in this paper. Bandwidth Imaging is implemented with a packetsize of 3, meaning that Bandwidth Imaging has a temporal and spatial resolution that is interesting for endocardial border detection.

An experiment is provided, where apparent error rates of Bandwidth Imaging and Second-Harmonic Imaging are compared. The results indicate that Bandwidth Imaging are better than Second-Harmonic Imaging in some segments, especially in apical and anterior regions. The test suggests that Bandwidth Imaging has less differences between segments and improves more by averaging. This votes for automatic routines using several time frames.

References

1. Cerqueira, M.D., Weissman, N.J., Dilsizian, V., Jacobs, A.K., Kaul, S., Laskey, W.K., Pennell, D.J., Rumberger, J.A., Ryan, T., Verani, M.S.: Standarized my-ocardial segmentation and nomencclature for tomographic imaging of the heart. Circulation, 539–542 (January 2002)
2. Olstad, B.: Active contours with grammatical descriptions. In: 6th International conference on Image analyses and Processing, Como, Italy (September 1991)
3. Bosch, J.G., Savalle, L.H., van Burken, G., Reiber, J.H.: Evaluation of semiau-tomatic contour detection approach to sequences of short axes two-dimensional echocardiographic images. J. Am: Soc. Echocardiogr 8(6), 810–821 (1995)
4. McEachenand-2nd, M.C., Duncan, J.S.: Shape-based tracking of left ventricular wall motion. IEEE Transactions on Medical Imaging 16(3), 270–283 (1997)
5. Bosch, H.G., Mitchell, S.C., Lelieveldt, B.P.F., Nijland, F., Kamp, O., Sonka, M., Reiber, J.H.C.: Active appearance-motion models for fully automated endocardial contour detection in time sequences of echocardiograms, International Congress Series, vol. 1230, pp. 941–947 (June 2001)
6. Dove, E.I., Phillip, K., Gotteiner, N.L., Vonesh, M.J., Ramberger, J.A., Reed, J.E., Standford, W., McPherson, D.D., Chandran, K.B.: A method for automatic edge detection and volume computation of the left ventricle from ultrafast computed tomographic images. Investigative Radiology 29(11), 945–954 (1994)
7. Malassiotis, S., Strintzis, M.G.: Tracking the left ventricle in echocardiographic images by learning heart dynamics. IEEE Transactions on Medical Imaging 18(3), 280–290 (1999)
8. Angelsen, B.A.: 7.4,9,3, 10.4. In: Ultrasound Imaging Wawes, Signals and Signal Processing, Emantec, Trondheim, Norway (2000)
9. Torp, H.: Clutter rejection filters in color flow imaging a theoretical approach. IEEE Transactions on Ultrasonics, Ferroelectriscs. and Frequency Control 44, 417–424 (1997)
10. Spencer, K.T., Bednarz, J., Rafter, P.G., Korcarz, C., Lang, R.M.: Use of harmonic imaging without echocardiographic contrast to improve two dimensional image quality. American Journal of Cardiology 82(6), 794–799 (1998)
11. Jensen, J.A.: 6.5 and 7.5. In: Estimation of Blood Velocities Using Ultrasound, Cambridge University Press, New York (1996)
12. Malm, S., Frigstad, S., Sagberg, E., Skjærpe, T.H.L.: Accurate and reproducible measurement of left ventricular volume and ejection fraction by contrast echocar-diography. Journal of the American College of Cardiology 44, 1030–1035 (2004)
13. Johnson, R.A., Wichern, D.W.: Applied Multivariate Statistical Analysis. Prentice-Hall Inc., Englewood Cliffs (2002)
14. Heimdal, A., Torp, H.: Ultrasound doppler measurements of low velocity blood flow limitations due to clutter signals form vibrating muscles. IEEE Transactions on Ultrasonics, Ferroelectriscs. and Frequency Control 44, 873–881 (1997)

Applications of the Visible Korean Human

Jun Won Lee[1], Min Suk Chung[1], and Jin Seo Park[2]

[1] Department of Anatomy, Ajou University School of Medicine, Suwon, Korea
orijjanga@ajou.ac.kr
[2] Department of Anatomy, Dongguk University College of Medicine, Korea

Abstract. Visible Korean Human (VKH) consisting of magnetic resonance, computer tomography, anatomic, and segmented images was created. In the VKH, several techniques were developed and numerous data were acquired. The VKH techniques mainly contributed to the generation of advanced segmented images, Visible Living Human, and Visible Mouse. Also, a software for viewing sectional anatomy, three dimensional images for virtual dissection and virtual endoscopy, was developed based on the VKH data distributed worldwide. The VKH technique and data are expected to promote development of other serially sectioned images and software, which are helpful in medical education and clinical practice.

Keywords: Visible Korean Human, Magnetic resonance images, Anatomic images, Segmented images, Three dimensional images.

1 Introduction

Visible Human Project was the first trial ever made to obtain serially sectioned images of cadaver's whole body. The data derived from Visible Human Project have contributed largely in the medical image field [16]. Furthermore, technique used for the Visible Human Project has been modified in Korea for Visible Korean Human (VKH) [9,10,13] and in China for Chinese Visible Human [18]. By using the improved technique for VKH such as magnetic resonance (MR) scanning, computerized tomography (CT) scanning, serial sectioning, photographing, and segmenting, the VKH team acquired better data consisting of MR images, CT images, anatomic images, and segmented images. The improved VKH technique was introduced through article [9, 10, 13], whilst the VKH data were distributed worldwide. The objective of this report is to promote new trials by other researchers to create other serially sectioned images applying VKH technique and three dimensional (3D) images with VKH data, which will be greatly helpful in medical education and useful in clinical practice. To achieve this objective, this report describes the ideas and experiences in applying the VKH technique and data to generate new image data contributing to the medical image field.

2 Materials, Methods, and Results

2.1 Application of VKH Technique for Detail Segmented Images of VKH

Three years ago, 13 structures (skin, bones, liver, lungs, kidneys, urinary bladder, heart, cerebrum, cerebellum, brainstem, colon, bronchi, and arteries) in the anatomic

X. Gao et al. (Eds.): MIMI 2007, LNCS 4987, pp. 243–251, 2008.
© Springer-Verlag Berlin Heidelberg 2008

images were outlined to obtain basic segmented images [9]. However, these basic segmented images were insufficient to produce various 3D images, therefore, advanced segmented images of the many more structures were decided to be made, in order to complement and replace the basic segmented images.

By using segmentation technique on Adobe Photoshop™ (version 7.0) [9], important structures identifiable in anatomic images were segmented as follows: 104 structures of head and neck including brain components, 15 structures of heart, and 84 structures of left upper limb as well as 114 structures of left lower limb including each bone, muscle, nerve, and artery. A few segmented structures such as skin were used as they stood, and other segmented structures such as bone were classified into each bone. Whereas some unsegmented structures such as muscles were newly outlined. According to the color difference of each structure in gross examination, segmentation was performed automatically, semi-automatically, or manually using Adobe Photoshop. Through stacking the segmented images, coronal and sagittal segmented images were made in order to verify segmentation. As a result, advanced segmented images of 317 structures were produced (Fig. 1).

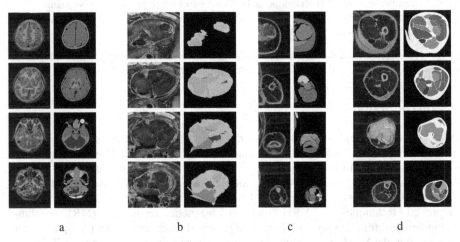

a   b   c   d

Fig. 1. Anatomic and segmented images of head (a), heart (b), left upper limb (c), and left lower limb (d)

2.2   Application of VKH Technique for Visible Living Human

Besides the VKH, Visible Living Human is newly planned to produce whole body MR images of living humans. While the Visible Living Human does not include anatomic images, it includes MR images of living human, whose body conditions are much better than those of cadaver. In order to carry out the Visible Living Human, MR images of a male adult, a female adult, and a male child are acquired and image processing is done as follows.

By utilizing MR scanning technique of the VKH, whole bodies of living humans were scanned by MR. The whole body of an adult can not be MR scanned at once. Through the experience from VKH, the first MR series from head to knees and the second MR series from knees to toes were scanned separately. Subsequently, both MR series were combined and aligned. Living humans' organs move contrary to cadaver, thus new technique was utilized for the Visible Living Human:.To minimize bowel movement, the volunteers had been starved for 12 hours prior to MR scanning. To compensate heart movement, electrocardiography sensor was attached. To compensate lung movement, lung movement sensor was worn by the volunteers. As a result, 613 MR images of male adult, 557 images of female adult, and 384 MR images of male child were acquired at 3 mm intervals (Fig. 2a,c,d) [8, 9].

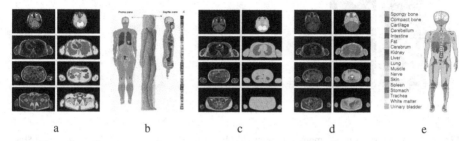

a   b   c   d   e

Fig. 2. MR and segmented images of male adult (a) [8], female adult (c) [9], and male child (d). 3D images of male adult (b) [6] and male child (e) with the color bar which indicates the segmented structures.

Through the same segmentation technique, anatomic structures in MR images were segmented. The Adobe Photoshop was adequate for segmentation not only in anatomic images (24 bits color) but also in MR images (8 bits gray). Yet MR images did not show definite anatomic structures, so that more knowledge of anatomists and radiologists was necessary for segmentation process. In the Visible Living Human, segmentation of the anatomic structures was performed, whose absorptance of electromagnetic wave is quite different, with 47 structures in male adult, 19 structures in female adult (segmentation in process), and 33 structures in male child (Fig. 2a,c,d) [6, 8, 9].

The segmented images of male adult were stacked and volume-reconstructed to produce 3D images of 47 structures. Electromagnetic wave was exposed on the 3D images in various ways to calculate influences of the electromagnetic wave on internal structures. In the same manner, the exposing simulation is being performed using the 3D images of the male child (Fig. 2b,e) [6]. In addition, the segmented images of male adult were stacked and surface-reconstructed to produce 3D images. A software on which the 3D images can be selected and rotated was produced for medical education [8].

2.3 Application of VKH Technique for Visible Mouse

Mouse anatomy is a fundamental knowledge for researchers who perform biomedical experiments with mice. So far the mouse anatomy has been educated through two dimensional images such as atlas, thus being difficult to be comprehended, especially the stereoscopic morphology of the mouse. In order to overcome this difficulty, it is necessary to produce 3D images made of Visible Mouse [12].

Through serial sectioning and photographing technique of the VKH, anatomic images of a mouse were obtained. The cryomacrotome with only 1 um error was designed for serial sectioning of any organism smaller than human. Using the cryomacrotome, a mouse was serially sectioned at 0.5 mm intervals to make sectioned surfaces. Every sectioned surface was photographed using a digital camera to produce 437 anatomic images. Distance between the sectioned surface and the digital camera could be adjusted closely to generate anatomic images with 0.1 mm pixel size. During photographing, the strobe light was flashed in the same condition to produce anatomic images with consistent brightness (Fig. 3) [10, 12].

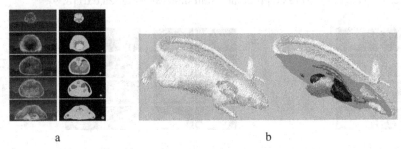

a   b

Fig. 3. Anatomic images, segmented images (a) [12], and 3D images (b) of the mouse with skin and internal structures

By practicing the same segmentation technique, 14 mouse structures in the anatomic images were segmented. The rodent structures were so small that exhaustive knowledge of mouse anatomy referred to mouse atlas was necessary for the segmentation process [5, 12]. From the segmented images, contours of the mouse structures were stacked on Alias™ Maya (version 7.0); stacked contours were volume-reconstructed on Autodesk™ AutoCAD (version 2007) (Fig. 3).

2.4 Application of VKH Data for Sectional Anatomy Education

Sectional anatomy is the course to learn anatomic structures on the sectional planes. The sectional anatomy has become much more important especially because medical students have to interpret MR and CT images. Because of the growing importance of sectional anatomy, browsing software of the VKH data was created. Raw data of the browsing software were 1,702 sets of MR, CT, anatomic, and segmented images (1 mm intervals) of the whole body. On the browsing software, a set of four images corresponding to one another was displayed. Different sets of images could be selected conveniently using graphic user interface. Names of the segmented structures in all images were also displayed. Among a set of four images, any image could be enlarged. The browsing software can be downloaded free of charge from our web site (anatomy.co.kr) (Fig. 4) [11].

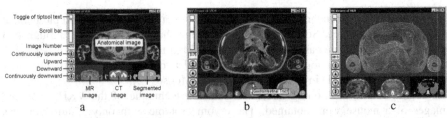

a   b   c

Fig. 4. Browsing software showing four images and graphic user interface (a), name of structure in CT image (b), and enlarged MR image (c) [11]

2.5 Application of VKH Data for Virtual Dissection (Volume-Reconstruction)

As the traditional method in educating anatomy, cadaver dissection is exceptionally important, but the cadaver dissection with time and place restriction can not be performed commonly. The problem can be compensated by virtual dissection. For the virtual dissection, volume-reconstruction was carried out primarily to produce 3D images out of the VKH data because volume-reconstruction enables users to section 3D images of structures with the same color as that of real-life human structures [14].

Virtual dissection software of whole body was created at Inha University, Korea. For this research, basic segmented images of 13 structures and corresponding anatomic images were used as materials. As the preprocess, intervals and pixel size of the anatomic and segmented images were increased from 0.2 mm to 1.0 mm because original image files were too large to be processed on a personal computer. Anatomic and segmented images were stacked and volume-reconstructed on Microsoft^{TM} Visual C++ (version 6.0) to produce 3D images. On programmed virtual dissection software, the 3D images with real color could be sectioned, selected, and rotated (Fig. 5a) [10].

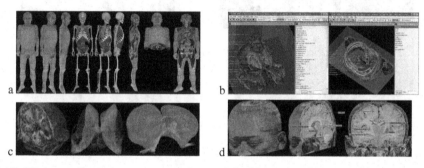

Fig. 5. 3D images by volume-reconstruction at Inha University, Korea (a) [10], University Medical Center Hamburg-Eppendorf, Germany (b), State University of New York at Stony Brook, US (c), and Texas Tech University, US (d)

Virtual dissection software of head and neck was produced at University Medical Center Hamburg-Eppendorf, Germany. For this research, advanced segmented images of 104 structures in head and neck were used as materials. Voxel-Man system was used for segmentation refinement and for volume-reconstruction [14]. On the virtual dissection software, the 3D images with real color could be stripped in sequence. The 3D images could be selected to display by names of structures. The 3D images could also be annotated. In the same manner, virtual dissection software of thorax including heart components was created (Fig. 5b). Additional virtual dissection software of head is being created at other institutes such as State University of New York at Stony Brook (Fig. 5c), Texas Tech University (Fig. 5d), Stanford University Medical Media & Information Technologies, Pittsburgh Supercomputing Center, and Upperairway Company, US, as well as in MAÂT3D, France.

2.6 Application of VKH Data for Virtual Dissection (Surface-Reconstruction)

After the trial of volume-reconstruction, surface-reconstruction was tried with segmented images of the VKH to produce 3D images of structures with outstandingly small file size. The surface-reconstructed 3D images can be selected to display, rotate, and transform themselves in real time. In addition, the 3D images can be easily distributed through the Internet [17].

3D images of urogenital tract were made by surface-reconstruction at University Paris V René Descartes, France. Contours of 42 structures including urogenital tract, its neighboring bones, arteries, and skin were stacked and surface-reconstructed using SURFdriver software to produce 3D images. The 3D images could be manipulated individually or in-group with the 3D images' transparency adjusted (Fig. 6a) [17]. Additionally by surface-reconstruction, 3D images of skull and 3D images of lower limb bones were made at University Malaya, Malaysia (Fig. 6b) and at Konrad-Zuse-Zentrum für Information Stechnik, Germany (Fig. 6c), respectively.

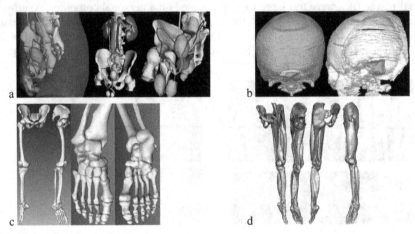

Fig. 6. 3D images by surface-reconstruction of University Paris V René Descartes, France (a) [17], University Malaya, Malaysia (b), Konrad-Zuse-Zentrum für Information Stechnik, Germany (c), and Ajou University, Korea (d) [15]

We tried to produce 3D images of left lower limb by surface-reconstruction on Maya and Rhino, which are both popular commercial software. Contours of 114 structures in left lower limb were stacked on Maya; gaps between contours were filled with non-uniform rational B-spline (NURBS) surfaces on Rhino; all NURBS surfaces were converted into polygon ones on Rhino; the surfaces were corrected to complete the 3D images on Maya. In this manner, surface-reconstruction can be done on the popular and commonly used software to produce 3D images in the Maya file format, thus be widely used by other researchers (Fig. 6d) [15].

2.7 Application of VKH Data for Virtual eEndoscopy

Virtual colonoscopy of a patient is becoming popular in diagnosing colon cancer. However, the virtual colonoscopy being based on the CT images, colon wall can not be displayed in real color. In the VKH, lumen of colon had been segmented. The anatomic and segmented images were stacked and volume-reconstructed to produce 3D image of colon wall's luminal surface, which held real color. Based on the 3D image, virtual colonoscopy was performed at Inha University, Korea. The virtual colonoscopy with real color was similar to real colonoscopy, so that educational effect could be enhanced. In the same manner virtual bronchoscopy and virtual arterioscopy were performed with the VKH data (Fig. 7) [13].

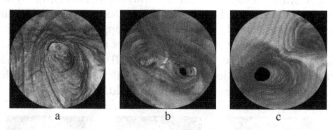

a   b   c

Fig. 7. Virtual colonoscopy (a), virtual bronchoscopy (b), and virtual arterioscopy (c) [13]

2.8   Application of VKH Data for Radiation Simulation

Just as Visible Living Human data were used for exposing simulation of electromagnetic wave, VKH data were used for radiation simulation at Hanyang University, Korea. The raw data from VKH were the segmented images of 22 structures at 2 mm intervals. The segmented images were stacked and volume-reconstructed to produce 3D images. Then the 3D images were exposed by broad parallel photon beams in various ways to calculate effects of radiation on each structure. These results could be used to prevent workmen in radiation-polluted environment from receiving radiation damage [4].

3   Discussion

Various applications performed with the VKH technique and data have been described. In discussion, further potential applications to be performed in the future are presented.

Segmented images of the VKH will be acquired to completion. For the VKH, it required a day and three months only to obtain MR images and anatomic images, respectively. Then it required three years to obtain segmented images of 317 structures (Fig. 1). Nevertheless, segmentation has not been finished yet [9, 10, 13]. It will take three more years to finish segmentation of the whole body. Three years later, the segmented images accompanied by corresponding anatomic images will be distributed worldwide free of charge. It is anticipated that other researchers reform some incorrect segmented images and make more detailed segmented images for their own purposes. In any case, the segmented images, which will be finished by authors, are expected to save precious time and effort of other researchers.

Female data of the VKH will be acquired. The female data, which are later than male data, need to be upgraded as follows. The female cadaver for the VKH needs to be of young age, good body contour, and with few pathologic findings. Anatomic images of whole body need to have 0.1 mm intervals, 0.1 mm pixel size, and 48 bits color depth. It seems that 0.1 mm voxel size of anatomic images is the last trial in this research, which belongs to gross anatomy. Additionally, the female data are desirable to be followed by the child data, fetus data, and embryo data. The systematic data according to sex and developmental age will be the main contents in the medical image library [10, 13].

Visible head data including 7.0 Tesla MR images will be made. State-of-the-art 7.0 Tesla MR scanner has been developed by Professor Zang-Hee Cho in Neuroscience Research Institute of Gachon University, Korea [3]. By using the 7.0 Tesla MR scanner, a cadaver's head were MR scanned recently. Surprisingly, several structures of brain (for example, cerebral arteries) appeared better in the MR images than in the anatomic images of VKH while the other structures appeared better in the anatomic images (Fig. 8). The cadaver's head will be serially sectioned to obtain anatomic images in correspondence to the MR images. These Visible Head data are expected to be milestone images in neuroscience field.

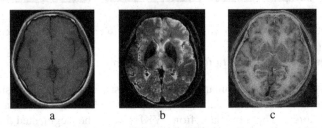

a   b   c

Fig. 8. 1.5 Tesla MR image with T1 (a), 7.0 Tesla MR image with T2 (b), and anatomic image (c)

Visible Patient data will be acquired by registration of the VKH data to a patient's data. For example, MR images of a patient are produced. Anatomic images of the VKH are transformed, thus be corresponding to the MR images of the patient. For the transformation, high level of registration technique and segmented images of VKH will be utilized. The anatomic images registered to the patient have color information and high resolution. Therefore, anatomic images can be used in production of realistic 3D images, which will be the basis for preoperative virtual surgery of the patient [7].

Pregnant female data of the Visible Living Human will be made. MR images of male adult, female adult, and male child have been scanned (Fig. 2) [8, 9]. Likewise, MR images of pregnant female will be scanned, including fetus images. The pregnant female data will be used for the exposing simulation of electromagnetic wave too [6].

Visible Rat data and Visible Dog data will be made. Like the Visible Mouse (Fig. 3) [12], Visible Rat and Visible Dog can be performed for biomedical experiment and veterinarian education by using the same cryomacrotome of VKH. In order to make better images than other Visible Rat [1] and other Visible Dog [2], micro MR machine and micro CT machine will be used for the rat; high level of serial sectioning and detail segmentation will be tried for both the rat and the dog.

In this report, our ideas from experiences to apply the VKH technique and data have been introduced. By applying the VKH technique, other images such as Visible Living Human (Fig. 2) [6, 8]. Visible Mouse (Fig. 3) [12] can be created; by applying the VKH data, sectional anatomy (Fig. 4) [11], virtual dissection (Figs. 5, 6) [9, 10, 17], virtual endoscopy (Fig. 7) [13], radiation simulation [4], and Visible Patient can be performed. Based on this report and the distributed VKH data, other researchers are expected to make better images and more progressive applications for use at medical education and clinical practice.

References

1. Bai, X., Yu, L., Liu, Q., Zhang, J., Li, A., Han, D., Luo, Q., Gong, H.: A high-resolution anatomical rat atlas. J. Anat. 209, 707–708 (2006)
2. Böttcher, P., Maierl, J.: Macroscopic cryosectioning. A simple new method for producing digital, three dimensional database in veterinary anatomy. Anat. Histol. Embryol. 28, 97–102 (1999)
3. Cho, Z.H., Jones, J.P., Singh, M.: Foundations of medical imaging. Wiley, New York (1993)
4. Choi, S.H., Lee, C.S., Cho, S.K., Chung, M.S., Na, S.H., Kim, C.H.: Construction of a high-definition 'Reference Korean' voxel phantom for organ and tissue radiation dose calculation. In: Proceedings WC 2006 Conf., pp. 4061–4064 (2006)
5. Iwaki, T., Yamashita, H., Hayakawa, T.: A color atlas of sectional anatomy of the mouse, Maruzen Co. LTD, Tokyo (2001)
6. Lee, A.K., Choi, W.Y., Chung, M.S., Choi, H.D., Choi, J.I.: Development of Korean male body model for computational dosimetry. ETRI J. 28, 107–110 (2006)
7. Li, L., Liu, Y.X., Song, Z.J.: Three-dimensional reconstruction of registered and fused Chinese Visible Human and patient MRI Images. Clin. Anat. 19, 225–231 (2006)
8. Lee, Y.S., Chung, M.S., Park, J.S., Hwang, S.B., Cho, J.H.: Three dimensional MRI and software for studying normal anatomical structures of an entire body. J. Korean Soc. Magn. Reson. Med. 9, 117–133 (2005)
9. Park, J.S., Chung, M.S., Hwang, S.B., Lee, Y.S., Har, D.H.: Technical report on semiautomatic segmentation using the Adobe Photoshop. J. Digit. Imaging 18, 333–343 (2005)
10. Park, J.S., Chung, M.S., Hwang, S.B., Lee, Y.S., Har, D.H., Park, H.S.: Visible Korean Human. Improved serially sectioned images of the entire body. IEEE Trans. Med. Imaging 24, 352–360 (2005)
11. Park, J.S., Chung, M.S., Choe, H., Byun, H.Y., Hwang, J., Shin, B.S., Park, H.S.: Serially sectioned images of the whole body (Sixth report: Browsing software of the serially sectioned images for learning sectional anatomy). Korean J. Anat. 39, 35–45 (2006)
12. Park, J.S., Chung, M.S., Hwang, S.B.: Serially sectioned and segmented images of the mouse for learning mouse anatomy. Korean J. Anat. 39, 305–312 (2006)
13. Park, J.S., Chung, M.S., Hwang, S.B., Shin, B.S., Park, H.S.: Visible Korean Human: Its techniques and applications. Clin. Anat. 19, 216–224 (2006)
14. Pommert, A., Höhne, K.H., Pflesser, B., Richter, E., Riemer, M., Schiemann, T., Schubert, R., Schumacher, U., Tiede, U.: Creating a high-resolution spatial/symbolic model of the inner organs based on the Visible Human. Med. Image. Anal. 5, 221–228 (2001)
15. Shin, D.S., Chung, M.S., Park, J.S.: Technique of the semi-automatic surface reconstruction of Visible Korean Human data on the commercial software. In: Proceedings SPIE Medical Imaging 2007 Conf. (in press, 2007)
16. Spitzer, V.M., Ackerman, M.J., Scherzinger, A.L., Whitlock, D.G.: The Visible Human Male: A technical report. J. Am. Med. Inform. Assoc. 3, 118–130 (1996)
17. Uhl, J.F., Park, J.S., Chung, M.S., Delmas, V.: Three-dimensional reconstruction of urogenital tract from Visible Korean Human. Anat. Rec. A Discov. Mol. Cell. Evol. Biol. 288, 893–899 (2006)
18. Zhang, S.X., Heng, P.A., Liu, Z.J.: Chinese Visible Human Project. Clin. Anat. 19, 204–215 (2006)

Preliminary Application of
the First Digital Chinese Human

Yuan Yuan, Lina Qi, and Shuqian Luo

College of Biomedical Engineering, Capital Medical University,
100069 Beijing P.R. China
yuanyuan1129@gmail.com

Abstract. A great deal of work has been attempted and accomplished based on VCH-F1 (the No.1 Virtual Chinese Human-Female) dataset these years. So far, the anatomic structures of the whole body have been 3D reconstructed and a varieties of further work such as health science education facilities, virtual acupuncture, image-guided neurosurgery, motion simulation etc. have also been developed and preliminarily implemented. In this paper, we will describe the application study of VCH-F1 dataset in our laboratory.

1 Introduction

Human body is a large complex system composed a hundred trillions cells. Though science and technology nowadays are developing fast, people still know little about themselves.

In 1994, the Visible Human Project (VHP) was established by the National Library of Medicine (NLM) [1] in USA. In 1994 and 1995, the first male and female dataset were published by the Health Sciences Center of the University of Colorado [2]. In March 2001, an anatomical cross-sectional image dataset of a male Korean (Visible Korea Human, VKH) was established by Anjou University in Korea and Korea Institute of Science and Technology Information successfully [3]. In November, 2001, the Chinese Digital Human research started with the support of National "863" Development Project of High-Tech Research [4, 5]. The data acquisition of the No.1 Virtual Chinese Human-Female (VCH-F1) was completed in February 2003 by Southern Medical University. The dataset was then sent to Medical Image Laboratory (MIL) in Capital Medical University for further process.

Much work has been attempted and accomplished based on VCH-F1 dataset these years. The anatomic structures and the major organs are segmented and 3D rendered. All these structures could be viewed independently or in combination. Based on this work, a variety of further applications have also been developed and preliminarily implemented for instance education facilities, virtual acupuncture, image-guided neurosurgery, motion simulation etc..

In this paper, we will describe the application study of VCH-F1 dataset and illustrate some related work of our laboratory.

X. Gao et al. (Eds.): MIMI 2007, LNCS 4987, pp. 252–261, 2008.

2 Early Works on Virtual Chinese Human-Female

The VCH-F1 dataset was acquired in Southern Medical University. The cadaver was CT scanned with the section thickness of 1.0 mm and 1718 serial images were obtained. It was MR scanned with the section thickness of 2.0 mm and 801 serial images were obtained. The specimen was then frozen at -70 ℃ and cryomacrotomed into 8556 slices. The thickness of each section is 0.2mm. Every slice was image captured with digital camera and the total dataset amounts to 149.7GB [6]. The parameters of CT, MR and anatomical images are shown in Table 1.

Table 1. Main parameters of VCH-F1 dataset

Items	Anatomic sections	CT	MRI
Sections	8556	1718	801
Section thickness	0.2 mm	1 mm	2 mm
Resolution	3024×2016	512×512	512×512
Data size	149.2GB	429.5MB	200.5 MB

The image preprocessing of VCH-F1 dataset includes image registration, background removal, image segmentation and 3D reconstruction [7]. Because of the size of the large data, it is extremely difficult to finish all the work with PC and traditional manual method. High realistic visualization of large dataset is of great importance and has raised the need of development of visualization methodology.

A series of visualization methods suitable for the large VCH-F1 dataset have been developed in MIL and brought us with approving results. Before the specimen was frozen, four fiducial markers were located in embedding agency to facilitate image registration. We designed a semi-automatic registration approach. Step1: Use rigid transform and shortest distance method to do coarse registration. Step2: Smooth the mark lines with a low-pass filter. Step3: Use affine transform to do precise registration. Powell method was used in this step as optimization algorithm. After image registration was finished, we implemented image segmentation in three steps. Step1: Convert the color space from RGB to HSI and complete the automatic segmentation. Step2: Improve the results with mathematical morphological operation. Step3: Do manual adjustment in case the auto method failed to segment some details. After all the steps above were completed, the dataset was normalized and ready for 3D visualization. Fig.1 shows an image browser produced in our lab. The upper left axial view is the normalized data while the upper right coronal view and lower left sagittal view is rendered from the normalized data in real-time. The lower right picture is from the CT data of VCH-F1. Besides traditional surface and volume rendering methods, we developed a new hybrid render method, which rendered surface from volume data. To improve the realism effect without much computational expense of the model, texture mapping is also introduced. The goal was to achieve high-resolution visualization of VCH-F1 dataset. Fig. 2 shows some 3D visualization results. So far, almost all the main anatomical structures of the whole body were segmented and reconstructed. Table 3 lists all the structure contained in our VCH-F1 3D model.

Table 2. Reconstructed anatomical structures of VCH-F1

Anatomical Structures	Components
Skin	
Bones	Skull, sternum, spine, ribs, clavicles, scapulas, humeri, radiuses, ulnas, palm bones, hip bones, femurs, patellae, fibulas, tibias, feet
Muscles	Temporalis, semispinalis capitis, splenius capitis, sternocleidomastoid , orbicularis oculi, orbicularis oris, masseter, levator labil superioris, latissmus dorsi, rhomboideus, teres major/minor, obliquus internus abdominis, obliquus externus abdominis, rectus abdominis, superaspinatus, infraspinatus, subscapularis, serratus anterior, erector spinae, trapezius, pectoralis major/minor, psoas major, biceps brachii, brachialis, triceps brachii, coracobrachialis, deltoid, branchioradialis, flexor carpi ulnaris, flexor pollicis longus, extensor carpi radialis longus&brevis, flexor carpi radialis, extensor digiti minimi, pronator teres, flexor digitorum superficialis/ profundus, extensor digitorum, anconeus, dorsal interossei, flexor pollicis brevis, abductor pollicis brevis, adductor pollicis, semitendinosus, semimembranosus, adductor longus, adductor magnus, sartorius, gracilis, quadriceps femoris, gluteus maximus, soleus, gastrocnemius, peroneus longus, flexor hallucis longus, tibialis posterior/ anterior, extensor digitorum longus, extensor hallucis longus
Brain	Cerebrum, cerebellum, brain stem, lateral ventricle, caudate nucleus, lentiform nucleus
Heart	Pericardium, ventricles
Spleen	
Urinary system	Kidneys, urinary bladder
Respiratory system	Lungs, Trachea, principal bronchi
Digestive system	Esophagus, stomach, liver, gallbladder, pancreas, intestine
Reproductive system	Uterus, ovaries, oviducts, folliculus
Arteries and veins	Ascending aorta, thoracic aorta, abdominal aorta, renal artery, femoral artery, obturator artery, superior vena cava, inferior vena cava, femoral vein, hepatic veins, renal veins

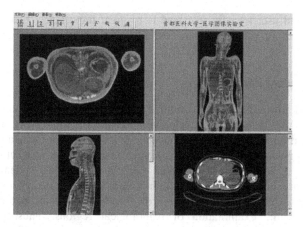

Fig. 1. Normalized dataset suited for 3D visualization was obtained after pre-processing of the raw images

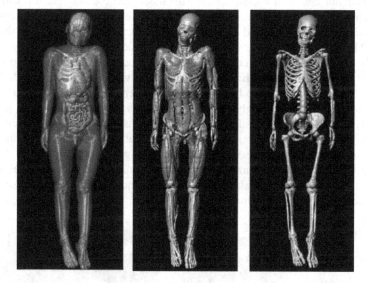

Fig. 2. Reconstruction of the main anatomical structures of VCH-F1, including the structures of organs (*left*), muscles (*middle*) and skeleton (*right*)

3 Applications

Virtual reality applications offer the possibility to visualize three-dimensional images, giving users the impression of real spatial perception [8]. Medical and biological applications of virtual reality technology serve a wide range of basic research, educational, diagnostic and surgical planning purposes [9]. In most of the medical applications, especially in education and training programs, models of the human anatomy usually play the main role. Thus the laborious model generation and refinement in visualization are necessary. Besides, human–computer interaction had to be achieved, and user-friendly interface is of great importance. Our applications of anatomical structure offered by the VCH-F1 3D model will be described in the following sections.

3.1 Health Science Education

Traditionally, knowledge about the human body is represented in books and atlases. Since 1990s, high IT technology development has allowed more powerful and versatile computer-based representations of knowledge [9]. Apart from the health information, the use of computer technology may provide an alternative instructional mode for health science teaching and learning. With the help of this atlas, students might obtain knowledge more efficiently. Further more, immersion into a virtual environment facilitates the exploration of a scene of three-dimensional medical objects or tomograms and the examination of pathological regions. Thus, physicians can recognize topological coherencies in a much faster and more natural way [10].

A 3D anatomy atlas based on Virtual Reality technology has been basically developed in our lab. In this atlas, not only the model representing general knowledge of gross anatomy is shown, with mouse click and movement, classical representations, such as pictures, movies, solid models and introductions could also be displayed (Fig. 3). The displaying mode, overall mode or specific mode, switches depending on the user's need. Under the overall mode, the surface model of the whole body is displayed. Any specific structure could be picked up with a single mouse click and a brief introduction of it will also be shown in the screen. Under the specific mode, the clicked structure is shown singly in full screen so as to facilitate users to get more details and a series of more detailed anatomical introduction will also be given.

Besides this, three health science education applications for popular health science teaching and learning were also developed including a slices browser of VCH-F1 dataset, a 3D skeleton jigsaw puzzle, and a demonstration of brain functional regions. These applications have been exhibited in China Science & Technology Museum, and gained visitors' universal acclaim.

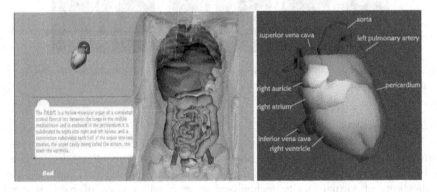

Fig. 3. Interfaces of the 3D atlas based on VCH-F1 under two displaying modes, the overall mode (*left*) and the specific mode (*right*)

3.2 Virtual Acupuncture

Acupuncture is an important aspect of Traditional Chinese Medicine. Because of its magic curative effect, simple operation, low cost, and few side effects, science of acupuncture has spread all over the world. An accurate description of the mechanism is quite necessary. The construction of the whole human dataset and the development of 3D visualization technology make it possible to integrate the traditional theory with modern medical information. An experiment was designed to explore it.

Based on the dataset of the female Virtual Chinese Human, serial axial images are marked according to the localization of acupuncture points in Chinese traditional medicine, and then a 3D atlas of acupuncture points and three meridian lines on lower limbs are marked.

The PET brain functional images of 7 normal subjects in the experiment shown that there are some excitation-enhanced regions and also some excitation-suppressive regions in the brain when Zu-San-Li (one of the most frequently used acupuncture points, and is also named STOMACH-36 or St 36) point was acupunctured. It explained that acupuncture may work by stimulating the central nervous system. Combined with 3D brain model, a demonstration was developed (Fig.4). In this demo, when Zu-San-Li (St 36) point was acupunctured, the excitation-enhanced and suppressive regions in brain were displayed in specific colors.

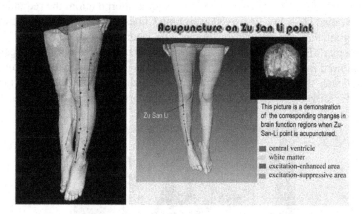

Fig. 4. The demonstration of virtual acupuncture on Zu-San-Li (*St 36*) point, which shows the Meridians on legs (*left*) and the reflection in brain regions when Zu-San-Li (*St 36*) point acupunctured (*right*)

3.3 Image Guided Neurosurgery

Image guided neurosurgery became indispensable over the last years. By using image guided technology, a neurosurgeon could preserve normal tissue while maximizing the resection of lesions during cortical surgery. Image Guided neurosurgery incorporates medical image process and analysis techniques, medical image 3D visualization techniques, modern robotics and modern medicine. Image guided neurosurgery strives to enhance the surgeon's capability to decrease the invasiveness of surgical procedures and increase their accuracy and safety. VCH-F1, as an integrated and detailed dataset of human body, offers us an opportunity in image-guided neurosurgery research.

A novel automatic segmentation algorithm for brain tissue segmentation was schemed out. This method integrates anisotropic diffusion filter, statistical threshold, mathematical morphological operations, fuzzy connectedness and geodesic active contour model (GACM). And we introduced a new idea for deformation driven by a Euclidean distance field of image edge in GACM. This method first generates a coarse segmentation of interest structure of brain using statistical threshold and mathematical morphology, and then refines the segmentation result using GACM driven by a Euclidean distance field of image edge. The algorithm was evaluated using Montreal Phantom Dataset of brain, and the results show that our method is effective and robust with random noise and intensity inhomogeneities existed.

Though VCH-F1 dataset includes detailed image data of the brain, as the specimen had no disease in brain, more pathological data is needed. It is generally recognized that the incorporation and effective utilization of MRA information in image guided surgery environment is very important [11]. To solve this problem, four MRA volume datasets from Navy General Hospital have been used to evaluate this algorithm.

For 3D reconstruction of labeled ROI data after segmentation, an improved Marching Cubes algorithm is presented. Only the boundary voxels are smoothed for surface normal calculation, this choice avoids using of Gaussian Filter in all image space. Using the edge flag buffer and point position interpolation, the redundant point storage is avoided [12]. The improved Marching Cubes algorithm has been practiced in the image-guided neurosurgery system of the neurosurgical department of Navy General Hospital, Beijing. Fig. 5 presents the visualization results of four vessel label datasets acquired from MRA images in which the conglobated blocked structures of the vessels indicate the location of cerebral hemorrhage, and such information is significant for surgeons while making surgical plan.

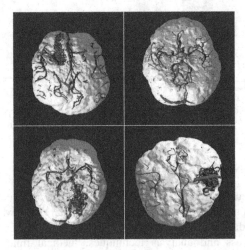

Fig. 5. Reconstruction of four vessel label datasets with the improved Marching Cubes algorithm, and the conglobated blocked vessels indicate cerebral hemorrhage

3.4 Motion Simulation

Physical Virtual Human is another step in the whole development of VCH-F1. Research on this regard has started in our lab recently. The motion of the 3D model is based on virtual skeleton, the controller of 3D model and different models have their respective controller. There are a variety of VR software and correlative technique to help us in research such as 3DSMax, Maya and Lightwave. We developed a motion simulation demo of the skeleton model of VCH-F1 with the software 3DSMax and Virtools Dev (Fig.6).

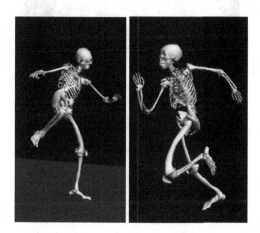

Fig. 6. Motion simulation of VCH-F1, including Chinese Kongfu (*left*) and running (*right*)

3.5 Other Application Works

3D Virtual Garment Design. Based on complete datasets of serial anatomical cross-sections, the digitalized virtual human can be used not only in medical science but also in 3D virtual garment design. Cross-section contours located at significant features (crotch, hips, waist, under bust, maximum bust) are extracted and cubic B-spline surfaces are then reconstructed interpolating points of these key contours. By texture-mapping images onto those parametric surfaces, virtual garments following the shape of the body can be directly obtained. Because B-splines are parametric and the surface is represented by a set of control points, further modification and deformation can be set freely.

Virtual Endoscopy. Virtual endoscopy (VE) describes a new method of diagnosis, using computer processing of 3D image datasets (such as those from CT or MRI scans) to provide simulated visualizations of patient-specific organs similar or equivalent to those produced by standard endoscopic procedures [14].

Conventional endoscope is invasive and often uncomfortable for patients and sometimes has serious side effects such as perforation, infection and hemorrhage. VE visualization avoids these risks and can minimize difficulties and decrease morbidity when used before actual endoscopic procedures. In addition, there are many body regions not suitable with real endoscope that can be explored with VE [13].

The VCH-F1 datasets allow us with good opportunity to set foot in this field. There are defects in the datasets that because the specimen dead of food-poison, clyster treatment made her intestines flat and virtual endoscopy will be very difficult from organs with so flat lacuna. However, most of the other organ models are available to practice this treatment. Fig.7. shows a flythrough in recta.

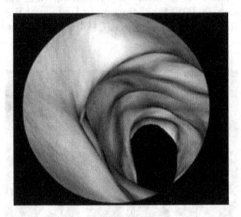

Fig. 7. A flythrough in the recta of VCH-F1

4 Summary

Based on previous work, a variety of applications including health science education facilities, virtual acupuncture, image-guided neurosurgery, motion simulation etc. have been developed and preliminarily implemented. All these are new technology of this time and with great significance. There are still large amount of works for us in these fields and as a good beginning has already been conducted, rapid progress will follow toward successful current solution and toward more vivid realization of the VCH-F1.

Acknowledgement

This research was supported by National "863" Development Project of High-Tech Research. The grant numbers are 2001AA231031 and 2002AA231021. We would like to thank Prof. Shizhen Zhong and his team for their excellent work on data acquisition of VCH-F1. Moreover, we express our acknowledgement to all the people involved in this project. It is their dedicated effort that makes the whole work possible.

References

1. Ackerman, M.J.: The Visible Human Project: A Resource for Education. Acad. Med. 74, 667–670 (1999)
2. Spizter, V., Ackerman, M.J., Scherzinger, A.L., et al.: The Visible Human Male: A Technical Report. J. Am. Med. Inform. Assoc. 3, 118-130 (1996)

3. Jin, S.P., Min, S., Ch., S.B.H., et al.: Visible Korean Human: Its Techniques and Applications. Clinical Anatomy 19, 216–224 (2006)
4. Zhong, S.Z., Li, H., Luo, S.Q., et al.: The Research of Chinese Digital Human. Xiangshan Science Conference 174, 4–12 (2001)
5. Zhong, S.Z., Li, H., Lin, Z.K., et al.: Digitized Virtual Human: Background and Meaning. China Basic Science 6, 12–16 (2002)
6. Zhong, S.Z., Yuan, L., et al.: Research Report of Experimental Database Establishment of Digitized Virtual Chinese No.1 Female. The Journal of First Military Medical University 23, 196–200, 209 (2003)
7. Du, G., Chai, H., Cao, H., Luo, S.: High Resolution Visualization of VCH-Female Dataset. In: Proceedings of SPE, vol. 5444, pp. 453–458 (2003)
8. Ellis, S.R.: What are virtual environments? IEEE Comp. Graph. Appl. 14, 17–22 (1994)
9. Camp, J.J., Cameron, B.M., Blezek, D., Robb, R.A.: Virtual Reality in Medicine and Biology. Future Generation Computer Systems 14, 91–108 (1998)
10. Krapichler, C., Haubner, M., Engelbrecht, R., Englmeier, K.-H.: VR Interaction Techniques for Medical Imaging Applications. Computer Methods and Programs in Biomedicine 56, 65–74 (1998)
11. Shattuck, D.W., Sandor-Leahy, S.R., Leahy, R.M., et al.: Magnetic Resonance Image Tissue Classification Using a Partial Volume Model. Volume Visualization of Magnetic Resonance Angiography. IEEE Comput. Graphics Appl. 12, 12–13 (1992)
12. Dale, A.M., Fischl, B., Sereno, M.I.: Cortical Surface-Based Analysis I. Segmentation and Surface Reconstruction. NeuroImage 9, 179–194 (1999)
13. Robb, R.A.: Virtual Endoscopy: Development and Evaluation Using the Visible Human Datasets. Computerized Medical Imaging and Graphics 24, 133–151 (2000)
14. Hajnal, J.V., et al.: A Registration and Interpolation Procedure for Subvoxel Matching of Serially Acquired MR Images. Comput. Assist. Tomog. 19, 289–296 (1995)

3D Head Reconstruction and Color Visualization of Chinese Visible Human

Fan Bao[1], Yankui Sun[1], Xiaolin Tian[2], and Zesheng Tang[1,2]

[1] Department of Computer Science and Technology, Tsinghua University,
Beijing 100084, P.R. China
[2] Faculty of Information Technology, Macau University of Science and Technology,
Macao, S.A.R.
syk@tsinghua.edu.cn

Abstract. Since visible human visualization using cryosection images is still a challenge for its own difficulties such as color inhomogeneity between adjacent images, most visible human visualizations use pseudo color. In this paper, we propose a method to make cross-section image along human surface homogeneous, and provide a method to reconstruct and visualize 3D visible human with an approximate and reasonable real surface color. The visualization method consists of three components, which are preprocessing (registering image series, obtaining color checkers' color and removing background), color correction (global color correction with the help of the color checker and local color correction by using adjacent image) and 3D visualization with color (smoothing model and generating color). The experiment on head data of Chinese Visible Human shows that our method is successful for the 3D reconstruction and color visualization.

Keywords: Color Correction, Homogenization, Human Visualization, Segmentation, Chinese Visible Human.

1 Introduction

Human visualization, which processes and reconstructs human's 3D graphics from thousands of human medical section images, is one of a world frontier cross discipline of information technology and medicine. The section images include CT, MRI or other grayscale image traditionally. Chinese Visible Human dataset (CVH), with world leading high precision, contains not only these grayscale images, but also color cryosection images. Because of the color inhomogenity of the cryosection images, 3D colored reconstruction and visualization of CVH is very difficult. To the best of our knowledge, most of visualization results, including National Library of Medicine's Visible Human Male and Chinese Digital Human Girl No. 1, use pseudo-color.

Color inhomogenity of cryosection images is resulted from two main reasons: one is the variation of light and camera condition, and the other is that the human organ or tissue's color may vary between different images because of the

X. Gao et al. (Eds.): MIMI 2007, LNCS 4987, pp. 262–269, 2008.
© Springer-Verlag Berlin Heidelberg 2008

irregular oxidation[1,2]. In order to generate 3D colored visualization results from CVH, color correction is required before reconstruction. [1] provides a method of homogenization to make cross-section image along depth axis homogeneous. In this paper, we propose a method to make cross-section image along human surface homogeneous. The 3D colored visualization of CVH is also provided.

2 Method

Here, a novel 3D colored reconstruction and visualization method is developed. It consists of the following three components: 1) Preprocessing: registering image series, obtaining color checkers' color and removing background; 2) Color correction: global color correction with the help of the color checker and local color correction by using adjacent image; 3) 3D visualization with color: smoothing model and extracting color.

2.1 Preprocessing

The preprocessing includes registering image, obtaining color checkers' color, and segmenting background.

For each cryosection image, there lie four marks, a color checker and a ruler, as illustrated in Fig. 1(a). With the help of the four marks on each cryosection image, we can register the image series correctly. Color checker's color, which is called as recorded color here, can be obtained manually from each cryosection image, as shown in Fig. 1(a). This information will be used in the following global color correction step.

In [3], we have proposed an automatic method to segment background of an image. The algorithm uses differences between color components to distinguish background from foreground. It can get good segmented results for most cryosection images, as depicted in Fig. 1(b).

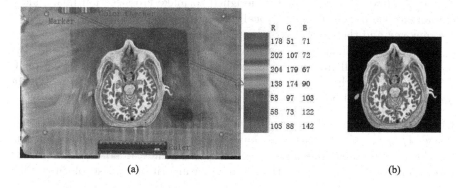

(a)   (b)

Fig. 1. (a) An example of cryosection color. The color checker's colors are also listed. (b) The result after segmentation.

However, the automatic segmentation algorithm is not always accurate. Thus, we need to adjust some segmentation results manually in certain cases so as to get good 3D colored reconstruction.

2.2 Global Correction by Color Checker

The objective of global correction is to correct the colors of cryosection images by color checker. Standard color checkers are put on every image during image acquirement of CVH. As mentioned above, for every image, its recorded color can be obtained. One representative color checker from all the images has been selected as reference color checker, which will be used as the standard color in global color correction.

The color checker of Chinese Visible Human data has its own feature, i.e., the hue of the colors on the checker covers the whole range, while the brightness is limited in a small range. Thus, we develop the following algorithm to determine the transformation from the reference color checker's colors and the recorded ones of each image, which will be used for correction later.

For each image, convert RGB values of recorded colors on the checker into HSV values. Denote the recorded colors as (H_i, S_i, V_i) $(1 \leq i \leq 7)$ and reference ones as $(H^r{}_i, S^r{}_i, V^r{}_i)$. The transformation between H and H^r can be determined by lookup table and interpolation method[4], and linear transformation between V and V^r can be obtained by least square fitting.

For each pixel in the image, by using above transformation on H and V (S will not be changed), we can get its corrected HSV. Thus, the image can be corrected when all its pixels have been adjusted.

After all the images have been global color corrected, colors of different images will be homogeneous in whole.

2.3 Local Correction by Histogram

A new local correction method is designed to make cross-section image along human surface homogeneous by local histogram when the images' background are removed and the colors have been global corrected.

To describe the method more clearly, this section will be divided into two parts. First, we will introduce how to correct one image with the help of its adjacent image in the series. Next, the order of the local correction for all the images in series will be discussed.

Correct one image. For every image I_i, it is corrected by one of its adjacent images I_j $(j = i \pm 1)$ to make the colors of the two images' edges homogeneous. For this purpose, we design a new algorithm, whose most important feature is to process only pixels on and near their edges. The algorithm consists of three steps:

Step1. For each point on the edge of I_i, find its corresponding point on the edge of I_j along the normal direction of the edge point on I_i, as shown in Fig. 2; these two points compose a point pair.

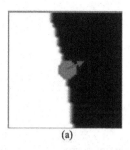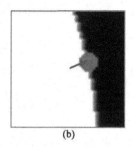

(a)   (b)

Fig. 2. The method to find the corresponding point. The white regions stand for the foreground, while the black regions mean the background. The red point in (a) is an original point on the edge of I_i, and its corresponding point on the edge of I_j is the red point in (b), which is found along the normal direction denoted as blue arrow.

Step2. In the foregrounds of I_i and I_j, more point pairs near their edges are found level by level, as illustrated in Fig. 3. These points are required by local histogram in next step and color generation in section 2.4, so they also need to be homogenized.

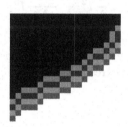

Fig. 3. Example of finding pixels near an edge. The gray pixels are the pixels on the edge, which are in the first level. The blue, green and red pixels near the edge are in the 2, 3 and 4 level accordingly.

Step3. For the point pairs of I_i and I_j obtained in above steps, calculate their local difference image and the histogram of the difference image for RGB components. In this histogram, the inhomogeneity that we need to reduce can be considered as a small shift of peak from 0 (err). Thus, a partial correction of amount $a \cdot err$ can be made on this point on $I_i[1]$, that is, $u' = u - a \cdot err$, where u, u' stand for one of the RGB components of the pixel before and after correction(Fig. 4).

Correct image series. Here we discuss the sequence of local color correction for all the images in series. The image series will be processed for three passes, that is, each slice will be corrected by its adjacent slice three times, as depicted in Fig. 5. In the first pass, an image with relatively high quality in the middle part of the series is selected as a seed image I_s. Then, the color correction is done in two directions: from I_s to I_0(the first image), which means that we first

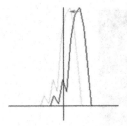

Fig. 4. Color correction by local histogram. A partial correction from blue to pink is needed in local color correction.

correct I_{s-1} with its adjacent image I_s, then correct I_{s-2} with I_{s-1}, and so on; and from I_s to I_{N-1}(the last image), which means that we first correct I_{s+1} with I_s, then correct I_{s+2} with I_{s+1}, and so on. The second pass is performed from I_0 to I_{N-1} while the third pass is from I_{N-1} to I_0. These passes both use the result of the image series after the first pass. Thus, two image series are obtained, and the final corrected image series is their weighted average

$$I_i = \frac{i}{N}I^2{}_i + \frac{N-i}{N}I^3{}_i .$$ (1)

In (1), i is the index of an image and its range is from 0 to $N-1$; I_i stands for the ith final corrected image, while $I^2{}_i$ and $I^3{}_i$ means the ith corrected images in the second and the third pass respectively.

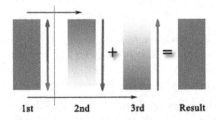

1st   2nd   3rd   Result

Fig. 5. Diagram of three passes. The first pass goes from a seed image in the middle part of the image series to the two ends. The second and the third pass both use the correction results of the first pass, and they process from one end to another. The ”+” and ”=” indicate that the final correction result is the weighted average of last two passes' result. The weight is indicated by grayscale.

2.4   Visualization

After color correction, we have got a set of homogeneous images without background. Now we will use these images to reconstruct and visualize a colored model.

The model is reconstructed from a binary volume, which can be obtained from the segmentation result. If we extract isosurface from this binary volume by marching cube algorithm directly, aliasing artifacts will exist. So the algorithm proposed in [5] is used to get a smooth model. The algorithm takes input data as a set of constraints on a deformable surface that iteratively seeks to minimize its surface area, and thus reduce the aliasing artifacts when marching cube algorithm is applied here.

The last step is to generate the color for each vertex of the model. The easiest way is to use the nearest data's color. However, although the images have been homogenized, the nearest color may still be inhomogeneous, since the segmentation has some error more or less, and this slight error will infect the surface color significantly. Our study shows that using weighted average of neighbors' data color can give us a better visualization result. The weights ensure that the nearer data's color has more influence to the result. In our experiment, $5 \times 5 \times 5$ neighbors have been used to generate color.

3   Experiments and Results

The dataset of our experiment is from the head part of Chinese Visible Human. The dimension of each image is 3072×2048 pixels, and the distances between adjacent images are from 0.1mm to 1.0mm. After the background removal step, to accelerate our experiment, the data have been trimmed and resized to $512 \times 512 \times 425$ before the homogenization step and visualization step. The experiment results are shown in Fig. 6.

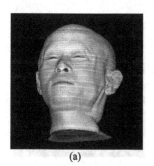 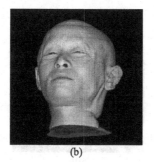 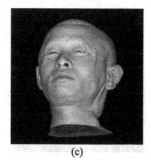

(a)   (b)   (c)

Fig. 6. 3D head model. (a) without color correction, (b) with global color correction, and (c) with both global and local color correction.

It is clearly that, without color homogenization, the head's color appears many layers, as shown in Fig. 6(a). After the process of global color correction, the layer structure weakens significantly as shown in Fig. 6(b). The final graphic in Fig. 6(c), where global and local color correction are done, gives us the best result of all. Compared with Fig. 6(b), the slight inhomogenity of horizontal layer is almost disappeared in Fig. 6(c). However, certain inhomogeneous are still hard to be eliminated, and most of them result from the inaccuracy of segmentation.

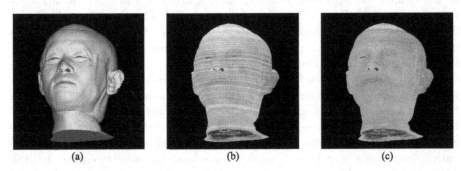

(a)   (b)   (c)

Fig. 7. 3D head model. (a) is the smoothed model with no color, (b) and (c) are the pure color before and after correction.

Fig. 7 illustrates the 3D head model without color. Fig. 7(a) shows that a high resolution head model can be reconstructed by our background removal method (Some flaws in the model, such as the one in the middle of nose, are due to some discontinuities in the cryosection images). Fig. 7(b) and (c) give only the color information to show the color correction result more clearly.

Note that if we do the experiment with the same cryosection images and the same processing algorithm but treat their distance between image slices as equal other than the real case mentioned above, the reconstructed head model will be different, as appeared in Fig. 8.

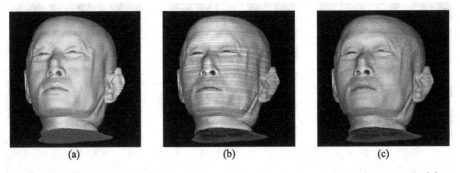

(a)   (b)   (c)

Fig. 8. 3D head model if distance between image slices are treated as equal. (a) is the smoothed model with no color, (b) and (c) are the color model before and after correction.

4   Conclusions and Future Work

On the basis of our automatic background removal for cryosection images, we propose a method to make cross-section image along human surface homogeneous, and provide a method to reconstruct and visualize 3D visible human with color. The experiments show that our method is effective.

Some future works to do include finding more accurate segmentation method, making the segmentation results of adjacent slices more homogenous, better color generation algorithm related to vertex's normal direction, hardware acceleration, and so on.

Acknowledgments. This work is supported by the National Nature Science Foundation of China (No. 30470487) and the National High Technology Research and Development Program of China (No. 2006AA02Z472). We would like to thank Prof. Shaoxiang Zhang, the principal of Chinese Visible Human Project Group, Third Military Medical University, China, for his providing us the experimental data.

References

1. Marquez, J., Schmitt, F.: Radiometric Homogenization of the Color Cryosection Images from the VHP Lungs for 3-D Segmentation of Blood Vessels. Computerized Medical Imaging and Graphics 24, 181–191 (2000)
2. Spitzer, V., Ackerman, M.J., Scherzinger, A.L., Whitlock, D.: The Visible Human Male: A Technical Report. Journal of the American Medical Informatics Association, 3(2), 118-30 (1996)
3. Zhao, Y., Tao, C., Tian, X., Tang, Z.: A New Segmentation Algorithm for the Visible Human Data. In: Proceedings of the 2005 IEEE, Engineering in Medicine and Biology 27th Annual Conference, pp. 1646–1649 (2005)
4. Hung, P.C.: Color Rendition Using Three-Dimensional Interpolation. In: Proc. SPIE: Imaging Applications in the Work World, pp. 111–115 (1988)
5. Whitaker, R.T.: Reducing Aliasing Artifacts in Iso-Surfaces of Binary Volumes. In: Proceedings of the 2000 IEEE Symposium on Volume Visualization, VVS 2000 (2000)

A Fast Method to Segment the Liver According to Couinaud's Classification

Shao-hui Huang, Bo-liang Wang, Ming Cheng, Wei-li Wu, Xiao-yang Huang, and Ying Ju

Computer Science Department, Xiamen University,
361005, Xiamen, Fujian, China
{hsh,blwang,chm,wwl,xyhuang,yju}@xmu.edu.cn

Abstract. For establishing a plan of Living Donor Liver Transplantation (LDLT), it is very important to estimate the volume of each liver segment. Usually Couinaud's classification is used to segment a liver, which is based on the liver anatomy. However, it is not easy to perform this method in a 3D space directly. In this paper, a fast segment method based on the hepatic vessel tree was proposed. This method was composed of four main steps: vasculature segmentation, 3D thinning, vascular tree pruning and classification, and vascular projection and curve fitting. This method was validated by application to a 3D liver from CT data, and it was shown to approximate closely Couinaud's classification with high speed.

Keywords: liver segment, Couinaud's classification, vessel tree, volumetric analysis.

1 Introduction

Nowadays liver surgery is a field in which computer-based operation planning has an enormous impact on the selection of a therapeutic strategy. For example before establishing a plan of Living Donor Liver Transplantation (LDLT), a computer must estimate the volume of each liver segment automatically. Usually Couinaud's classification is used to segment a liver[1], which is base on the liver anatomy and divides the liver into eight functionally independent segments, as shown in Fig.1.

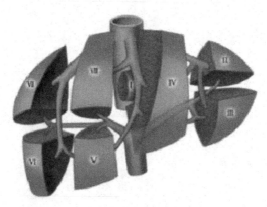

Fig. 1. Segmental anatomy according to Couinaud

X. Gao et al. (Eds.): MIMI 2007, LNCS 4987, pp. 270–276, 2008.

In this classification, each of segments has its own vascular inflow, outflow, and biliary drainage. Because of this division into self-contained units, each segment can be resected without damaging those remaining. In a LPLT, for the liver to remain viable, resections must proceed along the vessels that define the peripheries of these segments. In general, this means resection lines parallel the hepatic veins while preserving the portal veins, bile ducts, and hepatic arteries that provide vascular inflow and biliary drainage through the centre of the segment. Also in a LPLT, a volumetric analysis of the donor liver is of interest to achieving less complicated surgery, so classifying the liver correctly and quickly would be very helpful. According to this, we developed a fast method to segment a liver according to the Couinaud's classification. Our method is based on the hepatic vessel tree extracted from the liver CT images. This method was composed of four main steps: vasculature segmentation, 3D thinning, vascular tree pruning and classification, and vascular projection.

2 Liver Segmentation

2.1 Vasculature Segmentation

In the CT images, the Hounsfield units (HU) value of vessel is continuous and greater than value of the liver matter. Considering this, we can use threshold-based 3D-region-growing algorithm to segment the vessels. In this algorithm, the first step is that the seed point must be carefully chosen to ensure that it lies in the portal vein; the second step is the growing procedure. Here we grow this point under these two rules: 1. the grown point's HU value must be greater than a given threshold; 2. the grown point must be within a given distance from the seed point. Rule 2 ensures that our growing procedure may continue when it reaches some small holes.

Automatic determination of an appropriate threshold is possible. Our algorithm can be described as follows: When we decrease the threshold, the number of voxels may increase accordingly. Continue this procedure until we can finally get a threshold-voxel number curve, which is shown in Fig.2.

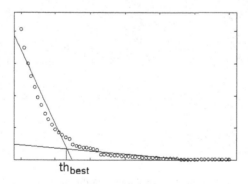

Fig. 2. Automatically detect an appropriate threshold. Here X-axis represents the number of voxels grown, Y-axis represents the threshold.

We then chose two lines to fit this curve, and minimize their sum of mean square. The x-coordinate of the intersection point of these two lines is just the appropriate threshold we need. Fig.3 shows the result of the vessel segmentation.

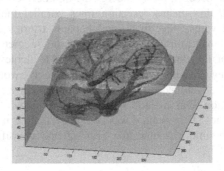

Fig. 3. Result of the 3D-region-growing algorithm

2.2 3D Thinning

Because the grown result usually contains many redundant points, thinning the final result is a necessary pre-process to analyze the vessel tree. This kind of thinning algorithm can be divided into two classes [2]: one is based on distance transform, by choosing the local extreme points as key points, and then connect these points as the skeleton; the other is based on the morphology, by repeatedly eroding the edge until we get an acceptable result. We chose the algorithm introduced by Ta-Chin Lee. This algorithm belongs to the second class. Details of this algorithm can be found in [3]. Here we only show the result of 3D-thinning in Fig.4. Note that this tree is only consists of discrete points, the line which connect every two points is added only for visualization.

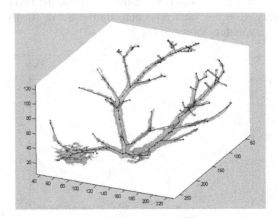

Fig. 4. Result of the 3D-thinning

2.3 Vascular Tree Pruning and Classification

The vascular system can be modelled as a tree. Unfortunately, due to the blur boundary of the vessels, especially in the twig of the vessels, the 3D-thinning result often contains some rings, or multiple edges. These rings may disturb our analyses, so we must get rid of them. Both the Prim algorithm and the Kruskal algorithm are good choices to reduce these rings. Reducing multiple edges is also simple, we only need to leave the shortest edge and exclude the others.

Classifying the tree is the main purpose of this step. In this procedure, a multi-resolution vessel tree must be generated to satisfy different purposes. We define the longest vessel from the root to the leaf as the first level vessel. The longest path from the first level vessel to the leaf is defined as the second level vessel, and so on. In practice, surgeons only care about the stems of the portal and venous, so the first three levels will be enough for them. If someone wants to know the total vascular system of the liver, we can show the entire tree. This trick helps us to reduce the rendering time of our system.

2.4 Vascular Projection and Curve Fitting

Couinaud divided a liver in a 3D space; in programming, it is not so easy to decide which segment a 3D-point lies in. To simplify this classification, we introduce a fast and easy method to divide the liver. We project the liver and the vessel tree to a plane. It is obvious that the projection of the vessel tree is a line segment, and the projection of different subsegments hold the different region of the plane. The classification is then transformed to how to classify a point in the projection plane. Of course, it is easy for us to do this.

The projection plane must been designed elaborately to get a reasonable result. Because the vessels inside the left hemiliver and the right hemiliver are quite different, we project the left part and the right part to different planes. To describe these planes, here we introduce some symbols. For convenience tet O stands for the venous point of intersection. Starting from vertex O, Let L stands for the nearest point of the left hepatic vein, M stands for the nearest point of the middle hepatic vein, R stands for the nearest point of the right hepatic vein, and we get three vectors $\overrightarrow{OL}$, $\overrightarrow{OM}$, and $\overrightarrow{OR}$. To simplify the equation of the projection plane, we let the point O lie on the plane, and then we choose $\overrightarrow{OL} + \overrightarrow{OM} + \overrightarrow{OR}$ as the normal. That is, the projection plane used to project the left hemiliver can be described as equation 1:

$$\overrightarrow{OP} \bullet (\overrightarrow{OL} + \overrightarrow{OM} + \overrightarrow{OR}) = 0 \tag{1}$$

Here P represents an arbitrary point on the projection plane, $\bullet$ means the dot-production of vectors, + means vector addition.

The right hemiliver can be classified like above, except that the normal of the plane must be re-chosen. To reduce the influence of the left part, in practice we use $\overrightarrow{OM} + \overrightarrow{OR}$ as the new normal, and this works well in practice. So the second projection plane can be described as equation 2:

$$\overrightarrow{OP} \bullet (\overrightarrow{OM} + \overrightarrow{OR}) = 0 \tag{2}$$

As shown above, the projection of the vessel tree is a line segment. In general, these segments are not smooth enough. That is not the fact. This error is caused by the poor contrast of the vessel in the CT slices. To reduce this error, we examine the projection of the middle hepatic vein on the projection plane and find that the trend of these points is near polynomial curve. Then we try a quadratic and a cubic polynomial curve to fit these points, and find that quadratic curve can fit these points very well. As shown in Fig.5, the mean square deviation is 2.09969.

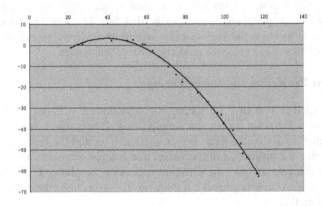

Fig. 5. Use quadric polynomial curve to fit the project points of the middle hepatic vein

We also check the other vessel's projection points, like right hepatic vein, left hepatic vein, and portal vein, only to find that quadratic polynomial is the best curve to fit their project points.

These polynomial curves divide the projection plane into several regions. To segment a liver, now we can project all the points of the liver on the projection plane, then decide which regions they lie in. It is an easier task to classify a point on a plane than in a 3D space. By this means we can segment the liver with high speed.

3   Volumetric Calculation

We run our method through a CT liver dataset, Fig.6 shows the classification result.

Table 1 shows the volume we get after the classification. Here we do not take into account the Segment I. Xu Min[4] calculated 22 male adults' liver volume and draw the conclusion that the average volume percent of segment II, III, IV, V, VI, VII, VIII is 9.9%, 11.6%, 16.6%, 17.0%, 14.6%, 14.7%, 15.6%, and the volume percent of left and right hemiliver is 38.1%, 61.9%. Stione[4] also concluded that the average volume percent of lateral segment left lobe, medial segment left lobe, anterior segment right lobe and posterior segment right lobe is 15%, 20%, 35% and 30%. It is

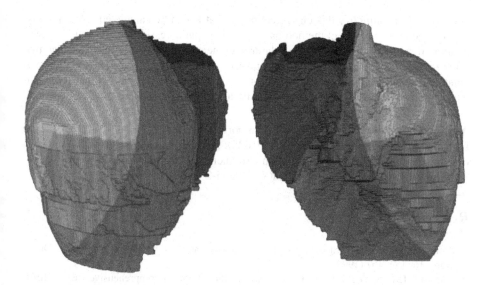

Fig. 6. Classification result. The left is visceral surface; the right is diaphragmatic surface. Different color represents different segment.

Table 1. Volumetric calculation result

	Num of voxels	Volume (ml.)	Percent (%)
Segment II: Lateral segment left lobe (superior)	79195	31.2	3.0
Segment III: Lateral segment left lobe (inferior)	293334	115.7	11.1
Segment IV: Medial segment left lobe	652201	257.2	24.7
Segment V: Anterior segment right lobe (inferior)	545543	215.2	20.6
Segment VI: Posterior segment right lobe (inferior)	161345	63.6	6.1
Segment VII: Posterior segment right lobe (superior)	417009	164.5	15.8
Segment VIII: Anterior segment right lobe (superior)	494519	195.0	18.7
Left hemiliver	1024730	404.1	38.8
Right hemiliver	1618416	638.3	61.2
Total liver	2643146	1042.4	100.0

obvious that our result fit well with their work. Their research proved that our method could produce a reasonable classification.

4 Conclusion

Resecting only specific liver segments is especially useful in patients with hepatocellular carcinoma. In practice, Couinaud's classification of liver anatomy is widely used. To simplify this classification so that is can be calculated more quickly, we designed a fast segment method based on the hepatic vessel tree. This method was composed of four main steps: vasculature segmentation, 3D thinning, vascular tree pruning and classification, and vascular projection and curve fitting. This method was validated by application to a 3D liver from CT data, and it was shown that the result closely approximated the Couinaud's classification with high speed.

Acknowledgments. This work was supported by the National Nature Science Foundation of China (6371012 and 60601025); And the Science Research Foundation of ministry of Health & United Fujian Provincial Health and Education Project for Tacking the Key Research, P.R.China(WKJ2005-2-001).

References

1. Couinaud, C.: Liver anatomy: portal (and suprahepatic) or biliary segmentation. Digest Surg. 16, 459–467 (1999)
2. Lam, L., Lee, S.-W., Suen, C.Y.: Thinning methodologies-a comprehensive survey. IEEE transactions on pattern analysis and machine intelligence 14, 869–883 (1992)
3. Lee, T.-C., Kashyap, R.L.: Building skeleton models via 3-D medial surface/axis thinning algorithm. Graph. Models Image Processing 56, 462–478 (1994)
4. Min, X., et al.: Study of the surgical anatomu and the volume of the liver in man. Chinese journal of general surgery 5, 1–3 (1996)

The Application of Watersnakes Algorithm in Segmentation of the Hippocampus from Brain MR Image

Xiang Lu and Shuqian Luo

College of Biomedical Engineering, Capital Medical University
Beijing, 100069 China
sqluo@ieee.org

Abstract. The application of watersnakes algorithm in segmentation of hippo-campus MR image has been investigated.This algorithm integrates the watershed transform and the active contour algorithm. The watershed transform, based on mathematical morphology, is powerful and flexible for segmentation. However, it does not allow the characteristics of region boundaries to be included in the way that active contour algorithm does. So, over-segmentation is shown in the result of watershed transform, this phenomenon is even worse for the segmentation of hippocampus. For watersnakes algorithm, the primitive contour of hippocampus can be obtained using watershed transform. Based on energy-driven, the contour of hippocampus can develop into the ultimate result. In the process of energy-driven, the information relating to characteristics of region boundaries is involved.

1 Introduction

The hippocampus is a critical structure in human brain, which plays a key role in memory performance [1, 2]. In clinical application, some reports have proved that some abnormalities in the volume and architecture of the hippocampus have close relation with some neurological and psychiatric illnesses, i.e. Alzheimer's disease [3]. So, how to segment hippocampus exactly in medical image analysis is critical in clinical aspects.

For MRI, hippocampus in tissue belongs to gray matter, which adjacent not only to white matter and cerebrospinal fluid but also to other gray matter. Moreover in MRI, the structure of hippocampus has relatively low contrast, low signal-to-noise ratio, and discontinuous edges. All these make the segmentation of hippocampus very difficult. The deformable model for hippocampus segmentation was reported in [4, 5]. However the method of deformable model is difficult to derive local minima.

The watershed transform [6, 7] has been proven useful and powerful for image segmentation. The intuitive description of this method is quite simple. A gray scale image is considered as a topographic relief, and the gray scale value of a pixel represents the height of a point in the topographic relief. Rain falling on the surface of the topographic relief will flow down until it reaches a region of minimum. All the points

X. Gao et al. (Eds.): MIMI 2007, LNCS 4987, pp. 277–286, 2008.
© Springer-Verlag Berlin Heidelberg 2008

of the surface, whose steepest slope path reaches a given minimum, constitute the catchments basin associated with this given minimum. Lines separating catchments basins are called watershed lines. And the watershed lines are thought as boundaries between the regions for segmentation.

An alternative to the rainfall model is to simulate a flooding process. The water comes up out of the ground and immerses the topographic relief into a lake without pre-determining the regional minima, and each regional minimum corresponds to a lake. Adjacent lakes meet at watershed lines as flooding continues.

2 Watersnakes

According to active contour algorithm, the concept of contour is thought as energy-based minimization. And, according to watershed transform, the watershed line is also thought as the contour. So, it seems that watershed transform has some relation with the active contour algorithm. Meyer [8] defined the watershed transform in terms of the topographical distance. In his method, the topographical distance can decrease the mistake brought by noise. If the energy can be described in terms of the topographical distance, it could not only decrease the mistake brought by noise, but also build a relation between watershed transform and active contour algorithm. For partitions $\Omega_1, \cdots, \Omega_k$, the energy can be defined in the following function:

$$E(\Omega_1, \cdots \Omega_k) = \sum_{i=1}^{k} \iint_{\Omega_i} ((f(\partial_i) + T(x, \partial_i)) dx \tag{1}$$

In this equation, ∂_i interprets the minima point of class Ω_i, $f(\partial_i)$ is the gray scale value of ∂_i, and $T(x, \partial_i)$ is the topographical distance between points x and ∂_i. k means the number of classes. $T(x, \partial_i)$ can be described by the following formula.

$$T(p, q) = \min_{\tau \in |p \sim q|} \sum_{n=0}^{l-1} cost(p_n, p_{n+1}) \tag{2}$$

Where $cost(p_n, p_{n+1})$ means the gradient between the point p_n and p_{n+1} when the water floods from the point p_n to p_{n+1} along a path $\tau = (p_0, \cdots, p_l)$.

For watershed [9], the values of the point in the image can be interpreted as in terms of the topographical distance.

$$L(x) = \min_{1 \le i \le k} \{f(\partial_i) + T(x, \partial_i)\} \tag{3}$$

Based on equation (1) and (3), for partitions $\Omega_1, \cdots, \Omega_k$, the energy formula can be described by the following formula.

$$E(\Omega_1, \cdots \Omega_k) = \sum_{i=1}^{k} \iint_{\Omega_i} (f(\partial_i) + T(x, \partial_i)) dx$$

$$\geq \sum_{i=1}^{k} \iint_{\Omega_i} L(x) dx \tag{4}$$

The active contour method is to search the minima of energy formula (4).

According to [10], for partitions $\Omega_1, \cdots, \Omega_k$, if and only if the partitions are watershed segmented, the minima of energy formula (4) can be obtained. Now, the task to search watershed line becomes equivalent with energy minimization.

So, for watershed segmentation the partitions $\Omega_1, \cdots, \Omega_k$ can be described to minimize the function as follows:

$$E(\Omega_1, \cdots, \Omega_k) = \min \sum_{i=1}^{k} \iint_{\Omega_i} L(x) dx \tag{5}$$

The segmentation method based on minimization of this energy function is called watersnakes algorithm.

3 Hippocampus Segmentation

The hippocampus segmentation can divided into six steps:

1) Selecting the seed points.
2) Obtaining gradient image.
3) Obtaining primitive partition using watershed transform.
4) Adjusting seed points.
5) Computing the topographical distance and obtaining the primitive contour.
6) Modifying the contour using watersnakes algorithm.

3.1 Selecting Seed Points

In the process of hippocampus segmentation, we need to select seed points twice. Firstly, we select seed points manually. Secondly, we select the regional minima as the seed points automatically according to the result of the first segmentation. The seed points we selected manually may be not the regional minima which can produce error in the processing of computing the topographical distance. The seed points to be selected automatically must meet two conditions. One, the seed point must have the same class as the corresponding seed point selected manually; the other, the seed point must have a small difference in gray scale value with the corresponding seed point selected manually. For this purpose, we can select the regional minima as the new seed point in one class. All these new seed points can decrease the mistakes in computing the topographical distance.

3.2 Computing the Topographical Distance

The topographical distance is the key of hippocampus segmentation. This method is based on the shortest path. In order to implement this method, we consider the physical model of a fluid flooding a terrain. The cost of flooding across the terrain can be computed. Ordered queues are used to limit flooding direction and to avoid unnecessary computing.

Firstly we put all the seed points into the ordered queues and suppose the cost of the seed points equals 0. Secondly we set the gray scale value in which the points coming from ordered queues propagate a wavefront. In order to keep the results smooth, the water can flood its 4-connented neighborhood. When the water floods from p to one of its 4-connented neighborhood q, if the gray scale value of the point exceeds pre-set gray scale value, or the point has been processed in some lower gray scale value, we don't need to count the cost. If the point q has not been processed, $cost(p,q)$ can be obtained as the cost of the point q .But if the point q has been processed, we suppose $cost(q)$ as the cost of the point q .

If $cost(p,q) < cost(q)$, then the value of $cost(q)$ is substituted by $cost(p,q)$.

If $cost(p,q) \geq cost(q)$, then the value of $cost(q)$ does not change.

Then the topographical distance which is computed, decides this point belonging to which class. For one point from ordered queues, all the points of its 4-connented neighborhood, which has been processed and isn't included in ordered queues, are sent to ordered queues, and the point which have greater value of cost has higher priority. If all the points of one point's 4-connented neighborhood have been sent to ordered queues, it must be removed from ordered queues. When all the points in ordered queues have propagated a wave-front to its 4-connented neighborhood, the gray scale value set for propagating a wavefront can be added. The point which all the points of its 4-connented neighborhood have been processed can be removed from ordered queues. When ordered queues are empty, the process of computing the topographical distance ends, and the primitive contour can be obtained.

3.3 Modifying the Contour

In order to obtain some satisfactory segmentation, we must modify the primitive contour with watersnakes algorithm. The watersnakes algorithm needs a partition of the image as starting point. Fortunately, the result of watershed transform can be used. An exchange of boundary pixels between the adjacent regions is performed for this purpose. The boundary pixels are defined as one having at least one neighbor with different class.

If a boundary pixel p is re-assigned to Ω_j from its adjacent region Ω_i, then the cost function can be defined as follows:

$$L_{i \rightarrow j, p} = min\{ f(\partial_j) + T(p, \partial_j)\} \qquad (6)$$

In such a circumstance, we can define the cost of energy by re-assigning p to Ω_j as follows:

$$\Delta E(p, i \rightarrow j) = L(p) - L_{i \rightarrow j, p} \tag{7}$$

If $\Delta E(p, i \rightarrow j) > 0$, we can re-assign p to Ω_j. Therefore, we call the value of $\Delta E(p, i \rightarrow j)$ the stability of p.

For our segmentation, the stages we modify the contour is stated as follows:

1) Computing the stability of the point in the primitive contour.
2) Selecting the point in the contour with highest stability. When this value is positive, perform the re-assignment and re-decide the contour.
3) Re-computing the stability in the new contour.
4) Iterating step 1 to 3 until no re-assignment is possible.

4 Results

Fig. 1 (left) is the result using traditional region growing by only selecting seed points once, Fig. 1 (middle) is the result using watershed transform by selecting seed points twice. Fig. 1 (right) is the result of watersnakes algorithm. From those results, we can see that over-segmentation is very serious in Fig. 1(left). In Fig. 1, over-segmentation exits in the regions the white arrows point to. Because region growing only selects seed points once, so it is hardly to select the true regional minima. Moreover, there is much noise in MR image, which disturbs the segmentation. The segmentation results in Fig 1(middle) shows a better effect than that in Fig. 1(left), but in some regions over-segmentation still exists. This phenomenon occurs because there are usually significant regional minima caused by noise other than objects of interest. In the result of fig 1(right), over-segmentation can be more restrained than the results of fig 1(left) and fig 1(middle).

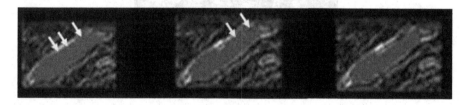

Fig. 1. Left: the result of region growing; Middle: the result using watershed transform by selecting seed points twice; Right: the result of watershakes

In order to obtain 3D hippocampus volumes, we applied our method to segment hippocampus on each slice. The segmentation approach has been tested on 3D MRI datasets of the human head acquired from six normal people subjects. The MRIs are acquired with 3.0 T. The image matrix of each people subject is $512 \times 512 \times 128$. The depth of slice is 1.3 mm. The size of pixel is 0.46875×0.46875 mm^2.

In the segmentation process of left hippocampus on each slice, firstly we select middle slice of left hippocampus to segment hippocampus. The hippocampus of this slice is clearer than others, and the segmentation of this slice is easier than that of others. Then, based on the segmentation results of this slice, we segmented hippocampus on each slice using watersnakes algorithm. Fig. 2 shows the results of hippocampus segmentation on each slice. This results show hippocampus has a big head and a small tail, and its shape looks like a bow.

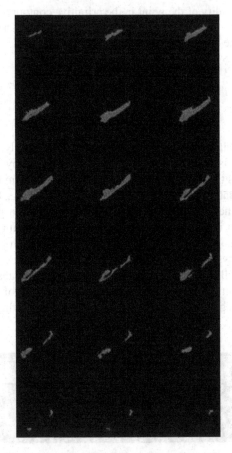

Fig. 2. The results of hippocampus segmentation on each slice

For 3D hippocampus segmentation, the hippocampus areas on each slice increase greatly and decrease slowly, and the shapes of the segmentation results of adjacent slices don't change greatly. The results using watersnakes algorithm meet this rule. Fig.3 shows the areas of hippocampus on each slice. Fig.4 shows overlaying region of the segmentation on the adjacent slices. The red region points in the segmentation results belong to the previous slice, the green region points in the segmentation results belong to the current slice, and the yellow region points are overlaying region.

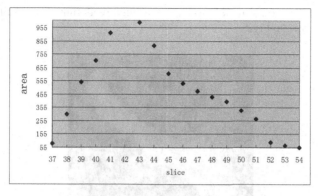

Fig. 3. The area of hippocampus on each slice

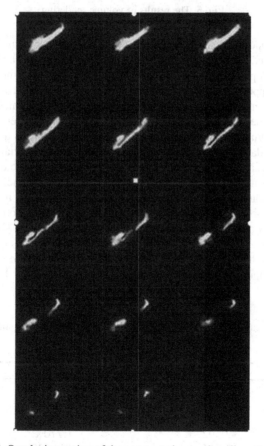

Fig. 4. Overlaying region of the segmentation on the adjacent slices

We use Analyze software [11] to realize volume rendering. The results of volume rendering is shown in Fig.5.

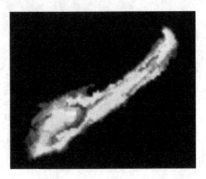

Fig. 5. The results of volume rendering

The aim of hippocampus segmentation is mostly used for quantitative analysis of hippocampus. Based on our segmentation we can obtain some data such as hippocampus volume and hippocampus areas on each slice. These data are important to quantitative analysis of hippocampus. We also can use these data to evaluate our segmentation results. Prior to quantitative analysis of hippocampus, we must normalize the segmented data to eliminate the mistakes brought by difference among deferent subjects. Table 1 shows the hippocampus volumes from six normal people subjects and some statistical index about these data. In table 1, we can see that the standard variance is 0.24cm³ and the average hippocampus volumes are 2.637 cm³. The max relative deviations between hippocampus volumes of one subject's dataset and mean volumes is 13.862%. The hippocampus data are very few which makes the mean possibly incorrect. Some parameters used to normalize the segmented data are calculated roughly from sagittal plane, which might bring mistakes in the process of normalization. Our research of this algorithm is just at a starting point, and the primitive segmentation algorithm can not be applied to process the blur contour. All these reasons make the max relative deviation between hippocampus volumes of one subject and mean volumes become larger than that expected.

Table 1. The hippocampus volume from six normal people and some statistical index about these data

	Hippocampus Volume(c m³)	RSD
1	2.889	8.691%
2	2.940	10.271%
3	2.636	0.056%
4	2.592	1.770%
5	2.316	13.862%
6	2.453	7.523%
Mean±SD	2.637±0.24	

Table 2 shows the hippocampus areas on some slices from different subjects. In this table, we set the slice serial number of the max hippocampus areas to zero, and the serial number of slices prior to this slice in turn minus one, the serial number of slices after this slice in turn plus one. From this table, we can conclude that the more close to the zero slices, the hippocampus areas on this slice among different subjects are more approximate.

Table 2. The hippocampus area on some slices of different subjects

slice	Hippocampus areas of 1 $(c\,m^2)$	Hippocampus areas of 2 $(c\,m^2)$	Hippocampus areas of 3 $(c\,m^2)$	Hippocampus areas of 4 $(c\,m^2)$	Hippocampus areas of 5 $(c\,m^2)$	Hippocampus areas of 6 $(c\,m^2)$	Mean ±SD $(c\,m^2)$
-4	1.6985	1.5029	0.6394	0.6702	0.3493	1.0986	0.9932±0.5315
-3	1.9006	2.1445	1.2217	1.2063	0.8108	1.6194	1.4839±0.4955
-2	1.9819	2.2631	1.2129	1.5557	1.2656	1.7798	1.6765±0.4114
-1	1.9819	2.0325	2.2500	2.0127	1.6633	2.1072	2.0079±0.1941
0	2.0874	2.3181	2.3862	2.3379	1.9072	2.2764	2.2189±0.1842
1	1.5908	2.0632	2.3840	2.1841	1.8215	2.2412	2.0475±0.2930
2	1.5007	2.0632	1.6963	1.8018	1.7820	1.8699	1.7805±0.1773
3	1.3140	1.9973	1.6897	1.3381	1.4854	1.9819	1.6344±0.3060
4	1.0789	1.9028	1.1052	1.1821	1.3359	1.5336	1.3564±0.3165
5	1.1272	1.4985	1.0811	1.0547	1.3689	0.7339	1.1440±0.2670
6	0.7075	0.7756	0.9294	0.9514	1.1646	0.5537	0.8470±0.2140
7	0.4966	0.3208	0.5515	0.8855	0.9514	0.4680	0.6123±0.2500
8	0.4482	0.1450	0.3428	0.7317	0.6987	0.3384	0.4508±0.2273
9	0.1472	0.0967	0.1846	0.5911	0.6262	0.1428	0.2980±0.2424
10	0.1384	0.0505	0.0769	0.2021	0.3889	0.1230	0.1633±0.1223

5 Conclusion

The MR images have some features such as much noise, low contrast and so on. The segmentation method based on traditional watershed transform is fast, flexible, and typically can be applied to gradient information, but it could bring unsatisfactory results due to noise. Moreover in some region low contrast makes the results even worse. The method based on active contour has power to track anatomic structure, but it needs the primitive contour points close to the true object boundary. In practice these points are hard to select. The watersnakes algorithm integrates the watershed transform and the active contour algorithm. This method combines the advantages of the watershed transform and active contour, and the advantage of active contour can constrain over-segmentation brought by watershed segmentation. Now our research on watersnakes algorithm is only in primary stage. In the near future, we will develop watersnakes algorithm to settle down the problem of blur boundary.

Acknowledgment

This project was supported by the National Natural Science Foundation of China (60472020).

References

1. Petersen, R.C., Jack, C.R., Xu, Y.C., Waring, S., O'Brien, P., et al.: Memory and MRI-based Hippocampal Volumes in Aging and AD. Neurology 54, 581–587 (2000)
2. Tisserand, D.J., van Boxtel, M.P., Jolles, J., Jolles, J.: The Relation between Global and Limbic Brain Volumes on MRI and Cognitive Performance in Healthy Individuals across The Age Range. Neurobiol Aging 21, 569–576 (2000)
3. Bobinski, M., Wegiel, J., Wisniewsky, H., Tarnawski, M., Bobinski, M., et al.: Neurofibrillary Pathology-correlation with Hippocampal Formation Atrophy in Alzheimer Disease. Neurobiol. Aging 17, 909–976 (1996)
4. Ghanei, A., Soltanian-Zadeh, H., Windham, J.P.: Segmentation of The Hippocampus from Brain MRI Using Deformable Contours. IEEE Trans. Pattern Analysis and Machine Intelligence 22, 203–216 (1998)
5. Lee, J.M., Kim, S.H., Jang, D.P., Ha, T.H., Kim, J.J., et al.: Deformable Model with Surface Registration for Hippocampal Shape Deformity Analysis in Schizophrenia. NeuroImage 22, 831–840 (2004)
6. Vincent, L., Soille, P.: Watershed in Digital Space: An Efficient Algorithm Based on Immersion Simulation. IEEE Trans. Pattern Analysis and Machine Intelligence 13, 583–598 (1991)
7. Roerdink, J.B.T.M., Meijster, A.: The Watershed Transform: Definition, Algorithm, and Parallelization Strategies. Fundamenta Informaticae 41, 187–228 (2001)
8. Meyer, F.: Topographic Distance and Watershed Lines. Signal Processing 38, 113–125 (1994)
9. Beare, R.: A Locally Constrained Watershed Transform. IEEE Trans. Pattern Analysis and Machine Intelligence 17, 1063–1074 (2006)
10. Nguyen, H.T., Worring, M., Boomggaard, R.: Watersnakes: Energy-driven Watershed Segmentation. IEEE Trans. Pattern Analysis and Machine Intelligence 25, 330–342 (2003)
11. Richard, A., Robb, K., Augustine, D., Bemard-Rhude, B., Cameron, J., et al.: Analyze 6.1 Verson, Staff of the Biomedical Imaging Resource. Mayo Foundation (2004)

Spiral MRI Reconstruction Using Least Square Quantization Table

Dong Liang, Edmund Y. Lam, George S.K. Fung, and Xin Zhang

Department of Electrical and Electronic Engineering
The University of Hong Kong, Pokfulam Road, Hong Kong
{dliang,elam,skfung,xinzhang}@eee.hku.hk

Abstract. Recently, the authors introduced least square quantization table (LSQT) method to accelerate the direct Fourier transform to reconstruct magnetic resonance images acquired using a spiral trajectory. In this paper, we will discuss the LSQT further in its adaptability, reusability and choice of the number of groups. The experimental results show that the LSQT method has better adaptability for the different reconstruction cases than the equal phase line (EPL) and Kaiser-Bessel gridding methods. Additionally, it can be reused for reconstructing different images of varied sizes.

Keywords: Image reconstruction; spiral trajectory; least square quantization table; adaptability; reusability.

1   Introduction

Recently, non-Cartesian scanning in k-space, such as spiral, has received increased attention in Magnetic Resonance Imaging (MRI). However, when the data is acquired using a non-Cartesian k-space trajectory, image reconstruction can no longer be accomplished with a direct FFT. Therefore, the problem of reconstructing image from a set of nonuniformly sampled data has drawn more attention in the past few years. The Kaiser-Bessel griding is the most widely used method to solve this problem, where nonuniformly sampled data are first resampled onto a Cartesian grid and then a FFT is applied to reconstruct the image. As the most straightforward and accurate solution, the direct Fourier transform [1] has some advantages over other methods. Unfortunately, the high computational demand makes it impractical compared with methods that use the fast Fourier transform (FFT) [2]. Two algorithms, Equal-Phase-Line (EPL) and look-up table (LUT), were proposed to solve this problem [3,4]. The EPL method does not take into account the actual distribution of phases for each data, and therefore may cause a large quantization error and consequently a large reconstruction quality loss. Meanwhile, the LUT method is only efficient for small size images due to the huge memory required for storing a large size look-up table.

More recently, the authors introduced a new algorithm for accelerating the direct Fourier transform to reconstruct MR images acquired using a spiral trajectory. The algorithm, called least square quantization table (LSQT) [5,6], reduces

X. Gao et al. (Eds.): MIMI 2007, LNCS 4987, pp. 287–293, 2008.
© Springer-Verlag Berlin Heidelberg 2008

the computation loads of direct Fourier transform with only a little quality loss. The results were shown to be more accurate than EPL and require less memory than LUT. In this paper, we will report further results in the LSQT method in terms of its adaptability, reusability and choice of the number of groups.

2   The Least Square Quantization Table Method

We summarize the LSQT method in this section. Further details can be found in [5]. When direct Fourier transform method is applied to reconstruct image I of size $N \times N$ from k-space data s with length L, the contribution of the pth data to the entire image space is [3] :

$$I_p (x, y) = s_p d_p \exp \left(j2\pi \left(xu_p + yv_p \right) \right). \tag{1}$$

where $x, y = [-N/2 : N/2 - 1]$ is image pixel and $u, v = [-1/2 : 1/2]$ is sampling position in k-space. d_p is the density compensation function. It can be seen from (1) that for a given $\{u_p, v_p\}$, if two pixels (x_1, y_1) and (x_2, y_2) have the same phase such that $2\pi \left(x_1 u_p + y_1 v_p \right) = 2\pi \left(x_2 u_p + y_2 v_p \right)$, the data s_p has the same contribution to the two pixel locations. Also, if we define $C_p = xu_p + yv_p$, because of the periodic property of the complex exponential function, C_p is also a periodic function with unity period and we can concentrate on the main phase band $[0, 2\pi)$, corresponding to the fractional part of C_p in $[0, 1)$, which we denoted as $\langle C_p \rangle$. If C_p is negative, we add an integer to it to bring it to between 0 and 1, and $\langle C_p \rangle$ then is the resulting fractional part. Thus, each pixel $\{x, y\}$ has a one-to-one correspondence to $\langle C_p \rangle$.

It is noted that if some pixels have the same $\langle C_p \rangle$, the acquired raw data in k-space have the same contribution to these pixels. Thus, all the pixels can be classified into groups, where each group is labeled by a different representative value and pixels in the same group receive the same contribution. If the contributions of the given data to all the groups are known, for a pixel, we only need to know which group it belongs to. Consequently, (1) is calculated only once for each group instead of for each pixel in the direct Fourier transform method. Therefore, the tradeoff between the reduction of computing loads and loss of image quality lies in the number of groups. Instead of requiring an exact value of $\langle C_p \rangle$ before two pixels can be classified into the same group, we use the Lloyd-Max quantization algorithm to classify all the pixels into only M groups where $M \ll N^2$. The group boundaries are calculated by quantizing the interval $[0, 1)$ into M bins in the least square sense of quantization error [7]. The representative value of each group is the centroid of the corresponding group, which is the optimal point to give the lowest quality loss.

Therefore, for the k-space data s with length L, we can pre-compute a least square quantization table (LSQT) Q of size $M \times L$. The construction of the table can be accomplished off-line and reused for the same k-space trajectory, being independent of the object being imaged. After loading the table, when a data arrives, the contributions of the data to all the groups can be calculated. Then for a pixel, we use binary-searching algorithm to map it to the corresponding group and set contribution directly . Considering the symmetric and periodic properties of $\langle C_p \rangle$, only pixels where $x \geq 0$ need to undergo mapping [3].

3 Results on Adaptability and Reusability

Our experiments are performed with the Shepp and Logan mathematical phantom [8] with three different sizes, 64×64, 128×128 and 256×256. Spiral trajectory used in [5] was applied to generate k-space data from phantoms. The size of k-space data is 13,392. Then there are three cases of image reconstruction: $L > N \times N$, $L \approx N \times N$ and $L < N \times N$. M takes the values 16, 32, 64 and 128 as in [5].

Similar to that in [5], the reconstructed image obtained with the direct Fourier transform is used as a standard. The normalized Root Mean Square (nRMS) error is calculated after reconstructed images are scaled to a range of gray levels [0,255] and the Maximum Absolute Difference (MAD) is normalized by dividing by 255.

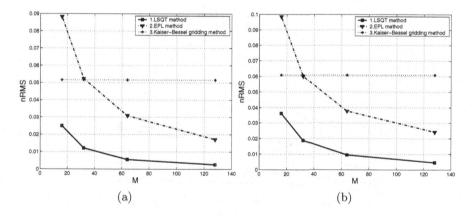

Fig. 1. (a) and (b) The nRMS of different methods against the number of groups for reconstructing N=64 and N=128 phantoms, respectively

Fig. 1 (a) and (b) shows the nRMS of different methods against the number of groups for reconstructing $N = 64$ and $N = 128$ phantoms, respectively. The performance of reconstructing $N = 256$ image from data acquired using this spiral trajectory can be found in [5]. For these cases, we can draw the same conclusion that the LSQT method can give more accurate reconstruction results than EPL and Kaiser-Bessel griding methods when M takes an appropriate value. Moreover, the LSQT method even when $M = 16$ performs better than the Kaiser-Bessel griding. The Kaiser-Bessel griding used here is the same as that used in [5].

Next we will explore the adaptability of different methods when facing different reconstructing cases, from oversampling to undersampling. Fig. 2 shows the nRMS against the size of reconstructed phantoms for the LSQT, EPL and grid-ing methods with different M, where the solid lines are for the LSQT, dashed lines for the EPL and dotted line for the Kaiser-Bessel griding. Theoretically, the nRMS error will become larger with increasing reconstructed image size while the number of k-space data is fixed, because the reconstruction case varies from $L > N \times N$ to $L < N \times N$. We can see from this figure that, the nRMS curves for the LSQT are flatter than those of EPL and Kaiser-Bessel griding methods with the same M in general. It means compared to other two methods, the LSQT has better adaptability for the different reconstruction cases. The reasons are because the actual distribution of $\langle C_p \rangle$ is taken into account and Lloyd-Max quantization algorithm is used.

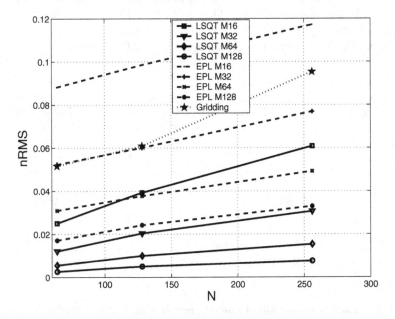

Fig. 2. The nRMS against the size of reconstructed Shepp and Logan phantoms for the LSQT and EPL methods with different M

As we described before, because constructing LSQT is only dependent on the k-space sampling positions and image pixel positions, the LSQT constructed for a given trajectory can be reused for reconstructing the different images with same size. It is affirmative because constructing LSQT is only dependent on the k-space sampling positions and image pixels positions. Moreover, another advantage of LSQT method is that the LSQT constructed in the case of $L < N \times N$ can be reused in the case of $L \approx N \times N$ and $L > N \times N$ where L is fixed. Fig. 3 (a) and (b) show the nRMS and MAD of LSQT method against the number of group for reconstructing different sizes of phantoms with different LSQTs. Here, LSQT256 N64/128 means reconstructing a 64×64 or 128×128

phantom from 13393 k-space data but with a LSQT constructed in the case of reconstructing 256×256 phantom from 13393 k-space data. LSQT64 N64 and LSQT128 N128 mean reconstructing a 64×64 or 128×128 phantom with their own LSQTs. It can be seen that reconstructing 64×64 and 128×128 phantoms with LSQT256 perform better than with their own LSQTs in nRMS and MAD. The reason is that each element of LSQT256 is obtained from 256×256 $\langle C_p \rangle$'s of interval $[0, 1)$ while each element of LSQT64/128 is obtained from 64×64 or 128×128 $\langle C_p \rangle$'s of interval $[0, 1)$. Obviously, the representative values stored in LSQT256 are more precise than those stored in LSQT64/128 when $\langle C_p \rangle$'s have the similar distribution. This advantage means the LSQT method can be reused not only for reconstructing the different images with same size, but for reconstructing the different images of reduced sizes.

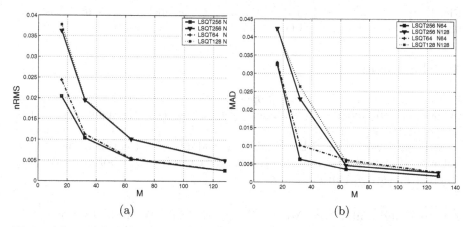

Fig. 3. (a) and (b) The nRMS and MAD of LSQT method against the number of group for reconstructing different sizes of phantoms with different LSQT's

As we know, the selection of the number of group controls the quantization precision and the size of LSQT and hence the reconstruction accuracy and required memory. Therefore, the selection of M is flexible in trading off required memory against reconstruction error in our method. It means the LSQT method can be customized for the particular application by selecting a predetermined number of groups that corresponds to the desired required memory. For example, if a high accuracy is desired, it is easy to implement by increasing the number of groups. Additionally, the selection of M avoids having the user choose more specific parameters of reconstruction like window width or neighborhood definition like other methods [2,9]. Fig. 4 illustrates the effect of the number of groups on the nRMS and MAD for reconstructing different sizes of Shepp and Logan phantoms when the size of k-space is fixed. The figure suggests that when $L > N \times N$, M can take a small value while when $L < N \times N$, M should take a large value to retain a substantial reduction in reconstruction error.

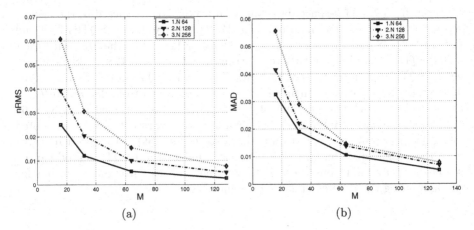

Fig. 4. (a) and (b) The nRMS and MAD against the number of groups for reconstructing different sizes of Shepp and Logan phantoms when the size of k-space is fixed

4   Conclusion

In this paper, the LSQT method proposed recently by the authors is explored in further detail in its adaptability, reusability and choice of the number of groups. The experimental results show further that LSQT performs better in reconstruction accuracy than EPL and has better adaptability than EPL when facing different reconstruction cases. Moreover, LSQT can be reused for reconstructing different images of reduced size.

Acknowledgments. This work was supported in part by the University Research Committee of the University of Hong Kong under Grant Number URC-10207440.

References

1. Maeda, A., Sano, K., Yokoyama, T.: Reconstruction by Weighted Correlation for MRI with Time-varying Gradients. IEEE Trans. Med. Imag. 7, 26–31 (1988)
2. Jackson, J.I., Meyer, C.H., Nishimura, D.G., Macovski, A.: Selection of a Convolution Function for Fourier Inversion Using Griding. IEEE Trans. Med. Imag. 10, 473–478 (1991)
3. Qian, Y.X., Lin, J.R., Jin, D.Q.: Direct Reconstruction of MR Images From Data Acquired on a Non-Cartesian Grid Using an Equal-Phase-Line Algorithm. Magn. Res. Med. 47, 1228–1233 (2002)
4. Dale, B., Wendt, M., Duerk, J.L.: A Rapid Look-up Table Method for Reconstructing MR Images from Arbitrary K-space Trajectories. IEEE Trans. Med. Imag. 20, 207–216 (2001)
5. Liang, D., Lam, E.Y., Fung, G.S.K.: Direct Reconstruction of Spiral MRI using Least Square Quantization Table. IEEE International Symposium on Biomedical Imaging: From Nano to Macro, 105–108 (2007)

6. Liang, D., Lam, E.Y., Fung, G.S.K.: A least square quantization table method for direct reconstruction of MR images with non-Cartesian trajectory. Journal of Magn. Res. 188, 141–150 (2007)
7. Gersho, A., Gray, R.M.: Vector Quantization and Signal Compression. Kluwer Academic Publishers, Boston (1992)
8. Shepp, L.A., Logan, B.F.: The Fourier Reconstruction of A Head Section. IEEE Trans. Nucl. Sci. NS-21, 21–43 (1974)
9. Rosenfeld, D.: An Optimal and Efficient New Griding Algorithm Using Singular Value Decomposition. Magn. Res. Med. 40, 14–23 (1998)

A Hybrid Method for Automatic and Highly Precise VHD Background Removal

Chen Ding[1], Yankui Sun[1], Xiaolin Tian[2], and Zesheng Tang[1,2]

[1] Department of Computer Science and Technology, Tsinghua University,
Beijing, China, 100084
syk@tsinghua.edu.cn
[2] Faculty of Information Technology, Macao University of Science and Technology,
Macao, China

Abstract. Background removal is a critical step in Visible Human Data (VHD) processing, which is the basic of all other researches. In this paper, a new segmentation algorithm based on the hybrid method for VHD background removal has been proposed, which combines a feature based segmentation method with a contour based one. The algorithm first determines the background part and the interested parts of an image at a coarse level by using its colour features, and then obtains a fine segmentation by using a Gradient Vector Flow (GVF) Snake model on the previous initial contour. Our test results on Chinese VHD show that the new algorithm is more robust and accurate than the previous methods.

Keywords: Image Segmentation, Background Removal, Hybrid Method, Snake model.

1 Introduction

The research into VHD is at the frontiers in medical image processing [1]. Background removal is a kind of image segmentation, which applies segmentation techniques to get the interested part in VHD and remove the background part. It is a fundamental step for all the processing on VHD and further research may depends on the accuracy of the background removal results.

Although background removal is important, it is difficult to get satisfactory results. The Chinese VHD is obtained in various conditions. Among these varieties, different illumination and coarseness of the ice make it difficult to be handled.

So far as we know, there are few published works on this topic. Most research on Chinese VHD hardly mention or even ignores this step. In [2], the background of more than 6000 digital human images are removed by hand; in [3], about 3000 images are processed by PHOTOSHOP, and adjusted manually. The fully automatic approach first appeared in [4]. It classifies a point as a background point if and only if the blue or green value of this point is not less than the red one. It is a rough estimation, which needs further complex post-processing, and thoroughly from the US Digital Human Project, so it is not very suitable to Chinese VHD. In [5], we use the colour feature of an image to distinguish its background and interested part, and then use Mathematic

X. Gao et al. (Eds.): MIMI 2007, LNCS 4987, pp. 294–303, 2008.

Morphology (MM) [6] to complete the final results. This method can get good results and is fit for most Chinese VHD images. But as mentioned before, Chinese VHD images are obtained in various conditions, so this simple approach may not handle all these images properly as illustrated in Fig.1.

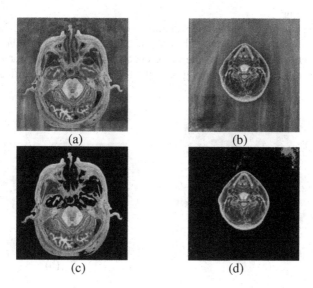

(a)   (b)

(c)   (d)

Fig. 1. (a) and (b) are two original images. (c) and (d) are the corresponding processing results. Some human body has been removed in (c) and some background part has not been removed in (d).

In this paper, we propose a more robust and finer algorithm based on hybrid methods [7] to segment the background. It first uses color feature to get a rough result, and further uses the GVF Snake model [8] to refine the initial result so as to get a more precise contour. It is a fully automatic method and can deal with all the CVHD we test effectively.

2 Algorithm

The algorithm is a hybrid method which combines a feature based segmentation method with a contour based one. It consists of the following steps:

1) Feature based segmentation

For every image, compute a global threshold of channel differences to distinguish the background and the interested part, and then remove the background and a small part of human body which cannot be distinguished by the differences;

2) Contour based segmentation

Use Mathematic Morphology to construct an initial contour and then design a Gradient Vector Flow Field to segment by using theSnake model.

2.1 Feature Based Segmentation

The background of a cryosection image may not be removed by the method in [5]. Here we adopt an aggressive approach to make sure that all its background part can be found.

1) Preprocessing

Every image contains a colour checker and a ruler as illustrated in Fig.2a. So in order to reduce computational complexity, the color checker block and ruler should be cut off firstly, as shown in Fig.2b. Since the color checkers and rulers appear in almost the same position of all cryosection images, cutting them off does not affect the human body part.

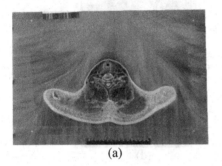 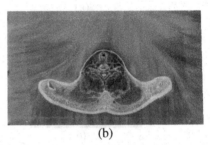

(a)   (b)

Fig. 2. An example of image cutting. (a) is an original image, and (b) is the image after cutting the color checker and ruler off.

2) Normalization of the intensity

For every image, compute the difference between channel R and channel G. Different from our previous method in [5], here we compute these differences by the normalized intensity value of channel R and channel G so that the influence of various illumination on background removal can be degraded. For a pixel (R, G, B), the normalized intensity R_{norm} and G_{norm} of its R, G components is:

$$G_{norm} = \frac{G}{R+G+B}, R_{norm} = \frac{R}{R+G+B}$$

3) Classification

By using the colour feature, we can classify pixels of an image into the background part and the interested one as follows.

```
if (G_norm - R_norm > T or I > I_o)
    classify the pixel (R, G, B) as background part;
else
    classify the pixel (R, G, B) as interested part;
```

where T and I_0 are two thresholds, and I stands for the intensity of a pixel. To make sure that all the background can be classified correctly, take T as a value slightly less than the threshold from the histogram. And I_0 is a parameter that marks all the highlight ice part as background.

2.2 Contour Based Segmentation

In the previous step, the whole background part of an image has been removed and a proper initial contour closing to the final result has been obtained, but a small part of human body may also been removed due to the aggressive approach. So a further processing is needed. Here we choose Snake model to complete the segmentation result because it works perfectly with the initial contour.

2.2.1 Gradient Vector Flow Snake Model

The Snake model is first proposed by Kass in [9]. The Snake process can be described as moving a curve, defined within an image domain, under the influence of internal forces coming from within the curve itself and external force computed from the image data.

In Mathematics, this model is a minimization problem.

Suppose that $x(s) = [x(s), y(s)], s \in [0,1]$ is a parametric curve, and define

$$E = \int_0^1 \left\{ \frac{1}{2} \left[\alpha |x'(s)|^2 + \beta |x''(s)|^2 \right] + E_{ext}(x(s)) \right\} ds$$

as an energy function, where α and β are weighting parameters that control the snake's tension and rigidity $x'(s)$ and $x''(s)$ respectively; the External Energy function E_{ext} is derived from an image.

The snake that minimizes E must satisfy the Euler equation

$$\alpha x''(s) - \beta x''''(s) - \nabla E_{ext} = 0$$

This function can be viewed as a force balance equation.

$$F_{int} + F_{ext} = 0 \tag{1}$$

where $F_{int} = \alpha x''(s) - \beta x''''(s)$ and $F_{ext} = -\nabla E_{ext}$.

Xu [8] further proposed a new external force, Gradient Vector Flow, to replace the traditional external force. The GVF can be obtained by solving the following minimization:

$$\varepsilon = \iint \left[\mu \left(u_x^2 + u_y^2 + v_x^2 + v_y^2 \right) + |\nabla f|^2 \, |v - \nabla f|^2 \right] dxdy$$

where f is the edge map derived from an image, which is large near image edges, μ is a weighting parameter and $v(x, y) = [u(x, y), v(x, y)]$ is the gradient vector flow.

It can be shown that the GVF field can be found by solving the following Euler equations

$$\mu\nabla^2 u - (u - f_x)(f_x^2 + f_y^2) = 0$$
$$\mu\nabla^2 v - (v - f_y)(f_x^2 + f_y^2) = 0$$

(2)

By solving equation (2), the GVF $v(x, y)$ is found. Then let $F_{ext} = V(x, y)$, $x(s)$ can be solved from (1) and this is the result of final segmentation.

2.2.2 Initialization of Snake Model

To apply the Snake model, we should specify an initial contour and an edge map derived from an image for it.

1) Extract the contour

The result of feature based segmentation may be fragmented due to the nature of feature based segmentation, so it cannot be used as an initial contour directly. To solve this problem, we use Mathematic Morphology to make the fragments be eliminated or merged into a big region, then extract the contour of this region and use it as the initial contour of the Snake model.

An image point is defined as a contour point if and only if there are both background points and non-background points in a small neighborhood around it (like 3×3).

After the Mathematic Morphology process, the non-background part should be several independent regions. Obviously, every region has a connected contour, which can be viewed as initial contour point set.

Firstly, remove all the single-connected contour points from the contour point set. A single-connected contour point is a contour point that connects with only one non single-connected contour point. Thus the remained contour points are connected with two other contour points at least.

Then select the left-most contour point as a starting point, so the non-background part should be on the right of this point, and traverse the contour along the direction which can maximize the area of non-background region.

Because each contour point has more than two connected contour points, the process can continue to find a new contour point one by one; and since the starting point is left-most, the searching always return to the starting point due to the maximizing criterion. So traversing in this way should stop when the correct contour is obtained.

Finally, the initial contour of the Snake model can be obtained by sampling along the contour.

The above procedure is shown in Fig.3. The contour point set obtained by feature based segmentation is in Fig.3a. Firstly, we remove all the single-connected contour points and start searching from point A and then we find the point B as illustrated in Fig.3b and Fig.3c. As the process continues, we reach point C, which has two unreached adjacent contour points marked as D and E. Then we choose the point E, which can maximize the area of non-background region, to be the next point in Fig.3d. The process finishes when we return to the point A, and the final contour is shown in Fig.3e.

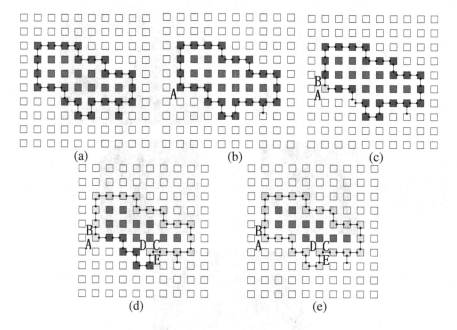

Fig. 3. The process of contour initialization

2) Compute the edge map

The edge map derived from an image is another issue. For any pixel, we define r as the ratio of the number of background pixels and total pixels in its small neighborhood (like 3×3). Because the edge separates the background part and the non-background part, a point with r close to 0.5 is more likely to be an edge point. Thus we define the edge map f as follow.

$$f = 1 - \left| r - \frac{1}{2} \right|$$

The edge map f can be used to compute the GVF in the Snake model.

3 Experiments and Results

We implement the new algorithm and test it on Chinese Visible Human Data. This data set has over 2000 slices cryosection images. The experimental results show that it can remove the background of all these images correctly.

Fig.4 illustrates the process of the algorithm. Fig.4c and Fig.4d demonstrate that some drawbacks of the initial contour have been adjusted by the Snake model.

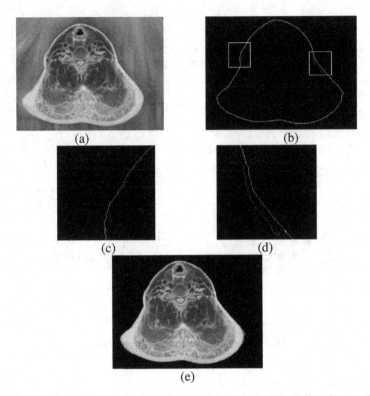

(e)

Fig. 4. (a) is an original image. (b) is its Snake model where the red line denotes the initial contour and the white line represents the final contour. Since the high resolution of (b), we magnify the detail of (b) in (c) and (d). (e) is the final result image of (a).

Our algorithm has the following prominent advantages.

3.1 Correctness and Accuracy

The images in Fig.1a and Fig.1b cannot be removed background well by [5], but they can be handled by our new algorithm correctly, as is shown in Fig.5.

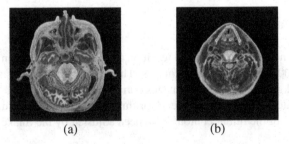

Fig. 5. The results by using the new algorithm. The original images are shown in Fig.1.

The background part of original image in Fig.1a is depicted in Fig.6. It is very accurate by human sight.

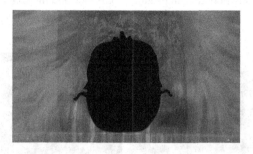

Fig. 6. The background part of Fig.1a

The hybrid method of feature based method and Snake model provides smoother contour than feature based method itself. Since the background removal is the basis of the further processes, an accurate and smooth segmentation result is very important to advanced research, such as visualization.

3.2 Robustness to Illumination Variation

Fig.7a and Fig.7b are two images with significant different illuminations. Fig.7c and Fig.7d are their background removal results. This shows that our algorithm can handle cryosection images with various illuminations effectively.

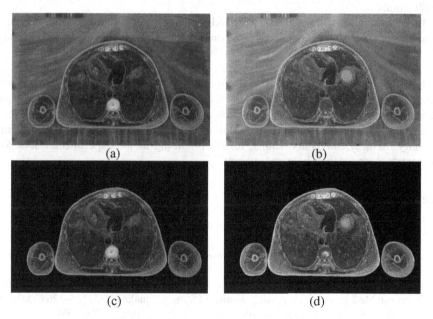

Fig. 7. (a) and (b) are two images with different illuminations. (c) and (d) are their background removal results.

3.3 Effectiveness for Images with Highlighted Background

Cutting the frozen human body can produce coarse ice and the coarse ice may introduce a highlighted area. For this kind of image, the algorithm can handle it properly as illustrated in Fig.8.

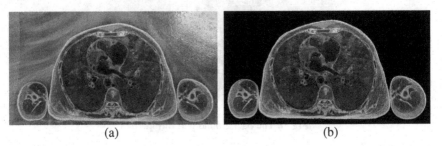

(a)   (b)

Fig. 8. (a) is an image with highlight part. (b) is the background removal result.

4   Conclusion

A new segmentation algorithm for VHD background removal has been proposed in the paper. It combines a feature based segmentation method and a contour based one. It can remove the background automatically and the test result shows that it can achieve satisfied accuracy and robustness. Since the parameters used in this algorithm are either computed from images or fixed to process all images, it can be easily used in practical applications.

In the future, we will use the background removal result to build a 3D human body model. Since the Snake model returns a contour rather than a simple image, we could use it directly.

Acknowledgments. This work is supported by the National Nature Science Foundation of China (No. 30470487) and the National High Technology Research and Development Program of China (No. 2006AA02Z472). We would like to thank Prof. Shaoxiang Zhang, the principal of Chinese Visible Human Project Group, Third Military Medical University, China, for his providing us the experimental data. We appreciate them for their help and support.

References

1. The U.S. National Library of Medicine: The Visible Human Project® Overview,
   http://www.nlm.nih.gov/research/visible/visible_human.html
2. Zhang, S., Heng, P., Liu, Z.: Atlas of Chinese Visible Human(Male and Femal). Science Press (2004)
3. Chai, H., Du, G., Cao, H., Luo, S.: The Method of 3D Rendering of Serial Anatomic Section Images in Medical Image Processing. Journal of System Simulation 15, 125–126 (2003)
4. Katz, W.T.: Segmentation and Visualization for the Digital Humans CD-ROM,
   http://www.nlm.nih.gov/research/visible/vhp_conf/katz/
   vishuman.html

5. Zhao, Y., Tao, C., Tian, X., Tang, Z.: A New Segmentation Algorithm for the Visible Human Data. Conf. Proc. IEEE Eng. Med. Biol. Soc., 1646–1649 (2005)
6. Castleman, K.R.: Digital Image Process. Prentice Hall. Inc., Englewood Cliffs (1995)
7. Imielinska, C., Metaxas, D., Udupa, J., Jin, Y., Chen, T.: Hybrid Segmentation of the Visible Human Data. In: Visible Human Project Conference III, Bethesda MD (2000)
8. Xu, C., Prince, L.J.: Snakes, Shapes, and Gradient Vector Flow. IEEE Transactions on Image Processing 7(3), 359–369 (1998)
9. Kass, M., Witkin, A., Terzopoulos, D.: Snakes: Active Contour Models. Intl. J. of Computer Vision 1(4), 321–331 (1988)

Analytic Modeling and Simulating of the Cornea with Finite Element Method

Jie-zhen Xie [1], Bo-liang Wang [1], Ying Ju [1], and Shi-hui Wu [2]

[1] School of Information Science and Technology, Xiamen University, Xiamen 361005, China
[2] Hospital of Xiamen University, Xiamen 361005, China
{xjz,blwang,yju}@xmu.edu.cn

Abstract. Finite element analysis is a useful tool for modeling surgical effects on the cornea and developing a better understanding of the biomechanics of the cornea. In this paper we proposed a method of building a physical model of the cornea with finite element method. Firstly, an individual 3D modal model of cornea was constructed. Then the finite element model was built up based on a nonlinearly elastic, isotropic formulation. Finally, the intra-ocular pressure and external pressure were simulated with results of cornea shape changes computed via finite element analysis.

Keywords: Cornea; finite element model; eye pressure.

1 Introduction

Eyes are the most complex organ in human body. The cornea is the transparent, dome-shaped window covering the front of the eye. It is a powerful refracting matter, providing 2/3 of the eye's focusing power.

The application of laser technology to correct myopia, hyperopia and astigmatism has become an every day practice during the last decade. Laser In-Situ Keratomileusis (LASIK) is a surgical procedure that utilizes the Microkeratome to create a corneal "flap" of about one-third of the total corneal thickness. The excimer laser is then used to reshape the exposed middle layer of the cornea. The flap is finally put back to assume a new shape created by the excimer laser.

The mechanical properties of the cornea are very important to the research on human eyes. Because of the lack of an adequate understanding of the shape, biomechanical properties and deformation mechanisms of the cornea, the analysis of the refractive state is difficult. Surgical interventions at human eyes are very difficult to plan and the final state depends highly on the surgical and individual parameters. So, the cornea behavior of the patient must be estimated before the interventions. This can be done by modeling and simulating the biomechanical effects before surgical acts. Surgical information and the different modeling aspects must be structured in a knowledge based manner.

Many descriptive 2D/3D models are available for the cornea. Some are based on shape patterns of the anterior surface curvature [1,2]. Some are based on mathematical geometric models [3-6]. These geometric models can be simple, with a few descriptive shape parameters, or more complicated with Zernike polynomial

X. Gao et al. (Eds.): MIMI 2007, LNCS 4987, pp. 304–311, 2008.

approximations [5,6]. Other eye models are developed based on the human cadaver eye [7,8]. The finite element model is usually based on the linear elastic theory [4].

In this paper, a finite element model of the cornea was implemented based on the nonlinear elastic deformation theory. Compared with the previous works, the proposed method is more practical, since all the parameters can be easily acquired in clinic. This model has the further advantage of providing automatic generation of eye models to represent patients. We consider the cornea as a nonlinearly elastic, isotropic geometry which is more approximate to the practice.

The model can be used to investigate factors influencing corneal shape. Cornea shape change was computed via finite element analysis. Both the inner pressure and external pressure were simulated.

The construction of the finite element model used in this work is described in section 2, along with the simulated application of deforming forces. Model deformation results are described in section 3. Finally, section 4 presents conclusions and plans future work.

2 Method

The finite element eye model in this study is designed to focus on the structural integrity of the cornea. The effect from the sclera is ignored. Our method is divided into three main steps, shown in the Fig.1. Initially, a geometric cornea model is developed based on the ellipsoid. The parameters of shape can be input. A finite element mesh is created based on a nonlinearly elastic, isotropic formulation and reported mechanical properties. Then simulation is done after input of the boundary condition and load.

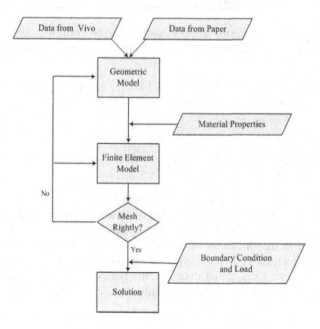

Fig. 1. Step of modeling and simulation

2.1 Geometric Model of the Cornea

An adult cornea is only about 1/2 millimeter thick and is comprised of 5 layers: epithelium, Bowman's membrane, stroma, Descemet's membrane and endothelium. The epithelium is layer of cells that cover the surface of the cornea. It is only about 5-6 cell layers thick and quickly regenerates when the cornea is injured. Boman's membrane lies just beneath the epithelium. Because this layer is very tough and difficult to penetrate, it protects the cornea from injury. The stroma is the thickest layer and lies just beneath Bowman's. It is composed of tiny collagen fibrils that run parallel to each other. This special formation of the collagen fibrils gives the cornea its clarity. Descemet's membrane lies between the stroma and the endothelium. The endothelium is just underneath Descemet's and is only one cell layer thick. This layer pumps water from the cornea, keeping it clear. If damaged or diseased, these cells will not regenerate. Tiny vessels at the outermost edge of the cornea provide nourishment, along with the aqueous and tear film.

The geometric model we constructed is also comprised of 5 layers. The ratio of layer thickness is in the Table 1.

Table 1. Ratio of the Cornea Layer Thickness

Layer of Cornea	Percent (%)
Epithelium	7
Bowman's membrane	1
Stroma	90
Descemet's membrane	1
Endothelium	1

The surface of the anterior cornea and posterior corneal surface are similar ellipsoid. The mathematical models of corneal surface are shown as following:

$$\frac{x^2}{a_0^2} + \frac{y^2}{b_0^2} + \frac{(z-c_0)^2}{c_0^2} = 1 \qquad (a_0, b_0, c_0 > 0) \qquad (1)$$

$$\frac{x^2}{a_1^2} + \frac{y^2}{b_1^2} + \frac{(z-c_1+d)^2}{c_1^2} = 1 \qquad (a_1, b_1, c_1, d > 0) \qquad (2)$$

Equation (1) is of the mathematical model of the anterior cornea surface and equation (2) is the posterior cornea accordingly. In the equation, a_i, b_i, c_i is respectively the long half-shaft of horizontal, vertical and longitudinal direction, which is about 7 to 8mm. And d is the thickness of central corneal. We have designed an anterior segment image analysis system to acquire these parameters in clinic [2]. The model can be modified using the actual data. So this type of model has the advantage of providing cornea models to represent patients' data. Fig. 2 shows an example of the geometric model of the cornea.

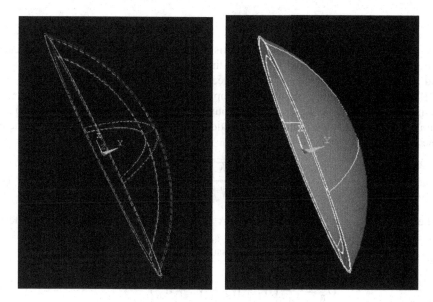

Fig. 2. Geometric Model of the Cornea

2.2 Material Properties of the Cornea

Investigations into the material properties of the cornea provide a basis for the development of biomechanical models. Such work includes an analysis of cornea strain distribution by Uchio, E. et al [7], or Yang Jian, et al [9].

The stroma is the thickest layer, and is the main load bearing part. The material parameter of the other layers is harder to get. In this paper, only the material parameter of stroma was considered.

Here we deal with the cornea as isotropic material. The material property constants are identified from the experimental data, which are obtained from mechanical tests on corneal strips and membrane inflation experiments.

The finite element model was based on a nonlinearly elastic, isotropic formulation. Material nonlinearity was modeled with a nonlinear stress–strain relationship given by

$$\sigma = \alpha(\varepsilon^{\beta\varepsilon} - 1) \qquad (3)$$

where σ is the stress and ε is the strain. The material constants α and β were equal to 17.5×10^{-4} N/mm^2 and 48.3, respectively [10].

The material temperature was 37 celsius degree. Further work needs to be done to characterize the thermal and thermomechanical effects in the corneal tissue, because the material properties will change when temperature increases or decreases.

Corneal tissue was assumed to behave as a nearly incompressible material with a Poisson's ratio equal to 0.49 [11].

2.3 Finite Element Model

The element of finite element model in this paper has six degrees of freedom at each node: translations in the nodal x, y, and z directions and rotations about the nodal x, y, and z-axes. Stress stiffening and large deflection capabilities are included.

If K_f, the foundation stiffness, is input, the out-of-plane stiffness matrix is augmented by three or four springs to ground. The number of springs is equal to the number of distinct nodes, and their direction is normal to the plane of the element. The value of each spring is:

$$K_{f,i} = \frac{\Delta K_f}{N_d} \tag{4}$$

Where: $K_{f,i}$ = normal stiffness at node i; Δ = element area; K_f = foundation stiffness; N_d = number of distinct nodes.

The output includes the foundation pressure, computed as:

$$\sigma_p = \frac{K_f}{4}(W_I + W_J + W_K + W_L) \tag{5}$$

Where σ_p = foundation pressure; W_I, etc. = lateral deflection at node I, etc.

Quad provides excellent representation of the eye's smooth curved surface geometry. To generate the mesh, several mesh densities were tested in order to ensure accurate and consistent convergence. The mesh of the cornea consisted of 8638 elements, and 8684 nodes. If the result of mesh is unsatisfied, mesh density can be modified reiteratively.

The boundary nodes at the edge of the cornea (i.e. at the limbus) through the thickness were assumed to be fixed in displacement. Any role played by the sclera was ignored.

In the original state, the cornea was loaded by a uniform pressure distribution, which was taken to be 0.002 N/mm^2, and was equivalent to a mercury column of 15 mm height [11,12]. It also is a parameter that can be input. The intra-ocular pressure was applied normal to the posterior surface of the model. The loading produced by the eyelids and the extra-ocular muscles was ignored.

A Newton–Raphson procedure, an iterative solution method with high quadratic convergence rate, was used in the nonlinear analysis.

3 Results

3.1 Deformation of the Cornea under Increasing Eye Pressure

The normal range for intra-ocular pressure is 10-21 mm Hg [12]. The application of intra-ocular pressure to the cornea model produced a deformed corneal surface, but further analysis was required to quantify the shape change. The shape change was analyzed by performing a least-squares fit of quadratic polynomial curves to the mesh nodes lying along the horizontal and vertical meridians of the deformed corneas. The radius of curvature of the quadratic curves was computed at the center point of the cornea.

The intra-ocular pressure is incrementally increased using time curves. Results are presented in the Fig.3 and Table 2.

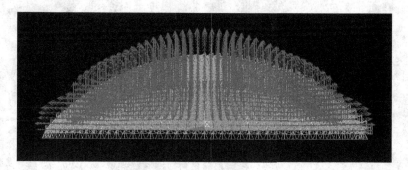

Fig. 3. The stress of cornea under intra-ocular pressure

Table 2. The Shape Deformation of Cornea under Increasing Eye Pressure

No	Intra-ocular Pressure(mmHg)	Displacement of the Center Node (mm)	Vertical Axis Radius of Curvature (mm)
1	16	2.185E-05	7.784
2	17	2.440E-05	7.780
3	18	2.590E-05	7.776
4	19	2.745E-05	7.773
5	20	2.895E-05	7.770
6	21	3.050E-05	7.767

3.2 Deformation of the Cornea under External Pressure

In employing a direct contact method of directly measuring the eye pressure, e.g. in Goldman applanation tonometry, a probe is pushed by a force f onto the eye until the eye flattens in a disc with the preset area of $A = \pi d^2/4$ with a diameter of $d = 3.06mm$. The pressure value $p = f/A$ is assumed to equal the inner eye pressure. If it exceeds 21mmHg, the eye pressure of a patient is said to be high, otherwise normal.

In the non-contact method, the surface of the eye is pushed by an air jet. The deformed area on the cornea is predefined by the shape of the air jet. The deformation of the eye is monitored by illuminating the eye by infrared light and using an optical sensor to measure the integrated reflected light intensity. When the detected amount of reflected light reaches its maximum, it indicates that the cornea is approximately flat in the predefined area. With the recorded force value at this time step and the size of the deformed area, the applied external and the inner pressure can be estimated.

In this simulation, external pressure was applied to the center part of the anterior cornea surface. Loads were used as the prescribed variables, and they were incrementally applied using time curves. The result was shown in the Fig. 4.

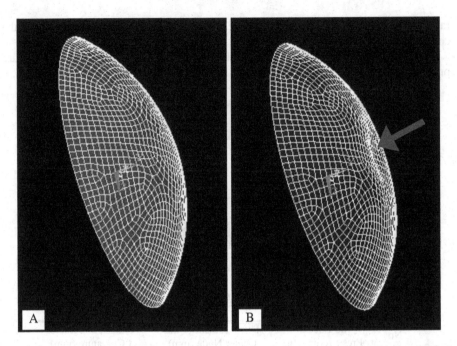

Fig. 4. A: view of a cornea model in original state. B: view of a cornea model being applied external pressure.

4 Discussion

In this paper, a nonlinearly elastic, isotropic, finite element model of the cornea has been presented and has been used to simulate. The individual model is implemented, which parameters are acquired from the data of patient, and deformations can be compared to the data on patient surgical outcomes. The model can be used to investigate factors influencing corneal shape.

Both the inner pressure and external pressure were simulated. Cornea shape change was computed via finite element analysis. The results suggest that this FEA model has potential usefulness as a simulation tool for cornea and it can provide useful information. The finite element model results indicate that the radius of the cornea is changed by forces from intra-ocular pressure.

Future work may expand on the current work in the following ways. The first one is generating cornea models with different thickness in different degrees and orientations. The role of sclera and muscle will be taken into account. The other future work is using the model of the cornea to simulate the effects of some usual surgical procedures.

Acknowledgments. This work was supported by the National Nature Science Foundation of China (60371012 and 60601025).

References

1. Laliberté, J.F., Brunette, I., Meunier, J.: 3D Average Human Corneal Models. In: Proceedings of the 26th Annual International Conference of the IEEE EMBS, San Francisco, CA, USA, pp. 1573–1576 (2004)
2. Ju, Y., Wang, B.L., Xie, J.Z., Huang, S.H., Wu, S.H., Wan, M.X.: A New Method Based on Slit Light Micrograph to Obtain Anterior Eye Segment Character. Chinese Journal of Biomedical Engineering 23, 193–198 (2004)
3. Zhang, Y.H., Shen, J.X., Hu, L.G., Liao, W.H.: Mathematical Models for Laser in Situ Keratomileusis and Photorefractive Keratectomy. Chinese Journal of Biomedical Engineering 22, 289–295 (2003)
4. Crouch, J.R., Merriam, J.C., Crouch, E.R.: Finite Element Model of Cornea Deformation. In: Duncan, J.S., Gerig, G. (eds.) MICCAI 2005. LNCS, vol. 3750, pp. 591–598. Springer, Heidelberg (2005)
5. Zhang, Y.H., Liao, W.H., Shen, J.X., Cao, Z.L.: Mathematical models for wavefront-guided refractive corneal surgery. Journal of Southeast University (Natural Science Edition) 34(15), 585–588 (2004)
6. Guo, H.Q., Wang, Z.Q., Zhao, Q.L., Quan, W., Wang, Y.: Eye Model Based on Wavefront Aberration Measured Subjectively. ACTA Photonica Sinica 34(11), 1666–1669 (2005)
7. Uchio, E., Ohno, S., Kudoh, J., Aoki, K., Kisielewicz, L.: Simulation model of an eyeball based on finite element analysis on a supercomputer. British Journal of Ophthalmology 83, 1106–1111 (1999)
8. Xie, J.Z., Wang, B.L., Ju, Y.: Research on Virtual Chinese Human Eye and its Application. In: Proceedings of the 27th Annual International Conference of the IEEE EMBS, Shanghai, China, pp. 2906–2909 (2005)
9. Yang, J., Zeng, Y.J., Li, Z.H.: Biomechanical Properties of Human Cornea. ACTA Biophysica Sinica 15(1), 208–213 (1999)
10. Fernandez, D.C., Niazy, A.M., Kurtz, R.M., Djotyan, G.P., Juhasz, T.: A Finite Element Model for Ultrafast Laser–Lamellar Keratoplasty. The Journal of the Biomedical Engineering Society 34, 169–183 (2006)
11. Wang, J.Q., Jiang, H.Y., Zheng, Y.J., Li, X.Y., Qi, L.: Study of computer simulation of radial Keratotomy using finite element method. Beijing Biomedical Engineering 18, 65–72 (1999)
12. Pinsky, P.M., Datye, D.V.: Microstructurally-based finite element model of the incised human cornea. Journal of Biomechanics 24, 907–922 (1991)

An Improved Hybrid Projection Function for Eye Precision Location

Yi Li, Peng-fei Zhao[*], Bai-kun Wan, and Dong Ming

Department of Biomedical Engineering and Scientific Instrument, College of Precision
Instrument and Opto-electronics Engineering, Tianjin University, Tianjin 300072, China
{Dong Ming,richardming}@tju.edu.cn

Abstract. An improved hybrid projection function (IHPF) for precise eye
location is presented in this paper. This algorithm combined the advantage of
variance projection function (VPF) and hybrid projection function (HPF) by
optimizing their weights in the traditional integral projection function (IPF).
Two different face databases, BioID face database downloaded from the
internet and PSFace database established by our laboratory, were used to test
the influence of different projection functions on correctness and relative mean-
error of eye locations. The results show that IHPF with optimized proportion
factors has a high eye location correctness of 96~100% and the lowest relative
error with better face feature location capability.

Keywords: facial feature location; eye precision location; projective function;
optimizing proportion factor.

1 Introduction

As a popular technique of biometrics recognition, face recognition has become a hot
topic in biomedical information detection fields for years, which still has a good
prospect of application[1],[2]. Facial feature location is an important component of
face recognition, whose goal is to search for the information of position, key points or
contours of facial features such as eyes, nose and mouth in a certain area of the face
image[3]. By now, facial feature location algorithms have been extensively used in
the fields of face detection, face location and face recognition etc.

Commonly used facial feature location algorithms consist of template-based, color-
based, knowledge-based, model-based, network-based and motion-based approaches.
Model-based face location is widely used for its advantage of high calculate speed,
high accuracy and wide applicability[4],[5]. The geometry projection function, which
is one of the model-based face location functions, contains two popular projection -
functions: integral projection function (IPF) and variance projection function (VPF).
Despite their widely application, both IPF and VPF have their limitation. IPF will fail
when the horizontal or vertical summation of the elements are unchanged in the
searching area, while VPF will fail in case of the same variance and different mean of
the elements.

---

[*] Supported by Key Discipline Construction Foundation of Tianjin.(2001-31).

X. Gao et al. (Eds.): MIMI 2007, LNCS 4987, pp. 312–321, 2008.

To rectify these shortcomings of IPF and VPF, a hybrid projection function (HPF) was recently introduced by Feng CG *et al*[6]. But, by simply summing IPF and VPF with an equal weight, this function cannot guarantee the best eye-location precision. This paper suggested an improved hybrid projection function (IHPF) by optimizing the weights of IPF and VPF based on experiments. The IHPF was tested on BioID face database and PSFace database on location correctness and relative mean-error in this paper to further verify its validity.

2 Rough Eye-Location

Some facial features other than eyes such as eyebrows, mouth are darker than their neighborhoods which will also respond to the projection function. Using projection function to do precise eye location in the whole facial region will reduce the eye detection accuracy greatly. So an eye-window that will only contain eyes regions must be found firstly. Eye position in the facial region can be located roughly by using binarize operation[7],[8],[9].

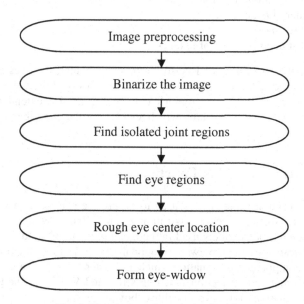

Fig. 1. Sketch map of rough eye-location

Figure 1 is the sketch map of rough eye-location. In the image preprocessing stage, the original image was smoothed to filter the noises. We used double-humped method to find a threshold value of the processed image and obtained a binary image. In the binary image, facial features, such as eyes, nose, mouth, were transformed into several isolated joint regions. These regions could be easily identified in a binary image by using label treatment algorithms and then forming an edge image. Along with the facial features regions, there would be some small regions coming from noises which are also labeled. So the edge image should be filtered for a second time to get rid of these noises. The threshold value of the filter was decided by experiment knowledge. Eye regions, which could be divided into left eye region (L) and right eye region (R), could be located by the laws below:

a). The centers of L and R are below the hair region H
b). The lowest pixels' position of L and R cannot be too low in the image
c). No other joint regions should be exist in a certain area below L and R
d). The distance between centre abscissas of L and R cannot be too short
e). The difference of the centre ordinates of L and R cannot be too big
f). L and R must be under the eyebrows regions

By experimental experience, eye regions were located by the method above and further described as formula(1).

$$Rng = \{(x, y) \mid B(x, y) = 0, \sum_{(i,j) \in \Omega} E_{(i,j)} > \theta\} \qquad (1)$$

Where Rng: region of eye dots volume
(x, y): a random pixel in the image
B : binary image
E : edge image
Ω: eight neighborhood of pixel (x, y)

Considering the barycenter of Rng to be the eye's center, the eyes centers can be rough located by calculating the barycenter of Rng from the edge image E. Eye-window containing double eyes regions can be formed by extending the region around eyes center to a certain area which will be further described in the sections below.

3 Geometrical Projection Function

Geometrical projection function was used to do precise eye-location within the eye-window in this paper. Projection algorithm is an efficient way for image feature extraction which has been widely used in the facial recognition fields. Usually one 2D image can be transformed into two orthogonal 1D projection functions containing relatively less complicated information which are easier for further analysis. The most widely used geometrical projection function is IPF and VPF[10]. The presently used HPF is the combination of the two functions above mentioned.

3.1 Integral Projection Function and Variance Projection Function

If $I(x, y)$ stands for the gray scale value of pixel (x, y), the vertical integral projection function $S_v(x)$ and the horizontal integral projection function $S_h(y)$ can be respectively described as formula (2) in interval $[x_1, x_2]$ and $[y_1, y_2]$.

$$S_v(x) = \int_{y_1}^{y_2} I(x, y) dy \ , \quad S_h(y) = \int_{x_1}^{x_2} I(x, y) dx \qquad (2)$$

Pixels in digital images are discrete, so the integral projection function can be transformed as formula (3):

$$S_v(x) = \sum_{y_i=y_1}^{y_2} I(x, y_i) \; , \; S_h(y) = \sum_{x_i=x_1}^{x_2} I(x_i, y) \qquad (3)$$

The average vertical integral projection function $M_v(x)$ and the average horizontal integral projection function $M_h(y)$ can be described as:

$$M_v(x) = \frac{1}{y_2 - y_1 + 1} \sum_{y_i=y_1}^{y_2} I(x, y_i)$$

$$M_h(y) = \frac{1}{x_2 - x_1 + 1} \sum_{x_i=x_1}^{x_2} I(x_i, y) \qquad (4)$$

$S_v(x)$ and $M_v(x)$ reflect the changes of the average gray value in a certain column of the image. And $S_h(y)$ and $M_h(y)$, in turn, reflect changes of the average gray value in a certain row of the image. Therefore the landmarks of an image can be identified through IPF. Fig.2 shows the projection functions' reflection to the gray scale changing in several image areas. In Fig.2, the curve of IPF changes at the boundaries of part 2, part 3 and part4, which can be used to distinguish different areas.

For the VPF, the vertical variance projection function $\sigma_v^2(x)$ and the horizontal variance projection function $\sigma_v^2(y)$ can be respectively described as formula (5) in interval $[x_1, x_2]$ and $[y_1, y_2]$.

$$\sigma_v^2(x) = \frac{1}{y_2 - y_1} \sum_{y_i=y_1}^{y_2} [I(x, y_i) - M_v(x)]^2$$

$$\sigma_h^2(y) = \frac{1}{x_2 - x_1} \sum_{x_i=x_1}^{x_2} [I(x_i, y) - M_h(y)]^2 \qquad (5)$$

When the variance of the gray level of a certain column or row in the image has changed, the variance projection function will also change, which can be used to analyze image character. For e.g. in Fig.2 the curve of VPF changes at the boundaries of part1 and part 2 as well as part 4 and part5. The jumps of the variance curve reflect exactly the changing of image gray scale in part 1, part 2, part 4 and part 5.

Although IPF and VPF can do eye location, both of them have their disadvantage. IPF will be invalid when the total gray value of the columns or rows in an image are the same while the gray value of each pixels are not, for the reason that essentially this function is only a simple sum of the gray values of the columns or rows. For instance, in Fig.2, part1 and part 2 are different in patterns but their total gray level are the same, so the curve of IPF cannot identify them, while VPF can distinguish these two parts. And VPF will be invalid when the variances of the pixels gray value

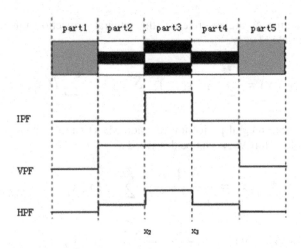

Fig. 2. The reaction of IPF、VPF and HPF to the areas with grey changes

in different parts are the same, for the reason that this function can only reflect the gray levels changes, while neglects other image information. For instance, in Fig.2, to different parts (part 2, part 3 and part 4) VPF can not show their difference, while IPF function can distinguish them.

3.2 Hybrid Projection Function

From the discussion above, we draw a conclusion that IPF and VPF are complementary in some ways. Hybrid projection function was presented from this knowledge for the improvement of these two projection functions. The HPF can be divided into vertical hybrid projection function $H_v(x)$ and horizontal projection function $H_h(y)$, defined as blow:

$$H_v(x) = \frac{1}{2}\sigma_v^{2'}(x) + \frac{1}{2}M_v'(x), H_h(y) = \frac{1}{2}\sigma_h^{2'}(y) + \frac{1}{2}M_h'(y) \qquad (6)$$

In which, $\sigma_v^{2'}(x)$、$\sigma_v^{2'}(y)$、M'$_v$(x)、M'$_h$(y) separately stand for the normalization results of $\sigma_v^2(x)$, $\sigma_v^2(y)$, $M_v(x)$ and $M_h(y)$ calculated by the formulas below:

$$\sigma_v'(x) = \frac{\sigma_v(x) - \min(\sigma_v(x))}{\max(\sigma_v(x)) - \min(\sigma_v(x))}$$

$$\sigma_h'(y) = \frac{\sigma_h(y) - \min(\sigma_h(y))}{\max(\sigma_h(y)) - \min(\sigma_h(y))} \qquad (7)$$

$$M_v'(x) = \frac{M_v(x) - \min(M_v(x))}{\max(M_v(x)) - \min(M_v(x))}$$

$$M_h'(y) = \frac{M_h(y) - \min(M_h(y))}{\max(M_h(y)) - \min(M_h(y))} \qquad (8)$$

As above has mentioned, HPF is the combination of IPF and VPF, which therefore has a quality of them both with higher image feature extraction correctness. For e.g. in Fig.2 the curve of HPF changes at the boundary of all the five parts (from part 1 to part 5). Using the HPF can effectively identify all the parts.

In the hybrid projection function defined as formula (6), the weights of IPF and VPF are the same (both of the weights are 0.5), which may not be a prefect value for facial feature location. So, it is necessary to find proper weights of the two projection functions in formula (6). An improved hybrid projection function (IHPF) described as formula (9), in which coefficient a, b were presented to determine the weights, was used for the improvement of the original HPF. The definition of vertical improved hybrid projection function (IH_v) and horizontal improved hybrid projection function (IH_h) are:

$$IH_v(x) = a \cdot M_v'(x) + b \cdot \sigma_v^{2'}(x), \quad IH_h(y) = a \cdot M_h'(y) + b \cdot \sigma_h^{2'}(y) \qquad (9)$$

In the formula (9), $0 \leq a \leq 1$, $0 \leq b \leq 1$, and a+b=1.

The value of a, b will be affirmed by experiments in this paper for the most accurate facial feature location using hybrid projection function. When a=1, b=0, formula (9) is transformed into $H_v(x) = M_v(x)$ and $H_h(y) = M_h(y)$, where HPF is equal to IPF. When a=0, b=1, formula (9) is transformed into $H_v(x) = \sigma_v^2(x)$ and $H_h(y) = \sigma_h^2(y)$, where HPF is equal to VPF.

4 Experiments and Results

In this paper, a standard eye model was firstly built for the precise eye center location (Fig.3). In the model, x1, x2 separately represented the X axel coordinates of the left canthus and right canthus. While y1, y 2 were the Y axel coordinates of the upper eyelid and nether eyelid. The vertical IHPF changed evidently at x1, x2; the horizontal IHPF changes evidently at y1, y 2. The position of eye center could be located by the X axel value of left canthus and right canthus and the Y axel value of upper eyelid and nether eyelid. Eye was considered to be a symmetrical structure in the model. So the coordinate of eye center, point $O(x_0, y_0)$, was:

$$x_0 = \frac{x_1 + x_2}{2}, \ y_0 = \frac{y_1 + y_2}{2} \qquad (10)$$

Twenty-one groups of a, b in formula (9) were given to optimize their values by experimental method. The optimized a, b values were the ones whose IHPF achieves the most accurate $O(x_0, y_0)$ value comparing to the actual eye center position as well as the lest error rate. The optimized IHPF can be described by this group of a, b.

In this paper two different databases — BioID face database [11] and PSFace face database — were used to do experiments. BioID face database contains 1521 gray level photos of 23 different people with the resolution of 384×268. The photos were taken in different seasons, different places with different background and lighting condition which could be used to test the universality of the IHPF. PSFace database is a face database established by Tianjin university for facial plastic surgery. It contains 21 pictures of different people with the same background and lighting condition, which was used to test the accuracy of IHPF in this paper.

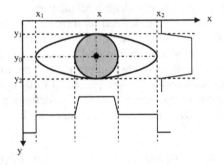

Fig. 3. Standard eye model

A standard must be established before calculating the eye-location accuracy of IHPF. We used the standard of Jesorsky to test the accuracy of IHPF with different a, b values[12]. The relative error of the eye-location was described as:

$$err = \frac{\max(d_l, d_r)}{d_{lr}} \tag{11}$$

In which: E_l and E_r separately stand for the true position of the left eye and right eye; E'_l and E'_r separately stand for the located position of the left eye and right eye; d_l is the distance between E_l and E'_l; d_r is the distance between E_r and E'_r; d_{lr} is the distance between E_l and E_r.

This method considers the located eye center is acceptable when it lies in the eye region. I.e. the longer one of d_l and d_r must be shorter than half of the eye's width.

Usually, d_{lr} is two times of the width of an eye. So, the reception threshold is 0.25. When err<0.25, the location result is considered to be right; otherwise, the location result is wrong.

After rough eye location, IHPF defined as formula (9) was used to do precise eye-location. In the experiments, a=i/20 (i=0, 1, 2...20), b=1-a. Fifty pictures of the experiments samples were picked out randomly from the BioID face database and twenty pictures of the experiments samples were picked out randomly from the PSFace database. And the experiment results were investigated in two ways: a) Correctness, i.e. the numbers of the pictures whose IHPF location error was less than 0.25. b) Relative mean-error, i.e. the average value of errors which were less than 0.25. The experiment results are presented as Table 1.

Table 1. Results of HPF with different a and b values tested on BioID and PSFace

coefficient / Results		Mean correctness		Relative mean-error	
a	b	BioID(%)	PSFace(%)	BioID	PSFace
0	1	92	100	0. 0840	0. 1001
1/20	19/20	92	100	0. 0812	0. 0955
1/10	9/10	92	100	0. 0801	0. 0955
3/20	17/20	96	100	0. 0848	0. 0941
1/5	4/5	96	100	0. 0870	0. 0941
1/4	3/4	96	100	0. 0873	0. 0855
3/10	7/10	96	100	0. 0904	0. 0855
7/20	13/20	96	100	0. 0959	0. 0820
2/5	3/5	94	100	0. 0970	0. 0808
9/20	11/20	94	100	0. 0971	0. 1102
1/2	1/2	96	100	0. 1004	0. 1200
11/20	9/20	96	95	0. 1121	0. 0803
3/5	2/5	94	95	0. 1129	0. 0128
13/20	7/20	94	90	0. 1231	0. 0982
7/10	3/10	90	90	0. 1287	0. 0982
3/4	1/4	88	90	0. 1314	0. 0953
4/5	1/5	88	95	0. 1351	0. 0881
17/20	3/20	90	95	0. 1308	0. 0881
9/10	1/10	90	100	0. 1217	0. 1250
19/20	1/20	92	100	0. 1112	0. 1248
1	0	94	95	0. 1060	0. 0777

The results from the Tab.1 indicate that the location results of IPF or VPF were not the perfect ones. And the original HPF stated as formula (6), although improved the location correctness, did not get the best results on relative mean-error.

Table.2 shows the mean-correctness and relative mean-error of IHPF eye location under the conditions of a<b, a=b and a>b. On the condition of a<b with VPF holding a better influence on IHPF, the location results were better than the circumstance of a>b under which IPF held a stronger influence. The reason was that in the eye regions the gray level was low and the grey scale change was high, which made VPF more effective.

The data of tab.1 suggests that the eye location correctness was the highest while the relative mean-error was relatively small on BioID and PSFace when a=1/4 and b=3/4. From this knowledge, the coefficients in IHPF could be optimized as a=1/4, b=3/4. Formula (9) could be described as formula (12).

$$H_v(x) = \frac{1}{4}M_v'(x) + \frac{3}{4}\sigma_v^{2'}(x) \ , \ H_h(y) = \frac{1}{4}M_h'(y) + \frac{3}{4}\sigma_h^{2'}(y) \qquad (12)$$

Table 2. Mean-correctness and relative mean-error on the condition that a<b, a=b or a>b

Results coefficient	Mean correctness		Relative mean-error	
	BioID(%)	PSFace(%)	BioID	PSFace
a<b	94.4	100	0.0885	0.0923
a=b	96	100	0.1004	0.1200
a>b	91.6	94.5	0.1213	0.0889

Fig.4 showed the location result using the IPHF defined as formula (12). In Fig.6, the round dots (O) represent the rough eye location position while the crossings (+) represent the precise eye location position. From Fig.4, we can draw a conclusion that the precise eye location can find the real position of the pupils.

Fig. 4. Result comparison of rough eye location (○) with accurate eye location (+)

5 Conclusion

In this paper, an improved projection function was presented to avoid the shortcoming of IPF, VPF and the original HPF while locating the image features in a circumstance with complicated gray scale distribution. The location effect of IHPF was tested on BioID face database and PSFace database, from which a correctness of 96~100% with the lowest relative error was obtained. The experiments results indicated that IHPF has a better facial feature location effect than IPF, VPF and HPF.

References

1. Li, D.H., Podolak, I.T., Lee, S.W.: Facial component extraction and face recognition with support vector machines. In: Proceeding of Automatic Face and Gesture Recognition, Washington, DC USA, pp. 76–81 (2002)
2. Wu, Y.K., Lai, S.H.: Locating facial feature points using support vector machines. In: Proceedings. 9th IEEE International Workshop on Cellular Neural Networks and their Applications, Hsinchu, Taiwan, pp. 296–299 (2005)
3. Yao, T.X., Li, H.D., Jin, Y.Q.: A fast and robust face location and feature extraction system. In: Image processing, 2002 proceedings, international conference, pp. I-157–I-160 (2002)

4. Kanade, T.: Picture Processing by Computer Complex and Recognition of Human Faces[D], Kyoto University, Japan (1973)
5. Feng, C.G., Yuen, P.C.: Variance projection function and its application to eye detection for human face recognition, Pattern Recognition Letters, pp. 899–906 (1998)
6. Geng, X., Zhou, Z.H., Chen, S.F.: Eye location based on hybrid projection function. Journal of Software, 1394–1400 (2003)
7. Trier, O.D., Jain, A.K.: Goal-directed evaluation of binarization methods, Pattern Analysis and Machine Intelligence, pp. 1191–1201 (1995)
8. Bai, J., Yang, Y.Q., Tian, R.L.: Complicated Image's Binarization Based on Method of Maximum Variance Machine Learning and Cybernetics. In: 2006 International Conference, pp. 3782–3785 (2006)
9. He, J., Do, Q.D.M., Downton, A.C., Kim, J.H.: A comparison of binarization methods for historical archive documents, Document Analysis and Recognition, 538 - 542 (2005)
10. Kumar, R.T., Raja, S.K., Ramakrishnan, A.G.: Eye detection using color cues and projection functions. In: Image Processing. 2002. Proceedings. 2002 International Conference on Publication, vol. 3, pp. III-337– III-340 (2002)
11. Web address, http://www.bioid.com/technology/facedatabase.html
12. Jesorsky, O., Kirchberg, K.J., Frisholz, R.W.: Robust face detection using the Hausdorff distance. In: Audio and video based Person Authentication. LNCS, pp. 90–95. Springer, Berlin (2001)

Spectropolarimetric Imaging for Skin Characteristics Analysis

Yongqiang Zhao, TieHeng Yang, PeiFeng Wei, and Quan Pan

The College of Automation, Northwestern Polytechnical University, Shannxi 710072, China
zhaoyq@nwpu.edu.cn

Abstract. Light scattering spectra and polarization states can provide important information about skin. To analyse the mechanisms of interaction between skin and light, and the relationship between the changes of light's characteristics and the variations of skin's states, a spectropolarimetric imaging system is proposed to acquire the spectral, polarimetric and spatial properties of the skin. After acquiring the spectropolarimetric imagery, an empirical line correction method is used to analyse the polarimetric spectra differences between normal skin and skin with a chicken pox scar. To enhance the visual difference between normal skin and skin with a chicken pox scar, and the polarimetric and spectral characteristics of the skin in different states, a false colour mapping based spectropolarimetric image fusion method is proposed that combines the intensity image, the degree of linearity of the polarization image, and the phase of the polarization image, with spectral imagery. We demonstrate experimentally that this imaging system can be used to discriminate between the different skin pathological conditions efficiently.

1 Introduction

Light scattering spectra can provide important information about the object of interest and it has been extensively used in physical science to study a great variety of materials. Although biological tissue is different from mineral surfaces, it can also be studied with light scattering spectra. It has been demonstrated that light scattering spectra can provide structural and functional information about biological tissue [1]. When light propagates through a biological tissue, another important characteristic of light, polarization states, will change due to the tissue's birefringence and scattering. It is the tissue's surface characteristics that determine how the polarization states of the incident light will change. Hence, a tissue can be characterized by the polarization states of light and light scattering spectra [2].

Considering the light scattering spectra and polarization states can provide quantitative, objective measurements of pathological parameters in real time without the need for tissue removal. Gurjar et al. [1] developed a new biomedical imaging modality based on polarized light scattering spectroscopy to provide morphological information about epithelial cells in situ. Backman et al. [7] used polarized light scattering spectroscopy to quantitatively measure epithelial cellular structures in situ.

X. Gao et al. (Eds.): MIMI 2007, LNCS 4987, pp. 322–329, 2008.

Jarry et al. [8] studied the randomization of linearly polarized light as it propagated through tissues and microsphere solutions, observing a surprising persistence of polarization when propagating through liver tissues despite multiple scattering of photons.

According to the image chain theory, by exploiting more information about the object of interest, better identification performance can be achieved [9]. The introduction of spectropolarimetic imaging has led to the development of techniques that combine spectral, polarimetric and spatial information. As spectropolarimetic imaging has become accessible, computational methods developed initially for remote sensing problems have been transferred to biomedical applications. Considering the spectral and polarimetric variability for different biological tissue states, spectropolarimetic imaging has the ability to improve the capability of automated systems for biological tissue analysis. Skin is the largest organ of the human body, and skin interactions with light often involve localized or diffuse changes in spectra and polarization states. Understanding the mechanisms of such interactions is therefore important in the study of skin physiology and pathology. This paper focuses on the use of spectropolarimetric imaging (in the visual light band, capturing linear polarization characteristics) to analyse the optical character of the skin. According to the characteristics of the spectropolarimetric image of the skin in different pathological conditions, a false color mapping based spectropolarimetric image combination method is proposed to make special characteristics of the skin more obvious.

2 Spectropolarimetric Imaging Systems

2.1 Spectropolarimetry

This section introduces the basic concepts of polarimetry and is not intended as an in depth analysis. A beam of homochromous incoherent radiation emitted or reflected from an object surface can be described by the four Stokes parameters [6]:

$$S=(I,Q,U,V) \tag{1}$$

where

$$I=(i_0+i_{45}+i_{90}+i_{135}) \tag{2}$$

$$Q= i_0 \text{-} i_{90} \tag{3}$$

$$U=i_{45} \text{-} i_{135} \tag{4}$$

where i_0, i_{45}, i_{90}, i_{135} are the intensity measured at the polarizer's four rotational positions 0^0, 45^0, 90^0, 135^0. In most polarization imaging systems, the individual Stokes components represent an entire two-dimensional image so the calculations are performed for each individual pixel.

An alternative (and more intuitive) form of the Stokes parameters is intensity, the degree of linear polarization (*DoLP*) and the phase of polarization (*Orient*) and they are related to the Stokes parameters as follows:

$$Int = I \tag{5}$$

$$DoLP = \frac{\sqrt{Q^2 + U^2}}{Int} \tag{6}$$

$$Orient = \frac{1}{2} arctan\left(\frac{U}{Q}\right) \tag{7}$$

2.2 Camera System

The camera system is schematically depicted in Figure 1. An incoherent white light source (halogen light source) is used. The light is collimated by a 20 cm focal length lens and delivered to the skin at an angle of 25° to the normal of the skin surface. The choice of angle is not critical and oblique angles of illumination beside 25° also work. The camera (Retiga Exi made by QImaging Corporation, 12-bit CCD camera) with macro lens only collected light that had entered the skin and been backscattered toward the camera. An analyzing linear polarizer and spectral filter (liquid crystal tunable filter made by Cambridge Research Instruments *(CRI)*, the full-width at half-maximum *(FWHM)* is 10nm when the center wavelength is 550nm, and the FWHM is proportional to the center wavelength squared, spectral range: 400nm-720nm) placed in front of the camera is manually aligned at four different angles 0^0, 45^0, 90^0, 135^0.

Four image sequences are acquired at every band, i_0, i_{45}, i_{90}, i_{135}. The imaging channels have unknown gains due to filter transmission and CCD response and unknown offsets due to dark current and stray light. These gains and offsets may change over time. Therefore, we devised a method to correct the raw images acquired by the spectropolarimetric camera to spectropolarimetric reflectance images for analysis. A spectralon panel and a spectrometer (spectral range: 350nm-2500nm, bandwidth between 350nm to 1050nm is 1.5nm, bandwidth between 1050nm to 2500nm is 11.5nm, total 640 channels) are used during calibration. The panel with approximately 99 percent reflectance is referred to as a white spectralon, it has nearly constant reflectance over the 0.3nm-2.5nm spectral range.

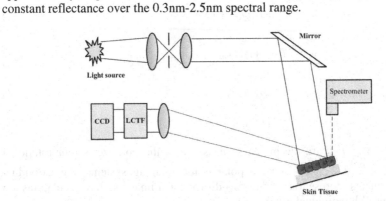

Fig. 1. Spectropolarimetric Imaging System where spectral span ranges from 400nm-750nm, there are a total 35 spectral bands of 10nm, and we get linear polarization characteristics: intensity, the degree of linear polarization, and the phase of polarization at every band.

2.3 Spectropolarimetric Correction

In spectropolarimetric imaging detection, the sensed light contains not only light scattered by tissue but also light scattered/reflected by the background and other materials. As the dark current of the detector, the variation of the filter's relative transmittance in different spectral bands and other non perfect factors will mean images contain an amount of noise, and mean a digital number value can not reflect real polarimetric spectra. These images must be corrected to make the acquired spectropolarimetric information more precise.

Traditional calibration uses several methods to convert measured digital number values to relative reflectance or absolute reflectance. Flat field calibration, logarithmic residuals and internal average relative reflectance (IARR) produce relative reflectance spectra. Empirical line calibration is a method for estimating apparent (absolute) reflectance. Empirical line calibration is used to force image data to match selected field reflectance spectra and requires a priori knowledge of a site. Specific pixels from the spectropolarimetric image are associated with these reference spectra and linear regression is used to calculate the gain and offsets which are needed to convert the digital number for each image band to reflectance. The instrument digital number values are then converted to reflectance using the acquired gain and offset values. By using empirical methods, the produced spectra can be made comparable with field or laboratory results.

3 Spectropolarimetric Imagery Combination Based on False Colour Fusion

Polarization is orthogonal to wavelength, and is a more general physical characteristic of light than intensity, it can carry additional information, thus providing a richer description of imaged tissues[4]. Figure 2 and figure 3 list the skin's images in different spectral bands and described by different polarimetric parameters.

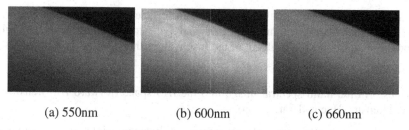

(a) 550nm   (b) 600nm   (c) 660nm

Fig. 2. Skin image in different spectral band

According to the meaning of intensity, the degree of linear polarization and the phase of polarization, and the representation of IHS color space, linear polarimetric information can be represented by a false color image. Fig.4 shows a mapping of the transmitted radiance sinusoid for partial linear polarization into an intensity-hue-saturation visualization scheme.

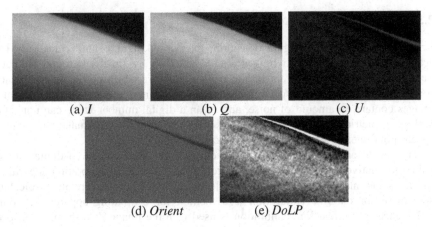

(a) *I*   (b) *Q*   (c) *U*

(d) *Orient*   (e) *DoLP*

Fig. 3. Skin image described by different polarimetric parameters

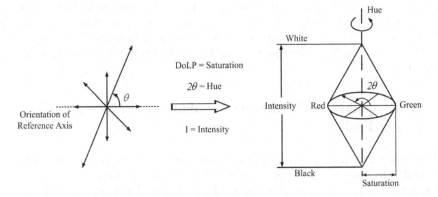

Fig. 4. Intensity-hue-saturation representation scheme for partial linear polarization

Based on this mapping method and the characteristics of multi-spectral imagery, a false color mapping based multi-spectral and polarimetric imagery fusion rule is proposed in algorithm 1. The detail of the fusion algorithm is listed as follows.

Algorithm 1:

1) Transform the multi-spectral image into the *IHS* space (forward *IHS* transform to get Intensity, Hue and Saturation).

2) Fuse the polarimetric intensity image and multispectral intensity component by wavelet image fusion to get a new *NInt* image.

3) Fuse the Hue with the degree of linear polarization to get a new *NDoLP* image.

4) Fuse the Saturation with the phase of polarization to get a new *NOrient* image.

5) Find the common part among the *NInt*, *NDoLP* and *NOrient* image:

$$Common = NInt \cap NDoLP \cap NOrient \tag{8}$$

6) Calculate the unique part in every image:

$$\begin{cases} DoLP^* = NDoLP - Common \\ Orient^* = NOrient - Common \\ Int^* = NInt - common \end{cases} \qquad (9)$$

7) Adjust the image by unique information:

$$\begin{cases} DoLP^{**} = NDoLP - Orient^* - Int^* \\ Orient^{**} = NOrient - DoLP^* - Int^* \\ Int^{**} = NInt - DoLP^* - Orient^* \end{cases} \qquad (10)$$

8) Reverse transformation of RGB to get final fused image.
$$F = RGB^{-1}(Int^{**}, DoLP^{**}, Orient^{**}) \qquad (11)$$

4 Experimental Results

We now present an experimental study to analyse the information provided by the spectropolarimetric imaging system and apply the empirical line calibration to produce relative reflectance polarimetric spectra of the area of interest and use the proposed false color spectropolarimetric image fusion method to combine the spatial, spectral and polarimetric information.

Figure 5 shows the unpolarized intensity images of normal skin (a) and skin with a chicken pox scar (b), polarization image of normal skin (c) and skin with a chicken pox scar (d). There is little difference between images (a) and (c) for normal skin. But between images (c) and (d) around the scar region, the image (d) is darker than image (b).

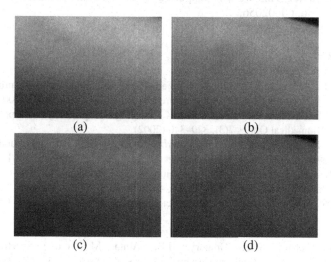

Fig. 5. Unpolarized intensity images of normal skin (a) and skin with chicken pox scar (b), polarization image of normal skin (c) and skin with chicken pox scar (d)

Figure 6 left shows the fused images for normal skin. Figure 6 right shows the fused images for the skin with a chicken pox scar. The fused images show the chicken pox scar as a darker region due to the strong backscatter from the collagen fibers induced by the trauma.

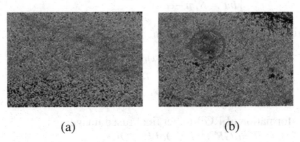

(a)   (b)

Fig. 6. Fused spectropolarimetric image of normal skin (a) and skin with chicken pox scar (b)

5 Conclusion

In this paper, we report a new spectropolarimetric imaging system for skin characteristics analysis and propose a method to fuse the spectral and polarimetric images using false color mapping. Through experiment, we conclude that this fusion algorithm can be well applied to maintain detail and spectral difference information. The fused images are therefore able to emphasize image contrast on the basis of light scattering in the superficial layers of the skin. The fused images also can visualize the disruption of the normal texture of the papillary and upper reticular dermis by skin pathology.

Acknowledgments. This work is supported by the National Nature Science Foundation of China no. 60602056.

References:

1. Gurjar, R.S., Backman, V., Perelman, L.T., et al.: Imaging human epithelial properties with polarized lightscattering spectroscopy. Nature Medicine 7(11), 1245–1248 (2001)
2. Jacques, S.L., Ramella-Roman, J.C., Lee, K.: Imaging skin pathology with polarized light. Journal of Biomedical Optics 7(3), 329–340 (2002)
3. Liu, G.L., Li, Y.F., Cameron, B.D.: Polarization-Based Optical Imaging and Processing Techniques with application to the Cancer Diagnostics. In: Steven, L.J., Donald, D.D., Sean, J.K. (eds.) Laser Tissue Interaction XIII: Photochemical, Photothermal, and Photomechanical, Proceedings of SPIE, vol. 4617, pp. 208–219 (2002)
4. Wolff, L.B., Mancini, T.A., Poluiquen, P., et al.: Liquid Crystal Polarization Camera. IEEE Transactions on Robotics and Automation 13(2), 195–203 (1997)
5. Stamatas, G.N., Balasb, C., Kolliasa, N.: Hyperspectral Image Acquisition and Analysis of Skin. In: Richard, M.L., Gregory, H.B., Anita, M.J. (eds.) Spectral Imaging: Instrumentation, Applications, and Analysis II, Proceedings of SPIE, vol. 4959, pp. 77–82 (2003)

6. Pajares, G.J., de la Cruz, M.: A Wavelet-based Image Fusion Tutorial. Pattern Recognition 37(9), 1855–1872 (2004)
7. Backman, V., Gurjar, R., Badizadegan, K., et al.: Polarized light scattering spectroscopy for quantitative measurement of epithelial cellular structures in situ. IEEE Journal of Selected Topics in Quantum Electronics 5(4), 1019–1027 (1999)
8. Jarry, G., Steimer, E., Damaschini, V., et al.: Coherence and polarization of light propagating through scattering media and biological tissues. Applied Optics 37(3), 7357–7367 (1998)
9. Schott, J.R.: Remote Sensing: Image Chain Approach, 3rd edn. Cambridge University Press, Cambridge (1996)

Image-Based Augmented Reality Model for Image-Guided Surgical Simulation

Junyi Zhang and Shuqian Luo

Biomedical Engineering College, Capital Medical University,
Beijing 100069, China
sqluo@ieee.org

Abstract. Image-based information is helpful for image-guided surgery therapy using medical imaging devices. In this paper, we present an image-based augmented reality model for potential medical application. Firstly, texture image is generated from two orthogonal images with multi-resolution technique. The surface of a 3D head based on MRI images is flattened onto 2D plane with cylindrical projection method. Then line-pair 2D warping method is used to determine the feature-based positional relationship between the texture image and the flattened image. The information of anatomical structure from medical images can be preserved for the future medical application. Experimental results show that the method can photo-realistically render 3D face with texture mapping. Finally, simple patient-to-model registration is used to obtain interactive augmented reality display of a surgical simulation for a simulated cyst in corpus callosum.

1 Introduction

3D face modeling has been an active area in computer images and graphic applications. However this kind of facial 3D data only include shape information without texture and internal structure information. Texture mapping is an effective way to improve the realistic effect of object rendering and can add more surface detail and internal structure information without much computational expense [1-7]. A series of reference features are determined to get the correspondence between every point of the 3D object and pixel of the texture image. The texture mapping of human face is used as an example with which the selected features are hairline, eyebrow, canthus, mouth, and chin. The polygon-based triangle-to-triangle texture mapping is computational expensive to apply these approaches based on computer vision. Besides, polygon-based data, preserving only the surface structure, are in nature not suitable for quantitative analysis. Therefore many research efforts have been made to generate realistic face modeling from photos taken with an ordinary video camera [8,9]. The role of medical imaging in establishing diagnosis and guiding therapy has been accepted along with technological advances. Image guidance can reduce the inherent invasiveness of surgery and improve the localization and target detection. Image-based information has always influenced the image-guided therapy by the improved quality and content of medical imaging.

X. Gao et al. (Eds.): MIMI 2007, LNCS 4987, pp. 330–339, 2008.

Until today, few texture mapping methods were designed solely for the applications of volume-based data. In this paper, we introduce an image-based approach to render 3D head model with two orthogonal photos. The proposed method is designed to directly map a texture onto the surface of 3D volume medical data. It provides an alternative way for fast texture mapping in computer graphics applications.

2 Image-Based Texture Mapping

The image-based texture mapping for a head model is composed of the following four steps.

1) Texture Generation. Generate the texture image from front view and side view facial images using multi-resolution technique.
2) Flattening. Flatten a 3D head model to a 2D map by cylindrical projection
3) Warping Texture Image. Determine the corresponding features on both the flattened and texture images, and then warp the images with line-pairs based methods.
4) Reconstruction. Reconstruct 3D head model from the warped texture images.

2.1 Texture Generation

Using the camera setup as shown in Fig.1, a frontal view and a side view images of nurse model (KAF-1) are simultaneously captured. The design mode of camera setup is similar to Ref. [10]. The type of optical camera is WAT-250D. The camera centers are separated by baseline distance b from each other, and are perpendicular to each other.

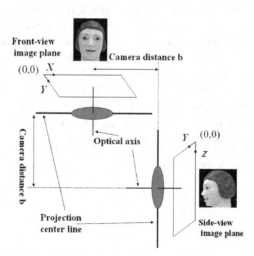

Fig. 1. Camera setup scheme, including nurse model (KAF-1) and optical camera (WAT-250D)

The intrinsic parameters of both cameras, such as the focus lengths, are assumed to be equal. Also the camera and image pixel coordinates are uniform without any

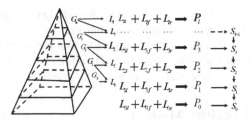

Fig. 2. Gaussian and Laplacian pyramid, both image size and resolution are decreased from level to level

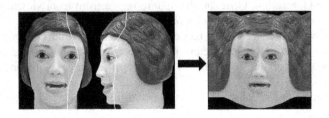

Fig. 3. Texture generation procedures, feature lines (*left*) and texture image (*right*)

camera calibration. The coordinates of a 3D point $p(x, y, z)$ can be provided by the calibrated (X, Y) coordinates in the front-view image and the (Y, Z) coordinates in the side-view image.

Suppose the human face is right-left symmetrical, three images including the front, the left and the right views are merged to form a complete face texture image. Firstly, reference feature lines (hairline, eyebrow, canthus, mouth, and chin) are determined on the front-view and the side-view images. Then these two images are merged to generate the texture image according to the matched reference lines.

Multi-resolution image pyramid decomposition method is used to remove boundaries and to smooth the texture image [11]. The method obtain the G_l (Gaussian image) and L_l (Laplacian image), where l is the level number. Both image size and resolution are decreased from level to level. An image G_l of each level on the pyramid is obtained from its lower level G_{l-1}.

$$G_{l+1}(i, j) = \sum \sum_{m,n=-2}^{2} w(m, n) \cdot G_l(2i + m, 2j + n)$$

$$l = 0, 1, 2 \ldots, N - 1$$

(1)

Where $w(m, n)$ is a weighting Gaussian-like function [12,13]. After the image pyramid is created as in Fig.2, three L_l images on each level are combined to obtain the P_l images. P_l is augmented with S_{l+1} to get S_l, which is the result of each level, and is constructed from its topper level by using Eq.(3). Finally, a final texture image (S_0 image) is obtained as shown in Fig.3.

$$L_l(i, j) = G_l(i, j) - \sum_{m,n=-2}^{2} w(m, n) \cdot G_{l+1}\left(\frac{i+m}{2}, \frac{j+n}{2}\right)$$

$$l = 0, 1, 2 \ldots, N - 1$$
(2)

$$S_l(i, j) = L_l(i, j) + \sum_{m,n=-2}^{2} w(m, n) \cdot S_{l+1}\left(\frac{i+m}{2}, \frac{j+n}{2}\right)$$

$$S_N = G_N, l = 0, 1, 2 \ldots, N - 1$$
(3)

2.2 Cylindrical Projection Flattening Procedures

In order to demonstrate the mapping of a 2D texture image to 3D volume medical data, the cylindrical projection and inverse cylindrical projection methods are used to map a photo-realistic face texture onto a MRI volume data of a human head.

Our medical data are MRI images. These images were acquired with a 3.0T MRI scanner according to DICOM3.0 format, the slice thickness is 2mm and the image size is 512×512 with totally 127 slices. Firstly, the profile of a human head is segmented from the gray-level tomography images. Because a disconnect pixel or an isolated pixel can confuse the final result of texture mapping, many image processing techniques, such as noise filtering, thresholding, region growing and morphology operation, have been used to obtain the integrated boundary. Finally, after these procedures are completed, polygon-based method is used to reconstruct a complete 3D head model based on medical images without fragment (Fig.5 (left)).

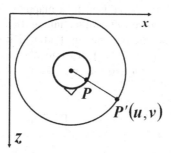

Fig. 4. The coordinates of u and v can be computed by cylindrical projection in one quadrant

The cylindrical projection which projects the images onto a cylindrical surface, defines the correspondence between $P(x, y, z)$ and $P'(u, v)$ (Fig.4).

If the center coordinates of cylindrical is (x_0, y, z_0), the mathematical expression of cylindrical projection is shown in Eq.(4).

$$u = \begin{cases} \arcsin(|x|/\sqrt{x^2 + z^2}) & x \le x_0, z \le z_0 \\ \pi - \arcsin(|x|/\sqrt{x^2 + z^2}) & x < x_0, z > z_0 \\ \pi + \arcsin(|x|/\sqrt{x^2 + z^2}) & x > x_0, z > z_0 \\ 2\pi - \arcsin(|x|/\sqrt{x^2 + z^2}) & x > x_0, z < z_0 \end{cases} \qquad (4)$$

$$v = y$$

After flattening the surface of a 3D head model, surface normal-vectors of the original surface are mapped onto the corresponding points of the flattened surface. Fig.5 (right) is the flattened model mesh of 3D head model.

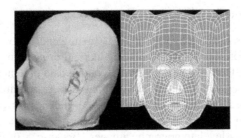

Fig. 5. 3D head model (*left*) reconstructed from MRI images, flattened model mesh (*right*) based on the surface of the 3D head model

2.3 Warping Texture Image and 3D Facial Reconstruction

After the texture image and the flattened image are obtained, mapping between a 3D head model and texture image is reduced to a mapping in 2D space. The line-pair based 2D warping method is a well-known technique used to find the correspondence of pixels between the texture image and the flattened image. The method was designed by Beier and Neely in 1992 [14]. It establishes the accurate correspondence with pairs of feature line between two images, and it is similar to the technique used in 2D metamorphosis.

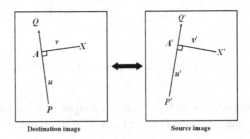

Fig. 6. Single line pair in line-pair based 2D warping method, including destination image and source image

In Fig.6, these two images are defined as source and destination images. The user-defined features are shown in the two images, and the features can be a single or multiple line pairs. The single line pair for the source and destination images are $\overline{P'Q'}$ and $\overline{PQ}$. This feature line pair finds the pixel X located the destination image that corresponds to X' in the source image. The warping field can be computed by Eq.(5).

$$
\begin{aligned}
u &= (X - P) \cdot (Q - P) / \| Q - P \|^2 \\
v &= (X - P) \cdot E (Q - P) / \| Q - P \| \\
X' &= P' + u \cdot (Q' - P') \\
&\quad + v \cdot E (Q' - P') / \| Q' - P' \|
\end{aligned}
\tag{5}
$$

The texture image is named as source image, and the flattened image is destination image. Firstly, the feature lines are determined on these two images respectively, including eyebrow, eye, nosewing, mouth, tragus and chin (Fig.7). Then the texture image is warped by line-pair based 2D warping method with respect to these feature lines.

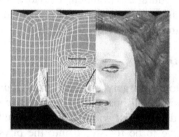

Fig. 7. Correspondence feature lines on mesh image (*left*) and texture image (*right*)

Because texture mapping is a feature-based approach, the selection of features will certainly affect the outcomes of texture mapping. Thus, selection and correspondence assignment have to be suitably determined in order to achieve desirable results. Though users can easily achieve good texture mapping with enough pairs of corresponding features, the feature-based methods needs provide proper feature selection and assignment by human interaction.

After the facial texture was warped, the correspondences between the flattened image and the texture image are achieved. The inverse cylindrical projection is used to render the 3D head model with texture mapping. Fig.8 shows the result of the proposed texture mapping methods.

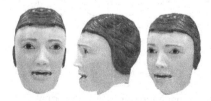

Fig. 8. Render the 3D head model with texture image and three different views of the resulted 3D head model

3 Image-Guided Surgical Planning and Simulation

During surgical treatment, surgeons prefer appropriately rendered and interactively displayed 3D data to comprehend more image-base information. Depending on particular application, surgical planning implies not only image reconstruction but also integration of various displays, image manipulation and visualization tools.

The role of surgical planning is to define the safest possible approach with the least possible damage to normal tissue. The optimal navigational paths and movements through the physical space are tested and analyzed using a preoperative model. Further expansion of surgical planning and simulation techniques requires more complex methods, such as soft tissue deformation, collision detection and haptic feedback, and more information about shape, position and orientation that may correct or account for unavoidable tissue deformations and organ shifts during surgery [15-18].

Using surgical planning to select optimal surgical strategies and to simulate lifelike invasive procedures not only facilitates training and encourages rehearsal but also supports the fundamental role of image guidance in actual execution of the plan. Establishing a simulated procedural environment is also a critical step for creating an image-based virtual and augmented reality environment that allows the user to actively enter the 3D environment and perform simulated procedures within it.

3.1 Augmented Reality Display

Patient-to-model registration is largely different from multimodality coregistration. Image fusion requires matching all image-based geometric data in one single coordinate system. The matched data coexist within a single virtual data base, but for image-guided procedures they have to be registered into the physical space of the patient, too. In addition, these data should be overlaid or projected to the patient's exposed surface if surgical guidance is necessary. We only used visual registration method to deal with the matched medical data in Maya software. Maya Embedded Language (MEL) scripting provides several advantages for animating these image guidance procedures [19].

As shown in Fig.9, skull and brain lobes models are reconstructed from VCH-female dataset [20,21]. By using Maya software, these two models are combined with

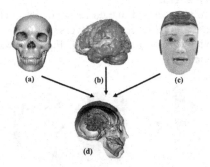

Fig. 9. (a) Skull model and (b) brain lobes model from Virtual Chinese Human (VCH) dataset, (c) 3D rendered skin surfaces head model, (d) Augmented reality display of the composite model

proposed 3D head model to obtain the interactive augmented view of the resulted composite model. The skin facial model is modified to fit the female skull and brain model. These models are manipulated to more clearly demonstrate anatomical relationships. These structures are overlaid on the skull models to complete representation of relevant head anatomy.

In MEL-scripted windows, MRI images can be browsed layer by layer. The median plane of brain is defined as "reference layer", such as the middle of frontal, parietal and occipital lobes, and then MRI images are subsequently mapped onto the corresponding plane created in 3D space in Maya. MRI images and 3D anatomical models are observed by difference orientation and position (Fig.10). At the same time, anatomical structures are clearly identified increasing layer level.

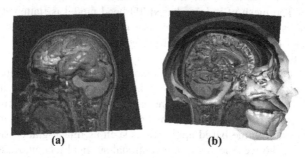

(a)   (b)

Fig. 10. Augmented reality display of Patient-to-model, (a) brain lobes model and MRI image, (b) the composite model

3.2 Image-Guided Surgical Simulation

A simulated cyst locates on the top of corpus callosum as in Fig.11, and the probe or instrument is put into the cyst (red) through the internal brain lobes.

Augmented reality visualization of surgical planning and simulation plays an important role in image-guided surgical therapy. It is easy to make surgeon see beyond the exposed surfaces and to maximally reduce surgical risk. But the limitation of surgical simulation is not able to simulate unavoidable tissue deformations and organ

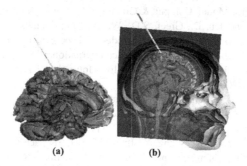

(a)   (b)

Fig. 11. Image-guided drainage of a simulated cyst using MRI guidance, (a) the orientation and position of cyst in brain lobes model, (b) the orientation and position of cyst in the composite model

shifts during surgery. Interactive visualization is sufficient for most percutaneous biopsy and intravascular interventional procedures but is not fully satisfactory for image guidance with near-real time, high contrast and spatial resolution volumetric images.

4 Conclusion and Future Work

The flattening and warping methods are integrated to achieve texture mapping efficiently and to establish good correspondence between every point of the 3D face model and pixel of the texture image. Firstly, two orthogonal images of a face are obtained by ordinary camera. Then multi-resolution image method is used to generate texture image. The mesh of volume-based 3D head model is flattened by cylindrical projection and is projected onto the texture image by line-pair based 2D warping method. Finally, the inverse cylindrical projection is used to render 3D head model with photo-realistic texture mapping.

Further research can be done towards a more accurate patient-to-model registration to establish the relationship between the patient and the images. We intend to find a good correlation between surface texture and internal anatomical structure information. Furthermore, it is shown that the method can be greatly convenient and accurate for the subsequent volume-based applications such as image-guided surgical simulation to overcome the weaknesses of conventional surgical techniques and the restrictions of minimally invasive or minimal access surgery.

Acknowledgements

This work has been supported by National Natural Science Foundation of China grant number 60472020.

References

1. Ip, H.H.S., Chan, C.S.: Script-based Facial Gesture and Speech Animation using a NURBS Based Face Model. Comput. & Graphics, Pergamon 20, 881–891 (1996)
2. Claes, P., Vandermeulen, D., Greef, S.D., Willems, G., Suetens, P.: Craniofacial Reconstruction using a Combined Statistical Model of Face Shape and Soft Tissue Depths: Methodology and Validation. Forensic Science International 159, 147–148 (2006)
3. Zhang, Y., Prakash, E.C., Sung, E.: Face Alive, Journal of Visual Language & Computing. 15, 125–160 (2004)
4. Faugeras, O., Quan, L., Sturn, P.: Self-calibration of a ID Projective Camera and its Application to the Self-calibration of a 2D Projection Camera. IEEE Transactions on Pattern Analysis and Machine Intelligence(PAMI) 22, 1179–1185 (2000)
5. Zhang, M., Ma, L., Zeng, X., Wang, Y.: Imaged-Based 3D Face Modeling. In: Proceeding of the international conference on computer graphics, Imaging and Visualization(CGIV 2004), IEEE, Los Alamitos (2004)
6. Weng, T.L., Lin, S.J., Chang, W.Y., Sun, Y.N.: Voxel-Based Texture Mapping for Medical Data. Computerized Medical Imaging and Graphics, Pergamon 26, 445–452 (2002)

7. Zhang, Y., Prakashb, E.C., Sunga, E.: Constructing a Realistic Face Model of an Individual for Expression Animation. Animation International Journal of Information Technology 8, 10–25 (2002)
8. Lee, W., Kalra, P., Magent Thalmann, N.: Model Based Face Reconstruction for Animation. In: Proc. Multimedia Modeling (MMM) 1997, Singapore, pp. 323–338 (1997)
9. Lee, W., Magenat Thalmann, N.: Fast Head Modeling for Animation. Joural Image and Vision Computing 18, 355–364 (2000)
10. Ansari, A., Mottaleb, M.A.: Automatic Facial Feature Extraction and 3D Face Modeling using Two Orthogonal Views with Application to 3D Face Recongnition. Pattern Recognition 38, 2549–2563 (2005)
11. Lee, W., Thalmann, N.M.: Head Modeling from Pictures and Morphing in 3D with Image Metamorphosis Based on Triangulation. In: Magnenat-Thalmann, N., Thalmann, D. (eds.) CAPTECH 1998. LNCS (LNAI), vol. 1537, pp. 254–267. Springer, Heidelberg (1998)
12. Burt, P.J., Adelson, E.H.: A Multiresolution Spline with Application to Image Mosaics. ACM Transactions on Graphics 2, 217–236 (1983)
13. Burt, P.J., Adelson, E.H.: The Laplacian Pyramid as a Compact Image Code. IEEE Trans. Commun. COM-31, 532–540 (1983)
14. Beier, T., Neely, S.: Feature-Based Image Metamorphosis. In: SIGGRAPH 1992, pp. 35–42 (1992)
15. Neil, G., Chris, W., John, M., Terry, P., Zhanhe, W.: Laser Projection Augmented Reality System for Computer Assisted Surgery. In: Ellis, R.E., Peters, T.M. (eds.) MICCAI 2003. LNCS, vol. 2879, pp. 239–246. Springer, Heidelberg (2003)
16. Jaime, G., John, F., James, J.: Three-Dimensional Surgical Planning for Maxillary and Midface Distraction Osteogenesis. The Journal of Craniofacial Surgery 14, 833–839 (2003)
17. Wusheng, C., Tianmiao, W., Zh, Y.: Augmented Reality Based Preoperative Planning for Robot Assisted Tele-neurosurgery. In: 2004 IEEE International Conference on Systems, Man and Cybernetics, pp. 2901–2906 (2004)
18. Eigil, S., Eirik, G., Murad, S.: 3D Graphical User Interface for Computer-Assisted Surgery, International Congress Series, vol. 1256, pp. 414–418 (2003)
19. Chris, M.: Maya Character Creation Modeling and Animation Controls (2004)
20. Guangwei, D.: High Resolution Visualization of VCH-Female Dataset. In: Processing of SPIE, vol. 5444, pp. 453–458 (2004)
21. Sh, Z., Zh, Z.S., Li, H., Lin, Z.K.: Digitized Virtual Human: Background and Meaning. China Basic Science 6, 12–16 (2002)

What ELSE? Regulation and Compliance in Medical Imaging and Medical Informatics

Penny Duquenoy[1], Carlisle George[1], and Anthony Solomonides[2]

[1] School of Computing Science, Middlesex University,
The Burroughs, London, NW4 4BT, United Kingdom
{p.duquenoy,c.george}@mdx.ac.uk
[2] CEMS Faculty, University of the West of England,
Bristol, BS16 1QY, United Kingdom
tony.solomonides@uwe.ac.uk

Abstract. The focus on the use of existing and new technologies to facilitate advances in Medical Imaging and Medical Informatics (MIMI), is often directed to the technical capabilities and possibilities that these technologies bring. In addition to discussing new methodologies, techniques and applications, there is need for a discussion of ethical, legal and socio-economic (ELSE) issues surrounding the use and application of technologies in MIMI. Such discussions are important because scientists need to be aware of the legal/regulatory framework which govern various new advances in MIMI research (especially to safeguard patients' interests), the ethical questions raised by such advances and the impact of these advances on society. This paper aims to discuss important ethical, legal and socio-economic issues related to MIMI and calls for an interdisciplinary approach to better address the increasing use of Information and Communication Technologies (ICT) in healthcare.

Keywords: Ethical principles, data integrity, material quality, usability, accessibility, training, data protection, confidentiality, electronic medical data, shared data processing, shared access, informed consent, standardisation, jurisdictional responsibility.

1 Introduction

The continuing rapid development of Information and Communication Technologies (ICT) has resulted in the increasing use of ICT in all aspects of human existence including healthcare. A major focus of such technological use is in Medical Imaging and Medical Informatics (MIMI). Medical Imaging (e.g. X-ray, Ultrasound, Magnetic Resonance Imaging - MRI, Computed Tomography - CT[1]) focuses on techniques to create and analyse images of the human body. It is an important part of making a medical diagnosis and planning a suitable treatment [1]. Image analysis is commonly used in medical processes such as the early detection of cancer, analysis of

---

[1] CT (Computed Tomography) involves the use of computers to generate a 3D image from flat (i.e., 2D) x-ray pictures.

X. Gao et al. (Eds.): MIMI 2007, LNCS 4987, pp. 340–357, 2008.
© Springer-Verlag Berlin Heidelberg 2008

neurological disorders (e.g. stroke), monitoring the progress of cardiovascular disease and the response to treatment [2]. Medical Informatics on the other hand is an umbrella term to describe the use of ICT and computing in the provision of healthcare.

One common feature of using ICT in MIMI is the generation and processing of electronic medical data for various activities including clinical practice and research. The term "electronic medical data" includes a wide range of data relating to a patient's health, including details of his/her past, current and future diagnoses, treatments and medication [3]. Electronic medical data also includes electronic/digital images such as an x-ray or mammography. Data processing includes collection, storage, organisation, retrieval, use, dissemination, consultation and transmission among others (EU Directive 95/46/EC). The processing of medical data is critical since misuse can have detrimental consequences for patients, medical professionals and researchers. Inaccuracies in a patient's medical data can result in misdiagnosis and disclosure of medical data can result in prejudicial treatment. Also medical professionals can face legal sanctions for malpractice due to inaccurate data, and researchers can be criminally liable for unauthorised disclosure of medical data. This means that adequate regulatory (ethical, legal) structures are needed to protect electronic medical data and hence safeguard patients, medical professionals and researchers alike. One must also be aware of the socio-economic impact of technologies in the provision of healthcare, since this will determine the viability and sustainability of particular uses. The discussion of ethical, legal and socio-economic (ELSE) issues related to ICT in healthcare is therefore important for the proper functioning of any healthcare system. This paper focuses on some ELSE issues relevant to MIMI.

The paper is structured to begin with abstract principles (in this case ethical principles), followed by the formalising of principles in legislation, and then gives a practical example of the impact of a new use of technology – grid computing – on the ELSE spectrum of issues. The following section discusses ethical principles and their application to medical imaging. Section 3 examines the legal issues relating to electronic medical data, and finally the paper discusses grid computing in the context of ELSE domains.

2   Principles to Practice: Ethics and Medical Imaging

The topic of medical imaging and ethics is often discussed in the context of the interaction between the medical practitioner (usually the radiologist) and the patient – for example as expressed in the Radiation Therapist Code of Ethics[2] – and matters concerning the safety aspects of radiation[3]. These are crucial ethical considerations that have, quite rightly, been addressed and are well documented. However, the issues that may arise from the use of technology in general, and the broadening scope allowed by ICT also need addressing. Technology has a mediating effect, not only through

---

[2] American Society of Radiologic Technologists, available from:
  http://www.asrt.org/content/RTs/CodeofEthics/Therapy_CodeOfEthics.aspx
[3] See for example the now complete European project Dimond at: http://www.dimond3.org/

capturing data and re-presenting it, but also in its capability of changing, storing, and disseminating information in ways that may either affect its interpretation, or be interpreted differently by different audiences. When this information relates to people and their health, consideration of the ethical implications of mediating technologies becomes vital.

This discussion takes the perspective of the technology impact on ethical considerations. To begin we highlight some high-level ethical principles, and then discuss how these might apply to medical imaging, and the types of ethical concerns that may be raised. The conclusion calls for open dialogue and training that aims to achieve a mutual understanding between technologists, ethicists and lawyers (as practitioners) as well as journalists and politicians (who will influence the debate).

2.1 Ethical Principles

A useful starting point for ethical principles concerning the medical domain is The Belmont Report[4], which is seen as a foundational document on ethical conduct of research that involves human subjects. This report lists three fundamental principles, which are considered to be universal:

- Respect for persons (i.e. acknowledging individual autonomy, choices)
- Beneficence (i.e. promoting well-being, reducing risks, protection of participant)
- Justice (i.e. equal benefits to all involved)

Writing in the field of biomedical ethics, Beauchamp and Childress [4] suggest the following principles, three of which follow those above but they add a fourth, which is the principle of non-malfeasance (do no harm).

- Beneficence
- Non-malfeasance
- Autonomy
- Justice

From these fundamental principles it is possible to derive more focused principles for the informatics setting, which centre on privacy – and associated personal data issues [5]. In broad terms the privacy-related principles follow the principles laid out in the Data Protection Act (UK) which in turn follows European directives on personal data. In more specific terms and in the context of this paper, Health Informatics Practitioners "have a duty to ensure that appropriate measures are in place that may reasonably be expected to safeguard:

- The security of electronic records;
- The integrity of electronic records;

---

[4] Department of Health, Education, and Welfare, Office of the Secretary, Protection of HumanSubjects. Belmont Report: Ethical Principles and Guidelines for the Protection of HumanSubjects of Research. Report of the National Committee for the Protection ofHuman Subjects of Biomedical and Behavioural Research. DHEW Publication No. (OS) 78-0013 and No. (OS) 78-0014. 18 April 1979.

- The material quality of electronic records;
- The usability of electronic records;
- The accessibility of electronic records." [5][5]

Taking the above points and transferring them to the context of medical imaging, we are adopting the position that the content (data) of medical images constitute an electronic record, and are personal data in that they represent information concerning a person (by virtue of the image and by virtue of its description embedded in the electronic file). However, this is not simply a discussion of personal data, and the rights of patients in connection with their data. It extends to issues of integrity and interpretation of data.

2.2 Transferring the Ethical Principles to Context of Use

The issue of security will not be discussed in this brief overview, as this is a familiar topic of general concern to those engaged in ICT and one that is being addressed. Of more interest in this context is the integrity of the image (i.e. the extent to which it matches its source), the material quality (which impacts on the integrity issue), its usability (which impacts on interpretation and usefulness), and accessibility (rights of access, and requirement for access). The following table gives an interpretation of these four aspects in relation to medical imaging.

Table 1. Relevant derivations of principles for Health Informatics Professionals and their interpretations

Integrity	the extent to which there is faithful reproduction of the original data source
Material quality	the extent to which a realistic interpretation can be made (i.e. related to image quality)
Usability	the ease with which the IT/human mediation can be made (without detriment to purpose)
Accessibility	the boundaries of access, the timeliness of access, and the presentation of material in a way that is accessible to those who need it

All of these aspects can be summarised as "the correct information at the right time, to the right people" which, for the purposes of the intention behind medical imaging, forms the basis for a strong ethical foundation. One only needs to consider the effects of the opposite – incorrect information at the wrong time, to the wrong people – to understand the importance of this. It should be noted that any combination of these aspects would result in an unwanted outcome (for example, correct information at the right time to the wrong people).

As mentioned above, the question of integrity is also tied in with quality, but they are not necessarily the same. The integrity of the data concerns its relationship to its

---

[5] The points listed are extracted from the handbook, and represent only a small portion of the complete book, they have been chosen for their specific relevance for the purposes of this short paper.

source – in particular that it actually relates to the person it claims to relate to, and that it has not changed in a way that could cause harm to that individual. That is, the image used should have a provenance directly related to the patient and not have been interfered with. However, the technical mediation and transmission may, of necessity, interfere with the original mapping which may in turn have an impact on all the other aspects.

Clearly the material quality of the image is important in order to be able to correctly identify any health issues, or to read associated and relevant text. Any ambiguity in the image (for example, caused by blurring, missing elements, etc.) may be detrimental to diagnosis, or other judgements – for example comparisons with other images for research purposes. Technical constraints of compression, reductions or enlargements of images may in some way add to material quality, but may have a detrimental affect on the other aspects of quality, usability and accessibility.

Some technical changes to the image may be necessary to aid usability. For example, compression to allow storage, or transmission, and subsequent decompression allow the exchange and sharing of data between users and across systems. Compatible file formats are important to reduce the need for more technical adaptations and risk of altering the quality and material content.

Accessibility and usability are of course linked to each other in terms of placing the 'human factor' within the scope of a successful 'human computer interaction'. The technical mediation of the image described although benefiting usability is likely to impact on accessibility, either beneficially (in the case of file sharing) or detrimentally. The enlargement of images, or changes in definition, for example may create difficulties when 'accessed' by their human interpreter (see e.g. [6]). Accessibility may not simply be a question of whether the image is physically accessible to whoever needs to see it at the time it needs to be seen. Cultural influences (not only national cultures but also work cultures) could prevent easy access. For instance, radiologists may be trained to interpret images presented in a different way, and may need training if they are presented in novel forms. Different approaches to medicine as practiced by different cultures may affect the perspective of the interpretation, or the ability to interpret. (Note the different approaches of eastern and western philosophies of medicine.)

It should be clear from the above discussion that the overriding aims of medical imaging meet the fundamental principles of Beneficence, Non-malfeasance, Autonomy, and Justice [4]. That is, the aims of the endeavour are to increase human well-being and not do harm (in aiming for improvements in imaging and understanding the medical condition of an individual), and to share knowledge in pursuance of those aims (meeting the justice criteria). Autonomy as a principle acknowledges individuals as having the right to make choices, and not to be used as "means to an end". Providing that patients are given a choice (duly informed) in having an image made in the first place, and that the images used for research do not treat the individual simply as a statistic and ignore their individuality – then the 'autonomy' principle is met.

The mediating role played by technology, and the developments continuously being achieved in the field, can allow changes that may impact on these principles.

The perspective taken here is essentially one of how computer technology is implemented to 'make life better', but that in order to achieve that objective consideration must be given to the context within which it is used – including scale and inter-connectedness. Experience has shown that not only can new technologies offer a new, often more efficient, way of doing things, they also offer a different context and concepts which are often difficult to understand (e.g. [7]).

This adaptation to new contexts, and the impact new contexts have on methods of working, are illustrated by the discussions in the next two sections. In the following section the transferring of patient records to the digital domain are highlighted by legislation on data protection (UK and EU) and the issues arising from the proposed introduction of electronic patient records in the UK. The technological move into grid computing changes the context once again (in terms of where the electronic data is held), and this is discussed in Section 4.

3 Legal Issues Regarding Electronic Health Data

The proliferation of electronic medical data has undoubtedly resulted in significant benefits (e.g. enhanced patient autonomy, better clinical treatment, and advances in health research), however, there are also important legal challenges such as: the privacy of health information; reliability and quality of health data; and tort-base liability [8]. These are also interconnected because the degree of privacy protection determines the reliability and quality of the data, which in turn determines tort-based liability for acts such as malpractice (e.g. due to inaccurate data) or privacy invasions (e.g. unauthorised access, modification or disclosure) of data [8].

This section of the paper discusses legal issues relevant to electronic medical data used for two main purposes namely: clinical practice and medical research. In clinical practice data is used to make diagnoses, decide on treatment and monitor such treatments. In medical research, data is used in order to analyse, investigate and develop new treatments and techniques to advance medical practice. For purposes of brevity, UK/EU legislation will be used as an example of a legal framework which regulates medical data.

In the UK the privacy of medical data is primarily protected by data protection legislation (e.g. The UK Data Protection Act 1988, based on EU Directive 95/46/EC), and the common law tort of breach of confidence.

3.1 Data Protection

The UK Data Protection Act 1988, regulates the processing of personal data[6]. The Act describes personal data as "data which relate to a living individual who can be

---

[6] Section 1(1) defines 'data' as: information which is being processed (or recorded to be processed) by equipment operating programmed to operate automatically; information recorded as part of (or with the intention of becoming part of) a relevant filing system; and information which forms part of an accessible record under Section 68. The Freedom of Information Act 2000 extended this definition to include all other recorded information held by a public authority.

identified (a) from the data or (b) from those data and other information which is in the possession of, or is likely to come into the possession of the data controller"[7]. The case of *Durant v Financial Services Authority (2003)*[8] established that data will 'relate to' an individual if it affects his/her privacy whether it be personal or family life, business or professional capacity. Further that information will affect an individual's privacy if it is biographical in a significant sense or if it has the individual as its focus. Processing of data refers to obtaining, holding or performing any operation or set of operations on data (e.g. consultation, disclosure, modification, destruction).

Under the Data Protection Act, information about the "physical or mental health or condition" (Section 2(e)) of an individual (i.e. medical data) is classed as "sensitive personal data" and hence is given a higher level of protection. The Act (Schedule I) stipulates eight data protection principles which must be observed (subject to various exemptions under the Act) when processing personal data, namely that personal data shall be:

- processed fairly and lawfully;
- obtained only for one or more specified and lawful purposes and not further processed in any manner incompatible with those purposes;
- adequate, relevant and not excessive in relation to the purposes of processing;
- accurate and kept up to date;
- not be kept longer then necessary;
- processed in accordance to rights of data subjects[9];
- kept secure from unauthorised access, unlawful processing, destruction or damage;
- not be transferred to a country outside the EU unless that country has an adequate level of data protection.

The Act also specifies at least nine criminal offences relating to the failure to comply with provisions of the Act. These include: processing without notification to the Information Commissioner[10] (Section 21(1)); unlawfully obtaining or disclosing personal data (Section 55(1)); and unlawfully selling personal data (Sections 55(4) and (5)).

In addition to the eight principles, the Act specifies various conditions (Schedule 3) relevant for the first principle (i.e. processing of sensitive personal data – which includes medical data). At least one of these conditions must be present. Among these conditions are:

---

[7] A data controller is the person who determines how personal data are to be processed.

[8] http://www.bailii.org/ew/cases/EWCA/Civ/2003/1746.html

[9] The Act gives data subjects (who are the subject of personal data) various limited rights in Part II such as the right of access to personal data subject to exemptions for example, if in the opinion of a relevant health professional such access would result in serious physical or mental harm to the data subject or any other person (*The Data Protection (Subject Access Modification) (Health) Order 2000*).

[10] Section 17 of the Data protection Act requires that all data controllers must register with the Information Commissioner and give notification of his processing activities. The Information Commissioner is the official responsible for supervising the enforcement of the Data Protection Act.

- the data subject must give explicit consent[11] to the processing of his/her personal data;
- the processing is necessary to protect the vital interests of the subject or another person where consent cannot be given (by or on behalf of the data subject) or the data controller cannot reasonably be expected to obtain the consent of the data subject or consent is unreasonably withheld;
- the processing is necessary for the purpose of any legal proceedings;
- the processing is necessary for the administration of justice;
- the processing is necessary for medical purposes (preventative medicine, medical diagnosis, medical research, treatment and healthcare management) and is undertaken by a health professional or a person who has a duty of confidentiality similar to a health professional.

The Act gives special provisions for research purposes (which includes statistical or historical purposes) subject to compliance with 'the relevant conditions' (Section 33) namely that: personal data are not processed in order to make decisions regarding the data subject, and will not cause damage or cause substantial distress to any data subject. Under section 33(2) data processed for research purposes (subject to compliance with 'the relevant conditions') are exempted from part of the second data principle, meaning that data not originally collected for research purposes, can be used for research however data subjects should be informed (due to the fair processing requirement) provided that contacting them does not involve a disproportionate effort[12]. In practice when collecting data from patients, they should be informed that their medical data may be used for treatment and research purposes (in order provide better medical care). Under Section 33(3), (subject to compliance with 'the relevant conditions') data processed only for research purposes are exempted from the fifth data principle, meaning that such data can be kept indefinitely. Further, Section 33(4)(b) allows for the publishing of research data provided that the data does not identify any data subject (i.e. it is anonymised).

3.2 Confidence: Duty and Breach

The law imposes a duty of confidence on anyone who receives information which he/she knows or ought to know should be regarded as being confidential. Information is deemed to be of a confidential nature (and hence attracts legal protection) if imparted in circumstances where there is an obligation of confidence between the parties (e.g. between medical practitioner and a patient). Medical data undoubtedly qualifies as confidential information. Medical professionals and researchers therefore have a 'duty of confidence' that obliges them not to disclose any medical information divulged to them unless authorised to do so. Disclosure will be authorised where the

---

[11] Consent means that the data subject gives his/her agreement to process his personal data. Consent must be informed, the person giving consent must have a degree of choice, and consent must be indicated either in an express manner (e.g. explicitly - orally or in writing) or it must be implied.

[12] A 'disproportionate effort' is determined on a case by case basis, taking into account factors such as the nature of the data, the time and cost involved in providing information to the data subject, and the effect on the data subject.

patient gives consent to disclosure or where disclosure is dictated by law such as in judicial proceedings or by statutory authority. Unauthorised disclosure of confidential information can result in the common law tort action of "breach of confidence" or in some circumstances negligence.

The conditions for establishing a "breach of confidence" action were formulated in *Coco v A N Clark (Engineers) Ltd [1969] RPC 41* and requires namely that: there is information of a confidential nature (e.g. medical data); which was imparted in circumstances importing an obligation of confidence (e.g. between patient and medical professional) and there was unauthorised use causing detriment (e.g. pain, suffering, public humiliation) to the party who originally imparted the information. A third party who receives information resulting from a breach of confidence also has a duty of confidence if he/she is aware or ought to be aware of the breach. An action in negligence can also result from a breach of the duty of confidence. For example where a medical professional or establishment fails to take reasonable care (e.g. adequate security) to prevent the disclosure of confidential information, and such disclosure results in injury (physical or psychological) to a patient.

It is worthwhile to note that The Health and Social Care Act 2001 (Section 60)[13], gives the Secretary of state the authority to temporarily suspend the duty of confidentiality (but not the Data Protection Act 1998), so that medical records can be used (without the consent of patients) for specified medical purposes where it is necessary or expedient to improve patient care or where there is an overriding public interest. Hence under Section 60, medical records can be used to carry out clinical audits, record validation and research without obtaining the consent of patients [9]. The rationale for Section 60 is that in some cases: consent cannot be obtained; it is impractical to obtain (e.g. where there are tens of thousands of patients); or excluding patients who refuse consent may devalue the data collected due to sample bias. In practice researchers need to apply for Section 60 exemption from the Patient Information Advisory Group,[14] of the Department of Health.

The issue of whether there is an overriding public interest needs to be made on a case by case basis, and can take into consideration factors such as the prevention of serious harm or abuse to others, national security, and the detection or investigation of criminal activity among others. Three court judgements in the UK regarding issues of disclosure of medical information to the public may shed some light on how the courts weigh the interest of the public against the duty of confidentiality.

In *X v Y [1988] 2 ALL ER 648*, the Court of Appeal prevented a national newspaper from publishing the names of two practising doctors suffering from AIDS. The Court concluded that: the risk of transmission of HIV from doctor to patient was minimal; there was a greater public interest in preserving the confidentiality of hospital records; and the information would be of minimal significance to the public in view of the wide ranging public debate on AIDS. In *W v Edgell [1990] 1 ALL ER 835*, a court considered whether a doctor who had sent confidential information (about the mental health of a dangerous patient) to the medical director of another hospital and to the Home Office, had breached the patient's confidentiality. The court

---

[13] The Health and Social Care Act 2001 (Section 60)[13]
    http://www.opsi.gov.uk/ACTS/acts2001/10015--g.htm#60
[14] http://www.advisorybodies.doh.gov.uk/piag/Index.htm

held that the public interest (protection from a dangerous criminal) justified the breach of confidence. Finally, in *H (A Healthcare Worker) v Associated Newspapers Ltd. & Ors [2002] EWCA Civ 195* the Court of Appeal prevented the public disclosure of the identity of a doctor who ceased medical practice after being diagnosed as HIV positive and suffering from AIDS. The Court of Appeal stated that "there is an obvious public interest in preserving the confidentiality of victims of the AIDS epidemic and, in particular, of healthcare workers who report the fact that they are HIV positive".

Two of the cases above illustrate that the public interest is not always best served by public disclosure. With regards to the cases on HIV infected health workers, maintaining confidentiality encourages workers who are infected in the future to identify themselves and seek treatment, hence preventing further harm to the public.

3.3 Protecting Electronic Medical Data in Practice

A main cause of concern regarding electronic medical data, is that such data is protected from unauthorised processing (especially unauthorised disclosure, alteration and use). A research study into the public reaction to implementing a UK Integrated Care Record Service (ICRS) to allow the electronic sharing of medical data (among health carers and patients), concluded that the only barrier to accepting ICRS was the perception that security of electronic systems was an issue [10]. Another study investigating the impact of the UK Program for IT (NPFIT[15]) in primary healthcare, on clinicians and medical staff, found that the biggest concern was the issue of patient confidentiality and security of electronic records [11].

In order to allay the fears of medical professionals and patients (regarding privacy), adequate measures (in addition to network security) must be in place to ensure compliance with data protection legislation, and the common law duty of confidence.

In the UK, with the introduction of the National Health Service (NHS) Electronic Card Record (in spring 2007) the Department of Health adopted various practices for the implementation and operation of this new healthcare system. These practices were approved by the Information Commissioner as being consistent with the requirements under data protection legislation [12]. The process begins with the uploading of information regarding a patient's current medication, known allergies and adverse reactions into a database to form a Summary Care Record (SCR). All patients will be notified before uploading of their SCR and given the option: to decline one; limit the future scope of information in the SCR; or to view the contents before uploading. The SCR, however will be uploaded without the explicit consent of the patient (but subject to notification and an opportunity to respond). After uploading, patients can remove any or all information uploaded to the SCR, and any subsequent additions to the SCR must be agreed between the patient and his/her doctor. Patients will also be able to limit the information which can be made visible without their consent. A wide range of access controls have also been adopted. Only staff with a legitimate relationship with a patient will be able to access that patient's SCR[16]. All access to an SCR will

---

[15] NPFIT includes care record systems, electronic booking service, electronic prescriptions and a national network infrastructure.

[16] This includes medical staff acting in an emergence such as staff working in an Accident and Emergency Department.

be via a smartcard and PIN, and is logged (providing an audit log). All patients will be able receive a copy of the audit log giving details of access to their SCR. The NHS also guarantees that information in the SCR will not be shared with any organisation without the explicit consent of the patient.

With specific regard to confidentiality, since November 2003 the NHS published a Code of Practice on Confidentiality [13] which sets out practical guidance for all workers within or under contract with the NHS. The Code uses a model which is aimed at providing a confidential service. This model has four requirements namely to: protect - patient's information; inform – patients of information use; provide choice - to a patient regarding disclosure or use of information and improve - the preceding three requirements.

The NHS also maintains a register of senior staff (healthcare or social professionals) who are responsible for protecting patient information called Caldicott Guardians[17]. The main responsibilities of a Caldicott Guardian are [14]: strategy and governance - championing confidentiality issues at the management level; confidentiality and data protection expertise, internal information processing – ensuring that confidentiality issues are reflected in organisational policies, strategies and procedures; and information sharing - overseeing arrangements, protocols and procedures for information sharing between organisations both external and internal to the NHS.

One of the challenges of protecting electronic data is that such data sometimes needs to be shared amongst organisations in order to assist medical professionals and researchers in making analyses, comparisons and deciding on diagnoses. Epidemiology[18] also occasionally requires larger or less uniform data sets than may be available from a single source. An example of this is in grid computing, which utilises many computers sometimes spread across organisations and geographical locations. The next section examines this aspect and discusses some of the ethical, legal and socio-economic issues related to grid computing.

4   Grid Computing: Ethical, Legal and Socio-economic Issues

4.1   Healthgrid

Grid computing ('the grid') is a new paradigm of distributed computing, offering rapid computation, large scale data storage and flexible collaboration by harnessing together the power of a large number of commodity computers or clusters of other basic machines. The grid was devised for use in scientific fields, but has also been used in a number of ambitious biomedical applications, while applications to health-care have been explored in research projects. There is some tension between the spirit of the grid paradigm and the requirements of medical or healthcare applications. The grid maximises its flexibility and minimises its overheads by requesting computations to be carried out at the most appropriate node in the network; it stores data at the most

---

[17] Caldicott Guardians are named after Dame Fiona Caldicott who chaired a 1997 report of the Review of Patient-Identifiable Information (called The Caldicott Report).

[18] The study of factors affecting health and illness in different groups of people. It is concerned with how often these diseases occur and why.

convenient node according to performance criteria. On the other hand, healthcare institutions are required to maintain control of their confidential patient data and to remain accountable for its use at all times. The ideal grid has been envisaged as the servant of a new collaborative paradigm, providing services to users who may, from time to time, join the grid, do some work and then leave, so that the transient alliances they form in their endeavours might be described as 'virtual organizations' or VOs for short. One approach to organizing the infrastructure for such collaboration is as a so-called 'service-oriented architecture' (SOA). In effect, it means that needed services – software applications – once constructed, are provided with a description in an agreed language and made available, or 'published', to be 'discovered' by other services that need them. A 'service economy' is thus created in which both ad hoc and systematic collaborations can take place. Medical data requires careful handling. Among the services required by healthcare applications are 'fine grained' access control – e.g. through authorization and authentication of users – and privacy protection through anonymization or pseudonymization of individual data or 'outlier' detection and disguise in statistical data.   Despite this apparent conflict in requirements, certain characteristics of the grid provide the means to resolve the problem: in the spirit of this paradigm in which "virtual organisations" arise ad hoc, "grid services" may negotiate ethical, legal and regulatory compliance according to agreed policy. In this section, we wish to discuss the implications of such advances in the ethical, legal and socio-economic (ELSE) domains in part through reference to two EU-funded healthgrid projects.

4.2 Breast Cancer

Areas of medicine and healthcare in which large databases – in both senses: with large numbers of records, and with large, multi-format records – are reasonable candidates for healthgrid applications. We consider one such example, the MammoGrid project, in the field of breast cancer.

Breast cancer is arguably the most pressing threat to women's health. For example, in the UK, more than one in four female cancers occur in the breast and these account for roughly 18% of deaths from cancer in women. Coupled with the statistic that about one in four deaths in general are due to cancer, this suggests that nearly 5% of female deaths are due to breast cancer. While risk of breast cancer to age 50 is 1 in 50, risk to age 70 increases to 1 in 15 and lifetime risk has been calculated as 1 in 9. The problem of breast cancer is best illustrated through comparison with lung cancer which also accounted for 18% of female cancer deaths in 1999. In recent years, almost three times as many women have been diagnosed with breast cancer as with lung cancer. However, the five year survival rate from breast cancer stands at 73%, while the lung cancer figure is 5%. [15] This is testament to the effectiveness of modern treatments, provided breast cancer is diagnosed sufficiently early. The statistics of breast cancer diagnosis and survival provide a powerful argument in favour of a universal screening programme. However, a number of issues of efficacy and cost effectiveness limit the scope of most screening programmes. The method of choice in breast cancer screening is mammography (breast X-ray). However, in younger women, the breast consists of around 80% glandular tissue which is dense and largely X-ray opaque. The remaining 20% is mainly fat. Through the menopause, this ratio is typically reversed. Thus in women under 50, signs of malignancy are far more difficult to discern in mammograms than they are in post-menopausal women. Consequently, most screening programmes, including the UK's, only apply to women over 50.

Electronic formats for radiological images, including mammography, together with the fast, secure transmission of images and patient data, potentially enables many hospitals and imaging centres throughout Europe to be linked together to form a single grid-based "virtual organization". While technological possibilities are co-evolving with an appreciation of their potential uses, it is generally agreed that the creation of very large "federated" databases of mammograms, which appear to the user to be a single database, but are in fact retained and curated in the centres that generated them, would yield several benefits in better diagnosis and epidemiology. Each image in such a database would have linked to it a large set of relevant information, known as metadata, about the woman whose mammogram it is. Levels of access to the images and metadata in the database would vary among authorized users according to their "certificated rights": healthcare professionals might have access to essentially all of it, whereas, e.g., administrators, epidemiologists and researchers would have limited access, protecting patient confidentiality and in accordance with European legislation.

This scenario raises some obvious and some rather subtle questions of ethics and regulatory compliance. Informed consent, in the usual sense of the term, cannot encompass uses of data which cannot be foreseen at the time the consent is being given. On the other hand, unconstrained consent is not even possible in some countries. And yet, the value of this approach lies precisely in what medical researchers may discover through extending their research questions as they analyse the data at their disposal. How to resolve this dilemma? It would appear that the best a healthgrid researcher can hope for is to highlight some valuable uses which are currently precluded and to look for political change.

A somewhat less obvious question concerns rights of access and confidentiality. How to reconcile, e.g. legal differences in what data a doctor may view in one country versus another? Does the constraint apply to an individual irrespective of their location or does it apply to a location? In other words, may a Scots doctor possibly view some data about her Scots patient (who has had some intervention in England) while visiting an English hospital which she would not be allowed to view in Scotland? What if that data is available to be viewed over a grid?

4.3 MammoGrid

The Fifth Framework EU-funded MammoGrid project (2002-05) [16] aimed to apply the grid concept to mammography, including services for the standardization of mammograms, computer-aided detection (CADe) of masses and 'microcalcifications', quality control of imaging, and epidemiological research including broader aspects of patient data. Clinicians rarely analyse single images in isolation but rather in a series or in the context of metadata. Metadata that may be required are clinically relevant factors such as patient age, exogenous hormone exposure, family and clinical history; for the population, natural anatomical and physiological variations; and for the technology, image acquisition parameters, including breast compression and exposure data.

The MammoGrid proof-of-concept prototype provides clinicians with a medical information infrastructure delivered in a service-based grid framework. It encompasses geographical regions with different clinical protocols and diagnostic procedures, as well as lifestyles and dietary patterns. The system allows, among other things, mammogram data mining for knowledge discovery, diverse and complex epidemiological studies, statistical analyses and CADe; it also permits the deployment of different versions of the image standardization software and other services, for quality control and comparative study.

We may now imaginatively consider what may happen in the course of a consultation and diagnosis using the MammoGrid system. A patient is seen and mammograms are taken. The radiologist is sufficiently concerned about the appearance of one of these that she wishes to investigate further. In the absence of any other method, she may refer the patient for a biopsy, an invasive procedure; however, she also knows that in the majority of cases, the initial diagnosis turns out to have been a false positive, so the patient has been put through a lot of anxiety and physical trauma unnecessarily. Given the degree of uncertainty, a cautious radiologist may seek a second opinion: how can the MammoGrid system support her? She may invoke a CADe service; the best among these can identify features which are not visible to the naked eye. Another possibility is to seek out similar images from the grid database of mammograms and examine the history to see what has happened in those other cases. However, since each mammogram is taken under different conditions, according to the judgement of a radiographer ('radiologic technician') it is not possible to compare them as they are. Fortunately, a service exists which standardizes and summarizes the images, provided certain parameters are available – the type of X-ray machine and its settings when the mammograms were taken. Perhaps at this particular moment the radiologist's workstation is already working at full capacity because of other imaging tasks, so it is necessary for the image to be transmitted to a different node for processing. Since our grid is distributed across Europe, it now matters whether the node which will perform the standardization is in the same country or not. Let us suppose that it is a different country. A conservative outcome is to ensure that, provided the regulatory conditions in the country of origin and in the country where the processing will take place are mutually compatible (i.e. logically consistent, capable of simultaneous satisfaction) that they are both complied with. If one set requires encryption, say, but the other does not, the data must be encrypted. If both sets of regulations allow the image to be transmitted unencrypted but one country requires all associated data transmitted with the image to be pseudonymized, this must be done. These are human decisions, but it is clear that they can be automated. Where will responsibility lie if something goes wrong in this process? In any case, the story has further ramifications: the whole idea of MammoGrid is to build up a rich enough database of images and case histories to provide a sound basis both for diagnostic comparison and for epidemiology. Once standardized and returned, is the image now to be stored and made available to others for comparative use, or is it to remain outside the system? This is now a question of informed consent. Will a service, in the sense we have already used the term, be trusted to determine whether such informed consent as the patient has given covers this question? There are, naturally, many more questions of a similar nature.

A further question arises in this context as to professional competencies in different countries. Imagine that a radiographer in one country, Italy say, is allowed to annotate an image (or to launch without medical supervision a CADe service to annotate an image) but then that mammogram with its annotation is used in another country, say the UK, by a radiologist to offer a second opinion. What should happen if in the UK a radiographer would not have had the 'professional competence' to annotate unsupervised? Is the radiologist at risk for having relied on an unauthorized annotation?

There is an almost invisible aspect of this initiative which deserves attention but will only be briefly touched on here. How is such a system to fit into the modern conception of evidence-based medicine, i.e. medicine that is based on scientific results? Evidence-based practice rests on three pillars: medical knowledge, as much as possible based on 'gold standard' (double-blind, controlled) clinical trials whose results have been peer reviewed and then published; knowledge of the patient, as complete as the record allows; and knowledge of the resources, procedures and protocols available in the setting where the encounter with the patient is taking place. However, the MammoGrid application we have described above plays a part in the 'dynamic' construction of knowledge. If images and histories are to be used as part of the diagnostic knowledge in new cases, it is imperative that they are collected with as much care and rigour as the cases in a controlled trial. Therefore, it is essential to know the 'provenance' of the data with precise details of how it has been handled (e.g. if standardized and subjected to CADe, which algorithms were used, set to what parameters, by whom, and if capture and interpretation were subject to appropriate practice standards). I have labelled this set of issues "the question of practice-based evidence for evidence-based practice". If this were to be accepted as an appropriate source of diagnostic information, the underlying grid services which maintain it would have to make quality judgements without human intervention.

4.4 The 'Whole Person' and Genetic Medicine

A major breakthrough in healthcare is anticipated from the association of genetic data with medical knowledge. This would suggest that genetic information would have to be accessed routinely in the course of healthcare. Viewing this as part of the information held on a patient raises a number of difficult problems. Among these are the predictive value and the shared nature of genetic information. Knowing a person's genome could mean knowing what diseases they may or may not be susceptible to. Knowing one person's genetic map also reveals that of his or her siblings' in large measure. This introduces a range of questions, from confidentiality to 'duty of care' issues. If physicians will be held liable both for what they do and what they do not do, is it necessary for the underlying knowledge technology to 'be aware' and to inform them of the possibilities?

The grid could provide the infrastructure for a complete 'electronic health record' with opportunities to link both traditional patient data and genetic information to bring us closer to the ideal of genomic medicine. Among many questions being investigated in current projects is a set concerning development and illness in childhood, especially conditions in which genetic predisposition is at least suspected and in the diagnosis of which imaging is also essential. Physicians want to know how certain genes impact the development of diseases and radiologists want to know what the earliest imaging signs are that are indicative of a disease. For example, the Health-e-Child project [17] is investigating paediatric rheumatology, cardiac dysmorphology and childhood brain tumours using this approach. Consider its aims:

(i) To gain a comprehensive view of a child's health by vertically integrating biomedical data, information, and knowledge, that spans the entire spectrum from genetic to clinical to epidemiological;

(ii) To develop a biomedical information platform, supported by sophisticated and robust search, optimization, and matching techniques for heterogeneous information, empowered by the Grid;

(iii) To build enabling tools and services on top of the Health-e-Child platform, that will lead to innovative and better healthcare solutions in Europe:
- Integrated disease models exploiting all available information levels;
- Database-guided biomedical decision support systems provisioning novel clinical practices and personalized healthcare for children;
- Large-scale, cross-modality, and longitudinal information fusion and data mining for biomedical knowledge discovery.

With major companies looking to translate research results into products, successful outcomes from this and other projects would bring the scenario described above closer to reality.

A less obvious outcome from this research may be a reduction in the degree of invasive genetic mapping that may be necessary to address certain paediatric conditions. If a strong association is established between an imaging feature and a genetic mutation, it may then be used to limit the need for blanket genetic screening, restricting attention to those with the give imaging telltale or eliminating the need entirely. This would be a case where technology would at least indirectly contribute to reducing data protection issues, although the implicit conflict between duty of care and data protection remains (for example, in cases where findings may have implications for the health of siblings).

5 Conclusions

In light of the increasing use of technology in healthcare, and the likelihood of further significant use of technology in the future, it is important to take into account the ethical, legal and socio-economic issues (ELSE). This paper has taken three levels of perspective: foundational principles, formalising principles in law, and an application domain in the context of the grid (representing a new technological context). Through this approach we have highlighted the ethical principles associated with healthcare practice and medical research (and, by extension, their rationale), how the law addresses issues pertinent to the medical profession in the digital domain, and how changes of context are relevant in the way they challenge existing cultural practice.

To fully exploit the benefits of developing technologies, and to facilitate the mutual understanding of the impacts of technology on ethical principles and consequent regulation and practice, there needs to be a mutual engagement and exchange between technology developers, ethicists, and above all, – in the light of issues raised in this article – the medical profession. Cross disciplinary (and interdisciplinary) training would aid understanding. At a minimum, technologists need to be educated in the basics of ethical, legal and social considerations; these are issues they are apt to be unaware of at first, and to wish to ignore once aware of them, not for any malicious reason but because they are, or at least appear to be, an obstacle to technical development.   On the other hand, ethicists, lawyers, journalists and politicians need to understand what the technology can do in a far more textured and nuanced manner than is common at present; this requires exposure to the culture of technology as well as to the basics of what current and foreseeable technologies can do.   This discussion, resulting from this paper, is an opportunity to begin the exchange, and to open a dialogue aimed at reducing the gap between disciplinary cultures, different understandings, and divergent long term aims and intermediate objectives.

References

1. Muller, H., Lovis, C., Geissbuhler, A.: The medGIFT project on medical image retrieval. In: Proceedings of first International Conference on Medical Imaging and Telemedicine (MIT 2005), Wuyi Mountain, China, August 16-19 (2005)
2. Yoo, T., Ackerman, J.: Medical image modeling tools and applications: Open source software for medical image processing and visualization. Communications of the ACM 48(2) (2005)
3. Lowrance, W.: Privacy and Health Research (1997),
   http://aspe.os.dhhs.gov/datacncl/PHR.htm
4. Beauchamp, T.L., Childress, J.F.: Principles of Biomedical Ethics, 5th edn., New York. Oxford University Press, Oxford (2001)
5. HEHIP: A handbook of Ethics for Health Informatics Professionals, The British Computer Society (endorsed by the International Medical Information Association) (2003)
6. Bankman, I.N. (Editor-in-Chief): Handbook of Medical Imaging Processing and Analysis. Academic Press, London (2000)
7. Moor, J.: What is computer ethics? Metaphilosophy 16(4) (1985)
8. Hodge, J.G., Gostin, L., Jacobson, P.: Legal Issues concerning Electronic Health Information. JAMA 282, 1466–1471 (1999)
9. Department of Health: Confidentiality: NHS Code of Practice (November (2003),
   http://www.dh.gov.uk/en/Publicationsandstatistics/Publications/
   PublicationsPolicyAndGuidance/DH_4069253
10. Health Which?: The Public View on Electronic Health Records, Health Which? And NHS National Programme for Information Technology (October 7, 2003),
    http://www.dh.gov.uk/prod_consum_dh/groups/dh_digitalassets/
    dh/en/documents/digitalasset/dh_4055046.pdf

11. Ndeti, M., George, C.E.: Pursuing Electronic Health: A UK Primary Health Care Perspective. In: Funabashi, M., Grzech, A. (eds.) Challenges of Expanding Internet: E-Commerce, E-Business, and E-Government: Proceedings of the 5th IFIP Conference on e-Commerce, e-Business, and e-Government (I3e 2005), Poznan, Poland, USA, October 28-30, 2005, Springer, Heidelberg (2005)

12. The Information Commissioner's view of NHS Electronic Care Records, `http://www.ico.gov.uk/upload/documents/library/data_protection/introductory/information_commissioners_view_of_nhs_electronic_care_reco%E2%80%A6.pdf`

13. Department of Health : Confidentiality: NHS Code of Practice, November (2003), `http://www.dh.gov.uk/en/Publicationsandstatistics/Publications/PublicationsPolicyAndGuidance/DH_4069253`

14. NHS: The Caldicott Guardian Manual (2006), `http://www.connectingforhealth.nhs.uk/systemsandservices/infogov/policy/resources/new_guidance`

15. Cancer Research UK factsheets for professionals, especially, Breast Cancer and Lung Cancer both (all accessed 12.06.07), `http://info.cancerresearchuk.org/ourpublications/healthprofessionals/factsheets/` see also female mortality data, `http://info.cancerresearchuk.org/cancerstats/mortality/females/`

16. The Information Societies Technology project: MammoGrid – A European federated mammogram database implemented on a grid infrastructure, EU Contract IST-2001-37614 (2001)

17. The Information Societies Technology Integrated Project: Health-e-Child – An integrated platform for European paediatrics based on a grid-enabled network of leading clinical centres, EU Contract Number IST-2005-027749 (2005)

CAD on Brain, Fundus, and Breast Images

Hiroshi Fujita[1], Yoshikazu Uchiyama[1], Toshiaki Nakagawa[1], Daisuke Fukuoka[2],
Yuji Hatanaka[3], Takeshi Hara[1], Yoshinori Hayashi[1], Yuji Ikedo[1], Gobert N. Lee[1],
Xin Gao[1], and Xiangrong Zhou[1]

[1] Department of Intelligent Image Information, Division of Regeneration and Advanced
Medical Sciences, Graduate School of Medicine, Gifu University, Gifu 501-1194, Japan
[2] Faculty of Education, Gifu University, Gifu 501-1193, Japan
[3] Gifu National College of Technology, Motosu City, Gifu 501-0495, Japan
fujita@fjt.info.gifu-u.ac.jp

Abstract. Three computer-aided detection (CAD) projects are hosted at the
Gifu University, Japan as part of the "Knowledge Cluster Initiative" of the
Japanese Government. These projects are regarding the development of CAD
systems for the early detection of (1) cerebrovascular diseases using brain MRI
and MRA images by detecting lacunar infarcts, unruptured aneurysms, and
arterial occlusions; (2) ocular diseases such as glaucoma, diabetic retinopathy,
and hypertensive retinopathy using retinal fundus images; and (3) breast
cancers using ultrasound 3-D volumetric whole breast data by detecting the
breast masses. The brain CAD system achieves a sensitivity of 96.8% at 0.71
false positive (FP) per image for the lacunar-infarct detection, and 93.8% at 1.2
FPs per patient for the small unruptured aneurysm detection. The sensitivity and
specificity for the detection of abnormal cases with arterial occlusions in MRA
images are 80.0% and 95.3%, respectively. For the glaucoma detection using
the retinal fundus CAD system, a sensitivity and specificity of 77.8% and
74.5% are obtained in the analysis of the optic nerve head and a sensitivity of
61.5% at 1.3 FPs per image is achieved in the detection of the retinal nerve fiber
layer defects. Hemorrhages and exudates in diabetic retinopathy diagnosis are
detected at a sensitivity and specificity of 84.6% and 20.6%, respectively, for
the former and 76.9% and 83.3%, respectively, for the latter. For hypertensive
retinopathy, the arteriolar-narrowing scheme can identify 76.2% of true
positives at 1.4 FPs per image. For the breast CAD system, the image viewer
that constructs the breast volume image data is developed, which also includes
the CAD function with a sensitivity of 80.5% at 3.8 FPs per breast. The CAD
schemes are still being improved for all the systems along with an increase in
the number of image databases. Clinical examinations will be started soon, and
commercialized CAD systems for the above subjects will appear by the
completion of this project.

Keywords: Computer-Aided Detection (CAD), Brain MRI, Brain MRA,
Cerebrovascular Disease, Lacunar Infarct, Unruptured Aneurysm, Arterial
Occlusion, Retinal Fundus Image, Glaucoma, Diabetic Retinopathy,
Hypertensive Retinopathy, Ultrasound Breast Images, Breast Cancer.

X. Gao et al. (Eds.): MIMI 2007, LNCS 4987, pp. 358–366, 2008.
© Springer-Verlag Berlin Heidelberg 2008

1   Introduction

Since 2002, eighteen knowledge clusters have been established in Japan under the "Knowledge Cluster Initiative" of the Japanese Government. These clusters are supported by the Ministry of Education, Culture, Sports, Science and Technology of Japan under a Grant-In-Aid for Scientific Research with a budget of USD 4.5 million per year per cluster over five years. The aim of the clusters is to promote industrial, academic and governmental cooperation in regional areas and to conduct innovative and technological research with a focus on the needs of industry. The clusters are based in universities and other research institutes in order to draw sources of advanced knowledge; hence, the name "knowledge cluster."

The Fujita Laboratory at Gifu University is part of the Gifu/Ogaki Robotics Advanced Medical Cluster with a focus on research in distinctive, new medical technologies and developing the state-of-the-art medical equipments such as surgery robots and medical diagnosis support equipments. Currently, there are three established cluster projects in the Fujita Laboratory, Gifu University, started since April 2004. These three projects are computer-aided detection (CAD) systems using brain magnetic resonance imaging (MRI) and magnetic resonance angiography (MRA) images, retinal fundus images and ultrasound breast images, and are described in the following sections.

2   CAD for MR Brain Images

2.1   Overview

Cerebrovascular disease is the third leading cause of death by disease in Japan [1]. Therefore, the screening system, which is named *Brain Dock*, has been widely used for the detection of asymptomatic brain diseases. The prevention of this disease is of paramount importance. MRI and MRA are very useful for the early detection of cerebral and cerebrovascular diseases. Lacunar infarcts, unruptured aneurysms, and arterial occlusions can be detected using MRI and MRA. These medical conditions indicate an increased risk of severe cerebral and cerebrovascular diseases. The presence of lacunar infarcts increases the risk of serious cerebral infarction, and a ruptured aneurysm is the major cause of subarachnoid haemorrhage (SAH).

It is important to detect lacunar infarcts, unruptured aneurysms, and arterial occlusions. However, visualization of these structures is not always easy for radiologists and neurosurgeons. For example, it is difficult to distinguish between lacunar infarcts and normal tissue such as Virchow-Robin spaces in MRI images. Small aneurysms in MRA studies are also difficult to distinguish from the adjacent vessels in a maximum intensity projection (MIP) image. CAD systems can assist neuroradiologists and general radiologists in detecting intracranial aneurysms, asymptomatic lacunar infarcts, and arterial occlusions and in assessing the risk of cerebral and cerebrovascular diseases. In this project, we use T1- and T2-weighted MRI brain images for the detection of asymptomatic lacunar infarcts [2, 3]. We also employ MRA brain images for the detection of intracranial aneurysms [4] and for developing a new viewing technique to facilitate the detection of intracranial aneurysms [5] and arterial occlusions [6].

2.2 Detection of Lacunar Infarct

The CAD scheme for detecting lacunar infarcts in MRI is shown in Figure 1. The cerebral region is first extracted from a T1-weighted image. Lacunar infarct candidates are extracted using a simple thresholding technique and a top-hat transformation on T2-weighted images. Twelve features are measured from each candidate and a neural network is used in the final classification of the lacunar infarcts [2, 3]. Using the above procedure for detecting lacunar infarcts, our developed CAD scheme can achieve a sensitivity of 96.8% at 0.71 false positive (FP) per image in a dataset of 132 studies.

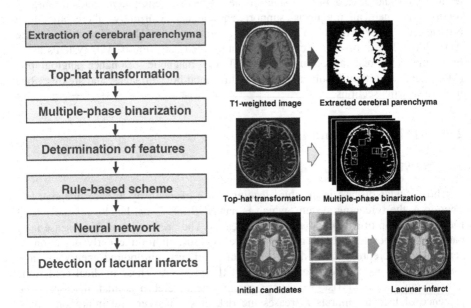

Fig. 1. Overall CAD scheme for the detection of lacunar infarcts [3]. Initial candidates are found in the three steps of image processing and then the FPs are reduced using the feature analysis of rule-based and neural-network techniques. The lacunar infarct(s) finally detected is marked with a small square on the T2-weighted image, in which it appears as tiny round-shaped object with a "white" color, as shown in the bottom-right image.

2.3 Detection of Unruptured Aneurysm

For the detection of unruptured aneurysm, vessel regions are first extracted from MRA images using linear gray-level transformation. A gradient concentration filter is then used to enhance the candidate aneurysms and quadratic discriminant analysis is used for the final detection of aneurysms [4, 5]. In a dataset of 100 MRA studies, our current CAD scheme achieves a sensitivity of 93.8% at an FP detection of 1.2 per patient.

2.4 Detection of Occlusion

The scheme for the detection of arterial occlusion in MRA studies consists of two parts, (1) classification of eight arteries based on the comparison of the target image with the reference image, and (2) detection of arterial occlusion(s) based on the relative lengths of eight arteries [6]. The sensitivity and specificity for the detection of abnormal cases with arterial occlusions are 80.0% and 95.3%, respectively, for the cases of 100 MRA studies including 15 arterial occlusions.

3   CAD for Retinal Fundus Images

3.1 Overview

Retinal fundus images are useful for the early detection of a number of ocular diseases which, if left untreated, can lead to blindness. Examinations using retinal fundus images are cost effective and are suitable for mass screening. In view of this, retinal fundus images are obtained in many health care centers and medical facilities during medical checkups for ophthalmic examinations. Glaucoma, diabetic retinopathy, and hypertensive retinopathy can be detected on fundus images and are the targets in this project. The increase in the number of ophthalmic examinations improves ocular health care in the population but it also increases the workload of ophthalmologists. Therefore, CAD systems developed for analyzing retinal fundus images can assist in reducing the workload of ophthalmologists and improving the screening accuracy.

3.2 Detection of Glaucoma

In a population-based prevalence survey of glaucoma in Tajimi City, Japan, one in 20 people who are aged over 40 was diagnosed with glaucoma [7, 8]. Around the world, the number of people with glaucoma is estimated to be 60.5 million in 2010 and 79.6 million in 2020 [9]. Glaucoma is the second leading cause of blindness in Japan and also worldwide. Although it cannot be cured, glaucoma can be treated if diagnosed early. Mass screening for glaucoma using retinal fundus images is simple and effective.

In the CAD system developed in this project, two different approaches are used for the detection of glaucoma. The first one is based on the measurement of the cup-to-disc (C/D) ratio. Blood vessels are first "erased" from the fundus image by image processing technique and the optical nerve head is located. The C/D ratio, which is the ratio of the diameter of the depression (cup) and that of the optic nerve head (ONH, i.e., disc), is evaluated for the diagnosis of glaucoma (Figure 2). Using 65 cases (47 normal and 18 abnormal), the sensitivity and specificity are reported at 77.8% and 74.5%, respectively.

We are also developing a method for measuring the depth of the cup by using our new digital stereo fundus camera along with an automatic reconstruction technique [10, 11] in an extended project, as a part of the Regional New Consortium Projects from Ministry of Economy, Trade and Industry, Japan.

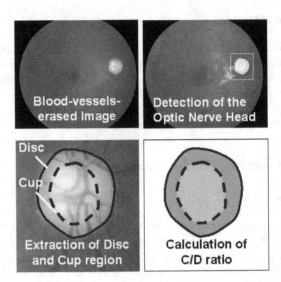

Fig. 2. Determination of the C/D ratio for the diagnosis of glaucoma. (Left to right; top to bottom) Blood vessels are first "erased" from the original image and the optic nerve head is located. A fundus image with a C/D ratio greater than 0.60 is considered to be abnormal.

The second approach developed in this project for the diagnosis of glaucoma is based on the detection of retinal nerve fiber layer defects (NFLDs) using image processing techniques [12]. Blood vessels in the original fundus image are erased and the optic disc is located as described previously. The fundus image is then transformed into a rectangular array before enhancing the NFLDs with Gabor filtering. Using 26 normal and 26 abnormal fundus images with 53 NFLD regions, this approach can identify 61.5% of true positives at 1.3 FPs per image.

3.3 Detection of Diabetic Retinopathy

In Japan, the number of people with adult diseases such as diabetes and hypertension is increasing every year. Diabetic retinopathy is the leading cause of blindness in Japan; this is a complication associated with diabetes. The probability for diabetic patients developing diabetic retinopathy within 10 years of the onset of diabetes is high. To prevent this disease, people aged over 40 or those who are at a risk should attend mass screening or have regular eye examinations. In an ophthalmologic examination, ophthalmologists look for the presence of hemorrhages (including microaneurysms) and exudates in the retinal fundus images.

For hemorrhage detection in the CAD scheme, the initial extraction includes both the hemorrhages and blood vessels. The blood vessels are subsequently identified and eliminated. In addition, the funicular shapes included in the initial extraction are also identified and eliminated. Further FP elimination is performed using feature analysis. A similar procedure is used in the exudates detection [13].

Using 113 fundus images (26 with hemorrhages and 87 normal), the sensitivity and specificity of the hemorrhage detection algorithm was evaluated to be 84.6% and

20.6%, respectively. Using 109 fundus images (13 with exudates and 96 normal), the sensitivity and specificity of the exudates detection algorithm was evaluated at 76.9% and 83.3%, respectively.

3.4 Detection of Hypertensive Retinopathy

Hypertensive retinopathy can also benefit from the analysis of retinal fundus images. With severe hypertensive retinopathy, the damage to the optic nerve or macula can be permanent. Figure 3 shows the hypertensive retinopathy detection scheme based on the measurement of the vascular diameter [14].

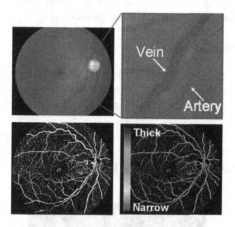

Fig. 3. Detection scheme of hypertensive retinopathy [14]. (Left to right, top to bottom) Original retinal fundus image; magnified view showing the difference in the diameter between a vein and an artery; extraction of blood vessels; the ratio of the size of the artery to that of the vein (A/V ratio) is determined. An A/V ratio >0.67 is considered as abnormal.

Our scheme comprises the extraction of blood vessels, classification of arteries and veins, and detection of arteriolar narrowing by the artery-vein diameter ratio (A/V ratio). An A/V ratio >0.67 is considered as abnormal. Using 39 normal and 44 abnormal fundus images with arteriolar narrowing, this approach can identify 76.2% of true positives at 1.4 FPs per image.

4 CAD for Ultrasound Breast Images

4.1 Overview

In Japan, breast cancer has the highest incidence rate among all the cancers in women [15]. It is also one of the most common causes of cancer death for women in many Western countries. Early detection of breast cancer is the key to simpler treatment and a better prognosis. In view of this, many countries, including Japan have introduced breast cancer screening programs. Mammography is widely used in breast cancer screening.

Its effectiveness in detecting breast cancer in women aged over 50, typically with less dense breast tissues, has been established. However, mammography is less effective for younger women or women with dense breast tissues.

In Japan, women typically have denser breast tissues than their counterparts in Western countries. Consequently, the image contrast between cancerous breast mass tissues and the dense breast tissues in mammographic images is low; thus, the detection of breast cancer over a background of dense breast tissue is difficult. Ultrasonography, on the other hand, is effective in distinguishing and characterizing breast masses set in a dense-breast-tissue environment. Currently, breast ultrasound is primarily used for the diagnosis of breast cancer, as opposed to the screening of breast cancer. There is a growing need for ultrasound examination to be available for breast cancer screening in women with dense breast tissues.

4.2 Whole Breast Scanner and CAD

Current diagnostic ultrasound breast images are obtained using conventional hand-held probes. Here, the results of the examinations are operator dependent and the reproducibility is poor. Moreover, the procedure is lengthy if the whole breast is to be scanned.

An ultrasound breast cancer screening was developed in this project. In the system, an automatic whole-breast scanner (ASU-1004, Aloka Co. Ltd, Japan) is used in acquiring and screening breast images. The scanner is an automated water path

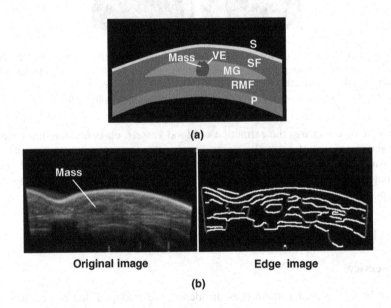

(a)

Original image   Edge image

(b)

Fig. 4. Illustration of the detection of a low-echo breast mass. (a) Schematic diagram of structures in a breast ultrasound image where S is skin layer, SF is subcutaneous fat, MG is mammary gland, RMF is the retro-mammary fat, P is pectorals and VE is a near-vertical edge of the mass. (b) The original breast ultrasound image and the processed edge image are shown [16].

system and can scan the whole breast in sweeps. A 3D volumetric whole breast data is reconstructed from the original scans in the workstation, which has a capability of the image viewer with CAD function [16].

Using a Canny's detector, the edge information in the ultrasound images is enhanced and analyzed (Figure 4). Normal structures in breast ultrasound images typically do not contain vertical edges. The detection of vertical edges in the image suggests abnormal structures [16]. Using 109 whole-breast ultrasound patient cases, our CAD system for breast-mass detection achieves a sensitivity of 80.5% at 3.8 FPs per breast. A CAD system that uses a bilateral subtraction technique to reduce the FPs detected by the mass detection scheme has also been developed [17]. It was found that a scheme for FP reduction based on the bilateral subtraction technique can effectively reduce FPs because 67.3% of the FPs was reduced without removing a true positive region.

5 Summary

In summary, all of the CAD projects are proceeding very well thus far and the clinical examinations will be started soon; according to our plan, commercialized CAD systems in the field of brain MR images, fundus images, and breast ultrasound images will appear by the completion of this project (March 2009).

Acknowledgements. The studies described above are supported mainly by a grant for the Knowledge Cluster Gifu-Ogaki (KCGO), referred to as the "Robotics Advanced Medical Cluster," from the Ministry of Education, Culture, Sports, Science and Technology, Japan. The study of the detection of glaucoma in retinal fundus images is supported in part by a grant for Regional New Consortium Projects from the Ministry of Economy, Trade and Industry, Japan. The authors are grateful to their many co-workers from universities, hospitals, and companies (TAK Co., Ltd., Konica Minolta Medical & Graphics, Inc., Kowa Co., Ltd., and Aloka Co., Ltd., Japan) who are involved in the "Big CAD projects" at KCGO.

References

1. Health and Welfare Statistics Association: Vital Statistics of Japan 2003. 1, 300–301 (2003)
2. Yokoyama, R., Zhang, X., Uchiyama, Y., Fujita, H., Hara, T., Zhou, X., Kanematsu, M., Asano, T., Kondo, H., Goshima, S., Hoshi, H., Iwama, T.: Development of an Automated Method for the Detection of Chronic Lacunar Infarct Regions in Brain MR images. IEICE Trans. Inf. & Syst. E90-D(6), 943–954 (2007)
3. Uchiyama, Y., Yokoyama, R., Ando, H., Asano, T., Kato, H., Yamakawa, H., Yamakawa, H., Hara, T., Iwama, T., Hoshi, H., Fujita, H.: Computer-Aided Diagnosis Scheme for Detection of Lacunar Infarcts on MR Images. Academic Radiology (in press)
4. Uchiyama, Y., Ando, H., Yokoyama, R., Hara, T., Fujita, H., Iwama, T.: Computer-Aided Diagnosis Scheme for Detection of Unruptured Intracranial Aneurysms in MR Angiography. In: Proc. of IEEE Engineering in Medicine and Biology 27th Annual Conference, Shanghai, China, pp. 3031–3034 (2005)

5. Uchiyama, Y., Yamauchi, M., Ando, H., Yokoyama, R., Hara, T., Fujita, H., Iwama, T.: Automatic Classification of Cerebral Arteries in MRA Images and Its Application to Maximum Intensity Projection. In: Proc. of IEEE Engineering in Medicine and Biology 28th Annual Conference, New York, USA, pp. 4865–4868 (2006)

6. Yamauchi, M., Uchiyama, Y., Yokoyama, R., Hara, T., Fujita, H., Ando, H., Yamakawa, H., Iwama, T., Hoshi, H.: Computerized Scheme for Detection of Arterial Occlusion in Brain MRA images. In: Proc. of SPIE Medical Imaging 2007: Computer-Aided Diagnosis, vol. 6514, pp. 65142C-1-65142C-9 (2007)

7. Iwase, A., Suzuki, Y., Areie, M., Tajimi Study Group, et al.: Japan Glaucoma Society: The Prevalence of Primary Open-angle Glaucoma in Japanese The Tajimi Study. Ophthalmology 111(9), 1641–1648 (2004)

8. Yamamoto, T., Iwase, A., Araie, M., Tajimi Study Group.: Japan Glaucoma Society: The Tajimi Study Report 2: Prevalence of Primary Angle Closure and Secondary Glaucoma in a Japanese Population. Ophthalmology 112(10), 1661–1669 (2005)

9. Quigley, H., Broman, A.: The Number of People with Glaucoma Worldwide in 2010 and 2020. Br. J. Ophthalmol. 90, 262–267 (2006)

10. Nakagawa, T., Hayashi, Y., Hatanaka, Y., Aoyama, A., Hara, T., Kakogawa, M., Fujita, H., Yamamoto, T.: Comparison of the Depth of an Optic Nerve Head Obtained using Stereo Retinal Images and HRT. In: Proc. of SPIE Medical Imaging 2007: Physiology, Function, and Structure from Medical Images, vol. 6511, pp. 65112M-1-65112M-9 (2007)

11. Nakagawa, T., Hayashi, Y., Hatanaka, Y., Aoyama, A., Hara, T., Kakogawa, M., Fujita, H., Yamamoto, T.: Cup Region Extraction of Optic Nerve Head for Three-Dimensional Retinal Fundus Image. Proc. of Asian Forum on Medical Imaging, IEICE Technical Report 106(510), 26–27 (2007)

12. Hayashi, Y., Nakagawa, T., Hatanaka, Y., Aoyama, A., Kakogawa, M., Hara, T., Fujita, H., Yamamoto, T.: Detection of Retinal Nerve Fiber Layer Defects in Retinal Fundus Images using Gabor Filtering. In: Proc. of SPIE Medical Imaging 2007: Computer-Aided Diagnosis, vol. 6514, pp. 65142Z-1-65142Z-8 (2007)

13. Hatanaka, Y., Nakagawa, T., Hayashi, Y., Fujita, A., Kakogawa, M., Kawase, K., Hara, T., Fujita, H.: CAD Scheme to Detect Hemorrhages and Exudates in Ocular Fundus Images. In: Proc. of SPIE Medical Imaging 2007: Computer-Aided Diagnosis, vol. 6514, pp. 65142M-1-65142M-8 (2007)

14. Hayashi, T., Nakagawa, T., Hatanaka, Y., Hayashi, Y., Aoyama, A., Mizukusa, Y., Fujita, A., Kakogawa, M., Hara, T., Fujita, H.: An Artery-vein Classification Using Top-hat Image and Detection of Arteriolar Narrowing on Retinal Images. IEICE Technical Report 107(57), 127–132 (2007) [in Japanese]

15. Minami, Y., Tsubono, Y., Nishino, Y., Ohuchi, N., Shibuya, D., Hisamichi, S.: The Increase of Female Breast Cancer Incidence in Japan: Emergence of Birth Cohort Effect. Int. J. Cancer 108(6), 901–906 (2004)

16. Ikedo, Y., Fukuoka, D., Hara, T., Fujita, H., Takada, E., Endo, T., Morita, T.: Development of a fully automatic scheme for detection of masses in whole breast ultrasound images. Medical Physics 34(11), 4378–4388 (2007)

17. Ikedo, Y., Fukuoka, D., Hara, T., Fujita, H., Takada, E., Endo, T., Morita, T.: Computerized mass detection in whole breast ultrasound images: Reduction of false positives using bilateral subtraction technique. In: Proc. of SPIE Medical Imaging 2007: Computer-Aided Diagnosis, vol. 6514, pp. 65141T-1-65141T-10 (2007)

CAD on Liver Using CT and MRI

Xuejun Zhang[1], Hiroshi Fujita[2], Tuanfa Qin[1], Jinchuang Zhao[1],
Masayuki Kanematsu[3],Takeshi Hara[2], Xiangrong Zhou[2], Ryujiro Yokoyama[3],
Hiroshi Kondo[3], and Hiroaki Hoshi[3]

[1] School of Computer, Electronics and Information, Department of Electronics and Information
Engineering, Guangxi University, Nanning City, Guangxi 530004, P.R. China
[2] Department of Intelligent Image Information, Division of Regeneration and Advanced
Medical Sciences, Graduate School of Medicine, Gifu University, Gifu 501-1194, Japan
[3] Department of Radiology, Gifu University School of Medicine & Gifu University Hospital,
Gifu 501-1194, Japan
xjzhang@gxu.edu.cn

Abstract. The incidence of liver diseases is very high in Asian countries. This paper introduces our computer-aided diagnosis (CAD) system for diagnosing liver cancer and describes the fundamental technologies employed in the system and its performance. The results showed that our system is useful for diagnosing liver cancer, and it is expected that employing CAD in clinical practice would reduce the mortality caused by liver cancer in Asian countries.

Keywords: Computer-aided diagnosis, Segmentation, Liver, Tumor, Cirrhosis, Multi-phase CT, Edge extraction, Subtraction method, Shape and texture analysis.

1 Introduction

Primary malignant liver tumors, including hepatocellular carcinoma (HCC), cause 1.25 million deaths per year worldwide. HCC is prevalent in Asia and Africa because of the presence of a large subclinical population with hepatitis C virus infection. Additionally, during the last 2 decades, the mortality rate from primary liver cancer is reported to have increased by 41%, and the proportion of hospitalization due to this disease has increased by 46% [1]. Although globally liver cancer is ranked 9th as the cause of death due to organ cancer, it is ranked from 1st to 3rd in many Asian countries, particularly in the coastal regions of Japan, Korea, China, and Southeast Asian countries. Early detection and accurate staging of liver cancer is an important issue in practical radiology. Although multidetector-row computed tomography (MDCT) or MRI is widely used for the diagnosis of liver tumors, the amount of information obtained from MDCT/MRI is very large, and it is currently difficult for inexperienced radiologists or physicians to interpret all the images within a short timespan.

The purpose of our study was to establish a computer-aided diagnosis (CAD) and surgery system for : aiding decision-making in regard to the diagnosis of liver cancer;

X. Gao et al. (Eds.): MIMI 2007, LNCS 4987, pp. 367–376, 2008.
© Springer-Verlag Berlin Heidelberg 2008

supporting radiologists and surgeons in the planning of liver resectioning anf facilating living donor transplantation using multiphase CT/MRI images.

2 Methods and Experimental Results

Three datasets from different hospitals were examined with different MDCT scanners. In the main dataset, an MDCT scanner (Aquilion; TOSHIBA, Japan) was used to scan a quadruple-phase protocol that included unenhanced, hepatic arterial, portal venous, and delayed phase images. Each patient received the contrast/bolus agent (Oypalomin370 or Optiray320) via a power injector at a rate of 3 ml/s, and the final average volume of the contrast material was 100 ml (range, 110–182 ml). Four complete acquisitions of the entire liver were obtained in a craniocaudal direction during one breath-hold with the following parameters: slice interval, 0.625–1.25 mm; bits stored, 16 bits; pixel-spacing, 0.50–0.625 mm; spatial resolution, 512 ×512; 165 mAs; and 120 kVp. Non-contrast scanning (i.e., the first pass) was performed in all patients. The final average start time for the hepatic arterial phase was 37-s (range, 35–40-s). The portal venous phase and the equilibrium phase (i.e., the third and fourth passes, respectively) scans were acquired at 65 s (range, 60–70 s) and 180 s, respectively, after the contrast material injection. These cases were categorized by experienced radiologists, as 12 normal cases, 32 cases with 44 HCC tumors, and 9 other tumor cases were confirmed.

Precontrast T1-weighted MR images are ordinarily obtained by using a spin-echo or gradient-recalled-echo sequence. In our experiment, the repetition time (TR)/echo time (TE) was set at 316 ms/11 ms. Further, fast spin-echo (FSE) T2-weighted imaging, which has been shown to play a key role in the characterization of liver lesions, was performed by using an FSE sequence. The signal intensities of metastases using T1- and T2-weighted images are variable but are usually prolonged. T2-weighted imaging is reported to be very effective in enabling radiologists to differentiate between cavernous hemangiomas and metastases. In this experiment, the effective TR/effective TE of an FSE T2-weighted image was set at 4615 ms/80 ms. We obtained the gadolinium-enhanced hepatic arterial and equilibrium phase images by using a phased-array body multicoil with the following settings: TE, 1.6 ms; TR, 150 ms; flip angle, 90°; matrix, 512 ×512; and breath-hold acquisition, 26-s. Images were obtained after administering an antecubital intravenous bolus injection of 0.1 mmol/kg gadopentetate dimeglumine (Gd-DTPA) (Magnevist; Schering AG, Berlin, Germany), followed by flushing with 15 ml of sterile saline solution. The scan timing was 18s and 3 min after initiation of the contrast injection. Using a 1.5 -T superconducting magnet (Signa Horizon; GE Medical Systems, Milwaukee, WI), 320 MR images of 80 patients (4 images per patient) with focal liver lesions were obtained. These cases were diagnosed by 2 experienced radiologists, and a majority of these cases were pathologically confirmed by biopsy or surgery. Although it was impossible to diagnose all lesions pathologically, the remaining patients underwent angiography-assisted ultrasonography, CT, or follow-up MRI to confirm the diagnosis. We followed a stringent criterion for diagnosing malignancy and excluded cases in which the lesion size was very small.

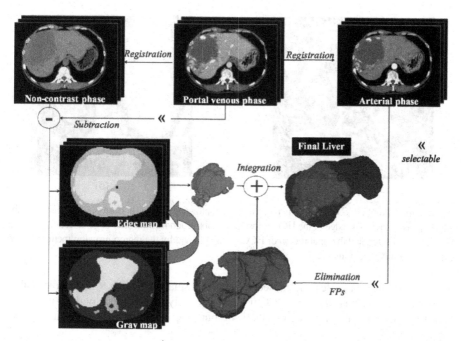

Fig. 1. Segmentation of an abnormal liver region from MDCT, based on the edge detection and subtraction method [2]

Based on the above CT/MRI datasets, our developed systems contained the following components:

2.1 Segmentation of the Liver Region from Tumor Tissues

We propose a fully automatic method to segment the liver and other organs on multi-phase MRI or CT images, regardless of the presence of cirrhosis or tumors such as hemangioma, HCC or cyst within the liver [2]. Our method is based on edge detection [3] and combined with a subtraction processing algorithm that is independant of the intensity or noise of the CT-MR images. In comparison to other methods [4– 8], this "Press-One-Button" system is extremely user-friendly and can be used without any training; moreover, it provides highly accurate 3D images of different organs within an average of 12 min of running on a PC (Pentium M 1.0 GHz with 512 MB RAM). This time is reasonable and acceptable for clinical applications. All the liver regions in 53 cases were successfully segmented by visual evaluation, without losing any part of the hepatic lesions. A comparison of the gold standard for liver regions prepared by radiologists with our experimental results revealed that in 6 cases of the entire dataset, the average error rate of liver segmentation was within 4.3%. Eleven hepatic tumors (3 hemangioma, 4 HCC, 3 metastasis, and 1 cyst) showing distinct intensity difference from the liver scanned in the portal venous MDCT images were extracted successfully and integrated into the final region. Figure 1 shows an extracted 3D liver

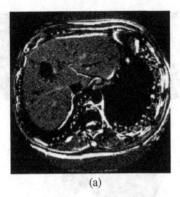 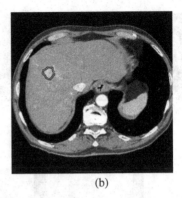

(a)   (b)

Fig. 2. Extraction of HCC candidates is performed by subtracting the equilibrium phase image from the arterial phase image. The edge of the HCC is lost in the subtraction map (a) after edge detection by Sobel filter and LoG filter, and the final region of HCC (b) is obtained by the region growing method on the extracted candidate regions [9].

tissue in which a large lesion, caused by hemangioma appears as a huge hole. Other cases such as a normal liver, or HCC tumors with only subtle intensity differences are performed with high and stable results using our proposed method without losing any hepatic tissues.

2.2 Computer-Aided Detection of Hepatocellular Carcinoma on Multiphase CT Images

Following the enhancement with the contrast material, the presence of HCC is indicated by high- and low-intensity regions in arterial and equilibrium phase images, respectively. We propose an automatic method for detecting HCC based on edge detection and subtraction processing [9]. Within a liver area segmented according to our scheme, black regions were selected by subtracting the equilibrium phase images with the corresponding registered arterial phase images. From these black regions, the HCC candidates were extracted as the areas without edges by using Sobel and LoG edge detection filters, as shown in Fig. 2a. The false-positive (FP) candidates were eliminated by using 6 features extracted from the cancerous and the surrounding liver regions. Other FPs were further eliminated by opening processing. Finally, an expansion process was applied to acquire the 3D shape of the HCC, as shown in Fig. 2b. In this experiment, we used the CT images of 44 patients with 44 HCCs. We successfully extracted 97.7% (43/44) HCCs successfully by our proposed method, with an average number of 2.1 FPs per case.

2.3 Application of an Artificial Neural Network to the Computer-Aided Differentiation of Focal Liver Diseases in MR Imaging

The differentiation of focal liver lesions in MR imaging is primarily based on the intensity and homogeneity of lesions with different imaging sequences. However, in some patients, these imaging findings may be falsely interpreted due to the involved

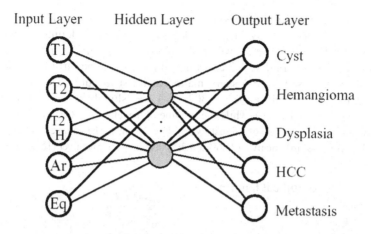

Fig. 3. A multi-layer feedforward network used in LiverANN [14-16] can automatically find the internal relationship between inputs and outputs by learning from samples and employing a backpropagation algorithm. Note: T2H = homogeneity of T2-weighted imaging. HCC = hepatocellular carcinoma.

complexity. Our aim was to establish a CAD system named LiverANN for classifying the pathologies of focal liver lesions into 5 categories by using the artificial neural network (ANN) technique, which has been proved useful in various medical fields [10–13]. On each MR image, a region of interest (ROI) in the focal liver lesion was delineated by a radiologist. The intensity and homogeneity within the ROI were automatically calculated to obtain numerical data that were analyzed by input signals to LiverANN. The outputs were the following 5 pathological categories of hepatic diseases, namely, hepatic cyst, hepatocellular carcinoma, dysplasia in cirrhosis, cavernous hemangioma, and metastasis. Of the 320 MR images obtained from 80 patients (4 images per patient) with liver lesions, LiverANN classified 50 cases of training set into 5 types of liver lesions with a training accuracy of 100% and 30 test cases with a testing accuracy of 93% [14–16].

2.4 3D Volume Analysis of Cirrhosis

Cirrhosis of the liver is one of the leading causes of death due to disease, killing more than 12,000 people in Japan each year. In the United States, about 26,000 people die from chronic liver diseases and cirrhosis each year. Liver MR imaging is useful for the diagnosis of cirrhosis. The enlargement of the left lobe of the liver and the shrinkage of the right lobe are helpful signs in MR imaging for the diagnosis of cirrhosis of the liver [17–20]. To investigate whether the volume ratio of left-to-whole (LTW) is effective in differentiating a cirrhotic liver from a normal liver, we developed an automatic algorithm for segmentation and volume calculation of the liver region in MDCT scans and MR imaging [21]. As shown in Fig. 4a, the 3D liver is divided into left and right lobes along the umbilical fissure. The volume (V) of each part is calculated slice by slice. The degree of cirrhosis is defined as the ratio of $LTW = Vleft/(Vright + Vleft)$, where $Vright + Vleft$ is the volume in Fig. 4b and $Vleft$ is the volume in Fig. 4c. 22 cases including normal and cirrhotic liver on MR and CT slices are used for 3D segmentation and visualization. The whole hepatic volume of the cirrhotic liver (931 ± 307 cm^3) was slightly lower than that of the normal liver (1070 ± 412 cm^3), while the volume of the left lobe in the cirrhotic liver (238 ± 53 cm^3) was larger than that of the normal liver (176 ± 69 cm^3). The volume ratio of LTW was relatively higher in the cirrhotic liver ($25.6\% \pm 4.3\%$) than in the normal liver ($16.4\% \pm 5.4\%$).

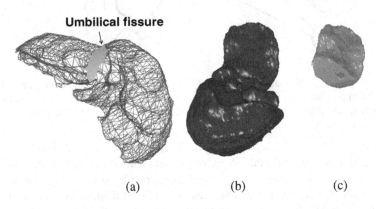

(a)   (b)   (c)

Fig. 4. 3D volume analysis of cirrhosis. (a) The liver is divided into left and right lobe by drawing an umbilical fissure. The volume ratio of LTW is defined as the ratio between the whole liver (b) and left lobe (c) volumes [21].

2.5 Improving the Classification of the Cirrhotic Liver by Shape and Texture Analysis

Two shape features were calculated from a segmented liver region, and 7 texture features were quantified using the grey level difference method (GLDM) [22] within the small ROIs. The degree of cirrhosis was derived by integrating the shape and texture features of the liver into a 3-layer feedforward ANN [23], as shown in Fig. 5. The liver was regarded as cirrhotic if the percentage of ROIs with a degree of cirrhosis of more than 0.5 was greater than 50%. The initial experimental result showed that the ANN-based method classified liver cirrhosis with a training accuracy of 100% on the 100 ROIs included in the training set. In the testing of the whole liver region, 82% (9/11) cirrhotic and 100% (7/7) normal cases were correctly differentiated from 18 test cases using the shape and texture analysis as compared to 55% (6/11) cirrhotic and 100% (7/7) normal cases using the texture analysis alone [24]. According to the ROC analysis, the Az value (the area under the ROC curve) improved from 0.57 to 0.84 by integrating the shape features into ANN inputs [25].

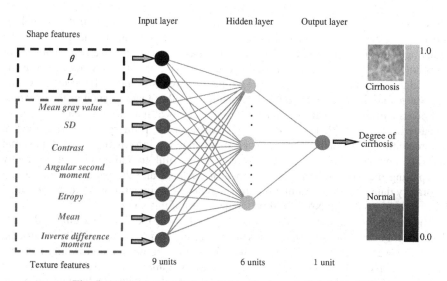

Fig. 5. ANN structure for calculating the degree of cirrhosis [25]

3 Discussion

The challenge of liver segmentation is to robustly extract the regions with lesions, or the regions that have received partial transplants. The liver not only has radiodensity that is similar to its surrounding structures, resulting in the common problem of connectivity to the heart, stomach, or kidney, but it is also affected by hepatic diseases that may change its shape and internal texture, or homogeneity. In addition, the image quality from different modalities varies in terms of signal-to-noise ratio, motion artifacts, etc. There are some reports on the segmentation of the abdominal organs on CT images using a thresholding method or, likelihood function. However, many reports address only the techniques involved in the segmentation of the normal liver tissue, and these techniques cannot usually be used for extracting the abnormal liver regions. In order to ensure that our software can be widely used in different hospitals for different modalities, we used edge detection in combination with a subtraction processing algorithm that is independent of the intensity or noise of the CT images or of the accuracy of the MR images.

Although our affine-based registration method was useful for liver segmentation, the position of cancer in arterial phase images might be different from that in equilibrium phase images when rigid transformation is used alone. In particular, if the tumor is small in size, the subtraction process cannot enhance the cancer region in the same position. Therefore, the small HCC candidate was eliminated as FP after edge detection. In our study, this HCC could be detected by using the nonrigid transformation method [26, 27], even if the patient changed the duration of breath-hold frequently during the period when the scanning was performed twice.

Focal liver lesions can be accurately detected and characterized by MR imaging. The misdiagnosis by LiverANN might have occurred because some HCCs are mildly hyperintense in T2-weighted images, moderately hypervascular in the hepatic arterial phase, and hypointense in the equilibrium phase. Hypervascular metastases such as renal cell carcinoma or carcinoid tumor have brisk arterial enhancement and may be indistinguishable from HCC. The broad spectrum of enhancement pattern or morphology of HCC makes it difficult to characterize this type of tumor using the CAD algorithm, and some overlap in imaging features is observed between HCC and metastasis in daily clinical practice. Information of other features such as the presence of fibrous capsules or cirrhotic changes around the focal liver lesions, elevated serum alpha-fetoprotein (AFP) level, or history of extrahepatic primary cancer is critical in differentiating HCC and metastasis; such supplementary information other than signal intensity and homogeneity of lesions is very helpful to radiologists in correctly interpreting the MR images. The presence of cirrhosis and the patient's clinical and laboratory data are helpful in making the diagnosis. The integration of such additional information into LiverANN would be the next step of this study.

The results of our study showed that the left lobe of the liver was enlarged while the right lobe was shrinked in patients with liver cirrhosis. No statistically significant difference was observed in the whole hepatic volume between the cirrhotic liver and the normal liver. However, the difference in the volume ratio of LTW between the cirrhotic liver and the normal liver was significantly improved by our proposed method, and the 3D feature performed better than the 2D feature [28, 29].

The two misdiagnosed cirrhosis cases had very similar shape feature values to those of the normal cases; this is because the shape of the liver may change in different sleeping postures, and the shape features may be affected by the scanning position when only one 2D slice is used. Our next step is to calculate the 3D shape features to solve this problem, since the dullness of the left lobe remains the same regardless of the variation in the shape. Furthermore, the CAD system is expected to differentiate micronodular cirrhosis, macronodular cirrhosis, and mixed types into different categories by using ANN.

4   Conclusion

In conclusion, we developed a CAD system for the detection and diagnosis of liver diseases on MR and CT images. The experimental results demonstrated that our system functioning as a computer-aided differentiation tool may provide radiologists with referential opinion during the radiological diagnostic procedure; the performance of our 3D segmentation technique was satisfactory for surgical use, and the agreement of the LTW ratio with shape and texture features may be effective for predicting cirrhosis on MR images. It is expected that employing CAD in clinical practice would reduce the mortality caused by liver cancer in Asian countries.

Acknowledgments. This research was supported in part by a Grant-in-Aid for Cancer Research from the Ministry of Health, Labour and Welfare, Japan; in part by a Grant-in-Aid for Scientific Research from the Ministry of Education, Culture, Sports, Science and Technology, Japan; in part by the National Natural Science Foundation of China (No. 60762001); in part by the Program to Sponsor Teams for Innovation in the Construction of Talent Highlands in Guangxi Institutions of Higher Learning; and in part by a research foundation project of Guangxi University (No. X071036). The authors would like to thank Gobert Lee, Hiroki Kato, Huiyan Jiang, Wenguang Li, Chao Gao, Tetsuji Tajima, and Teruhiko Kitagawa for their assistance in a part of the LiverCAD project and Shigeru Nawano and Kenji Shinozaki, who provided a part of the MDCT data used in this study.

References

1. El-Serag, H., Mason, A.: Rising incidence of hepatocellular carcinoma in the United States. N. Engl. J. Med. 340, 745–750 (1999)
2. Zhang, X., Tajima, T., Kitagawa, T., Kanematsu, M., Zhou, X., Hara, T., Fujita, H., Yokoyama, R., Kondo, H., Hoshi, H.: Segmentation of liver region with tumorous tissues. In: Proc. of SPIE Medical Imaging 2007: Image Processing, vol. 6512, pp. 651235-1-651235-9 (2007)
3. Marr, D., Hildreth, E.: Theory of edge detection. Proc. Royal Society of London B207, 187–217 (1980)
4. Hitosugi, T., Shimizu, A., Tamura, M., Kobatake, H.: Development of a liver extraction method using a level set method and its performance evaluation. Journal of Computer Aided Diagnosis of Medical Images 7, 1–9 (2003) (in Japanese)
5. Gao, L., Heath, D., Kuszyk, B., Fishman, E.: Automatic liver segmentation technique for three-dimensional visualization of CT data. Radiology 201, 359–364 (1996)
6. Masumoto, J., Hori, M., Sato, Y.: Automated liver segmentation using multislice CT images. IEICE J84-D-II, 2150–2161 (2001) (in Japanese)
7. Bae, K., Giger, M., Chen, C.: Automatic segmentation of liver structure in CT images. Med. Phys. 20, 71–78 (1993)
8. Park, H., Bland, P.H., Meyer, C.R.: Construction of an abdominal probabilistic atlas and its application in segmentation. IEEE Trans. on Med. Imaging 22, 483–492 (2003)
9. Tajima, T., Zhang, X., Kitagawa, T., Kanematsu, M., Zhou, X., Hara, T., Fujita, H., Yokoyama, R., Kondo, H., Hoshi, H.: Computer-aided detection (CAD) of hepatocellular carcinoma on multiphase CT images. In: Proc. of SPIE Medical Imaging 2007: Computer-Aided Diagnosis, vol. 6514, pp. 65142Q-1-65 142Q-10 (2007)
10. Asada, N., Doi, K., MacMahon, H., Montner, S.M., Giger, M.L., Abe, C., Wu, Y.: Potential usefulness of an artificial neural network for differential diagnosis of interstitial lung disease: pilot study. Radiology 177, 857–860 (1990)
11. Fujita, H., Katafuchi, T., Uehara, T., Nishimura, T.: Application of artificial neural network to computer-aided diagnosis of coronary artery disease in myocardial SPECT bull's-eye images. J. Nucl. Med. 33, 272–276 (1992)
12. Zhang, W., Doi, K., Giger, M.L., Nishikawa, R.M., Schmidt, R.A.: An improved shift-invariant artificial neural network for computerized detection of clustered microcalcifications in digital mammograms. Med. Phys. 23, 595–601 (1996)
13. Seki, K., Fujita, H., Hirako, K., Hara, T., Ando, T.: Detection of microcalcifications on mammograms using neural networks. Med. Imag. Tech. 15, 639–651 (1997) (in Japanese)
14. Zhang, X., Kanematsu, M., Fujita, H., Hara, T., Hoshi, H.: Computerized classification of liver disease in MRI using artificial neural network. In: Proc. of SPIE-Medical Imaging 2001: Image Processing, vol. 4322, pp. 1735–1742 (2001)
15. Kako, N., Zhang, X., Kanematsu, M., Fujita, H., Hara, T., Li, W.: Study of computer-aided diagnosis on MR imaging. Radiology 255, 749 (2002) (abstract)
16. Kako, N., Zhang, X., Li, W., Kanematsu, M., Fujita, H., Hara, T.: Artificial neural network method for differentiation of focal liver disease in MR imaging. Radiology 255, 646 (2002) (abstract)

17. Ito, K., Mitchell, D.G.: Hepatic morphologic changes in cirrhosis: MR imaging findings. Abdom. Imag. 25, 456–461 (2000)
18. Harbin, W.P., Robert, N.J., Ferrucci, J.T.: Diagnosis of cirrhosis based on regional changes in hepatic morphology: A radiological and pathological analysis. Radiology 135, 273–283 (1980)
19. Torres, W.E., Whitmire, L.F., Gedgaudas, M.K.: Computed tomography of hepatic morphologic changes in cirrhosis of the liver. J. Comput. Assist. Tomogr. 11, 47–50 (1986)
20. McNeal, C.R., Maynard, W.H., Branch, R.A., Powers, T.A., Arns, P.A., Gunter, K., Fitzpatrick, J.M., Partain, C.L.: Liver volume measurements and three-dimensional display from MR images. Radiology 169, 851–864 (1988)
21. Zhang, X., Li, W., Fujita, H., Kanematsu, M., Hara, T., Zhou, X., Kondo, H., Hoshi, H.: Automatic segmentation of hepatic tissue and 3D volume analysis of cirrhosis in multi-detector row CT scans and MR imaging. IEICE Trans. Inf. & Syst. E87-D(8), 2138–2147 (2004)
22. Haralick, R.M., Shanmugam, K., Dinstein, I.: Texture features for image classification. IEEE Trans. Syst., Man,Cybern. SMC-3, 610–621 (1973)
23. Rumelhart, D.E., McClellend, J.L.: Learning representations by back-propagating errors. Nature 323, 533–536 (1986)
24. Kato, H., Kanematsu, M., Zhang, X., Saio, M., Kondo, H., Goshima, S., Fujita, H.: Computer-aided diagnosis of hepatic fibrosis: Preliminary evaluation of MRI texture analysis using the finite difference method and an artificial neural network. American Roentgen Ray Society 189, 117–122 (2007)
25. Zhang, X., Fujita, H., Kanematsu, M., Zhou, X., Hara, T., Kato, H., Yokoyama, R., Hoshi, H.: Improving the classification of cirrhotic liver by using texture features. In: Proc. of the 2005 IEEE-EMBS (Engineering in Medicine and Biology), pp. 867–870 (2005)
26. Bookstein, F.L.: Principal warps: Thin-plate splines and the decomposition of deformations. IEEE Trans. on Pattern Analysis and Machine Intelligence 11, 567–585 (1989)
27. Wells, W., Viola, P.I., Atsumi, H., Nakajima, S., Kikinis, R.: Multi-modal volume registration by maximization of mutual information. Med. Image Anal. 1, 35–35 (1996)
28. Awaya, H., Mitchell, D., Kamishima, T.: Cirrhosis: Modified caudate-right lobe ratio. Radiology 224, 769–774 (2002)
29. Wang, Y., Itoh, K., Taniguchi, N., Toei, H., Kawai, F., Nakamura, M., Omoto, K., Yokota, K., Ono, T.: Studies on tissue characterization by texture analysis with co-occurrence matrix method using ultrasonography and CT imaging. J. Med. Ultrasonics 26, 825–837 (1999)

Stroke Suite: Cad Systems for Acute Ischemic Stroke, Hemorrhagic Stroke, and Stroke in ER

Wieslaw L. Nowinski, Guoyu Qian, K.N. Bhanu Prakash, Ihar Volkau,
Wing Keet Leong, Su Huang, Anand Ananthasubramaniam, Jimin Liu, Ting Ting Ng,
and Varsha Gupta

Biomedical Imaging Lab, Agency for Science, Technology and Research, Singapore
wieslaw@sbic.a-star.edu.sg

Abstract. We present a suite of computer aided-diagnosis (CAD) systems for acute ischemic stroke, hemorrhagic stroke, and stroke in emergency room. A software architecture common for them is described. The acute ischemic stroke CAD system supports thrombolysis. Our approach shifts the paradigm from a 2D visual inspection of individual scans/maps to atlas-assisted quantification and simultaneous visualization of multiple 2D/3D images. The hemorrhagic stroke CAD system supports the evacuation of hemorrhage by thrombolytic treatment. It aims at progression and quantification of blood clot removal. The clot is automatically segmented from CT time series, its volume measured, and displayed in 3D along with a catheter. A stroke CAD in emergency room enables rapid atlas-assisted decision support regarding the stroke and its location. Our stroke CAD systems facilitate and speed up image analysis, increase confidence of interpreters, and support decision making. They are potentially useful in diagnosis and research, particularly, for clinical trials.

Keywords: stroke, infarct, hemorrhage, penumbra, brain atlas, anatomy, blood supply territories, MR, CT.

1 Introduction

Stroke, or brain attack, is a sudden onset of neurological injury, vascular in origin disturbing cerebral perfusion. It is the second-leading cause of death in the world and the major cause of permanent disability. It has a great effect on public health and generates high costs for primary treatment, rehabilitation, and chronic care. In the US it happens every 45 seconds and its direct cost in 2006 was $58 billion. Despite a critical need, there is no computer-aided diagnosis (CAD) system for stroke, although there are a number of CAD systems in other fields including mammography [1], colonoscopy [2], chest [3] and brain cancer [4], among others.

There are two types of stroke: ischemic and hemorrhagic. Ischemia is an effect of parenchymal hypoperfusion due to arterial occlusion existing long enough. The infarct (or core) is that part of the ischemic area that is irreversibly injured. The penumbra is a hypoperfused region at risk of infarction, which still can be saved by treatment. Hemorrhage develops as a result of bleeding directly into the brain.

X. Gao et al. (Eds.): MIMI 2007, LNCS 4987, pp. 377–386, 2008.

Each type of stroke requires a different treatment. Thrombolysis is the main treatment for acute ischemic stroke by administering tissue plasmiongen activator (t-PA) intravenously and/or intra-arterially through a microcatheter. This procedure is allowed provided that the thrombolysis conditions are met and our acute ischemic stroke CAD checks them rapidly.

There are several ways to treat hemorrhagic stroke. One of them is to evacuate the hemorrhage. This can be done surgically by performing craniotomy. This preferred approach additionally facilitates decompression. A less invasive approach is to insert a catheter into the ventricular system and lyses the blood clot by administering t-PA. Our hemorrhagic stroke CAD system supports the latter procedure.

Neuroimaging plays a central role in stroke management. To make diagnosis and therapeutic decision, Computerized Tomography (CT) and/or Magnetic Resonance (MR) imaging are employed to: 1) Differentiate stroke from stroke mimicking conditions, such as brain tumor, brain abscess or encephalitis. 2) Distinguish between an ischemic and hemorrhagic stroke. 3) Identify any chronic infarct(s). 4) Identify in acute ischemic stroke the infarct, penumbra, and vessel occlusion, if any.

CT scanning usually involves unenhanced CT first, followed, if necessary and available, by CT angiography (CTA) and CT perfusion. In addition, perfusion maps have to be calculated from the CT perfusion including cerebral blood flow (CBF), cerebral blood volume (CBV), mean transit time (MTT), and time to peak (TTP).

Conventional and advanced MR multiple studies are usually acquired depicting anatomy, angiography, diffusion, and perfusion. They include MR diffusion-weighted imaging (DWI), MR perfusion imaging (PI), MR angiography (MRA), T1-weighted, T2-weighted, T2* GRE, and/or fluid-attenuated inversion recovery (FLAIR). Similarly as for CT, perfusion maps have to be calculated from the perfusion images.

The current practice is to process all these studies individually by visual inspection. This causes the process to be time consuming in the situation when "time is brain" and not quantitative, while certain conditions have to be calculated accurately to make the therapeutic decision.

The design and development of a CAD system, particularly in a research environment, is a difficult task. For acute ischemic stroke this difficulty amplifies as "time is brain". It is estimated that during stroke about 1.9 million nerve cells and 14 billion synapses die each minute, and the ischemic brain ages about 3.6 years each hour. Therefore, the speed of processing is a key requirement for this kind of a CAD system.

Our focus is on research, design, development, and deployment of a suite of CAD systems for stroke. At present, three systems are at various stages of development:

- CAD for acute ischemic stroke from MR and CT
- CAD for hemorrhagic stroke
- stroke CAD in emergency room (ER).

The goal of this paper is to describe the progress in the design, development, and deployment of these CADs systems.

2 Methods

Though each of the stroke CAD systems has its own functionality specific to its role, they are designed to have common software architecture to enable sharing of a library with core technology, brain atlases, and common tools.

2.1 Software Architecture

A common stroke suite software architecture is shown in Figure 1.

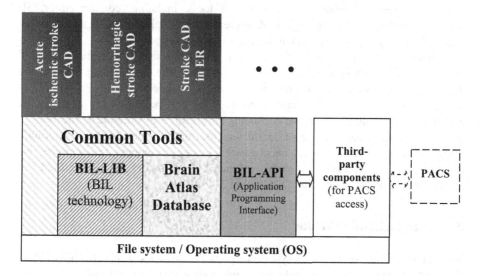

Fig. 1. Common software architecture of the stroke suite CAD systems

This architecture includes the BIL-LIB library, brain atlas database, and common tools. A key component is the BIL-LIB library which contains core algorithms developed in our lab (BIL) for stroke image processing. It is written in C++ to ensure high performance. Other fundamental components are the brain atlas database and common tools applicable across various stroke applications. To facilitate use in a clinical setting, third-party components for PACS access are also included.

2.2 Brain Atlas Database

The brain atlas database for stroke contains three brain atlases previously constructed by us: atlas of anatomy, atlas of blood supply territories (BSTs), and atlas of cerebral vasculature. For anatomy, the Cerefy brain atlas [5], derived from Talairach-Tournoux (TT) [6], is employed. This atlas is fully labeled with 138 white and gray matter structures including cortical areas. The construction of the Cerefy brain atlas and its enhancements were addressed earlier [7-9]. The BST atlas fits the atlas of anatomy [10]. It is parcellated into seven BSTs: penetrating branches of anterior cerebral artery (ACA), terminal branches of ACA, penetrating branches of MCA, terminal branches of MCA, penetrating braches of posterior cerebral artery (PCA) and posterior communicating artery (PCoA), terminal branches of PCA, and anterior choroidal artery. The cerebrovascular atlas with arteries, veins and sinuses has been constructed from high resolution angiographic data [11, 12].

2.3 Common Tools

The architecture comprises several common tools, including contour editor, 3D surface modeler, symmetric region of interests (ROIs) placement, histogramming, ellipse fitting for registration, and algorithm validation support.

A powerful yet easy to use contour editor allows the user to edit the segmented structures, such as an infarct, penumbra, or blood clot. The user can edit interactively the outline of a structure by creating, moving and deleting contours as well as moving, adding and deleting contour points. This can be done very precisely by zooming into the edited region and enhancing the accuracy of structure delineation.

A 3D surface model can be reconstructed from the 2D contours by generating a binary volume from the voxels encompassed by these contours and applying the Marching Cubes algorithm [13] to this volume. The 3D model can be displayed and manipulated (rotated, zoomed and panned) in 3D.

3 Acute Ischemic Stroke

The acute ischemic stroke CAD system supports thrombolysis. It checks rapidly three thrombolysis conditions on multiple individual studies. Our approach shifts the current paradigm from a 2D visual inspection of individual scans and maps to an atlas-assisted quantification and simultaneous visualization of multiple 2D and 3D images.

3.1 Concept

The method supports the thrombolysis algorithm [14], and provides quantitative image analysis and decision making support by checking the following conditions: 1) The presence of diffusion-perfusion mismatch. 2) The size of the infarct versus that of the MCA territory. 3) The site of vessel occlusion, if any.

The presence of a considerable diffusion-perfusion mismatch predicts treatment response, while a large infarct (taken in [14] as greater than a half of the MCA territory) predicts hemorrhagic transformation. These two conditions are quantitative and our method calculates them rapidly.

The infarct and penumbra are segmented speedily by a combination of automatic and interactive approaches. 3D models of the infarct and penumbra are reconstructed and their volumes and mismatch measured. The brain atlases are employed to provide and quantify the underlying anatomy and BSTs.

3.2 Workflow

The acute ischemic stroke CAD system supports the following workflow: 1) Open case (which may contain multiple studies). 2) View individual studies (to exclude hemorrhage and/or identify any previous infarct). 3) Process diffusion (to segment and quantify the infarct). 4) Process perfusion (to segment and quantify the penumbra). 5) Process MRA/CTA (to identify or exclude vessel occlusion). 6) Quantify the diffusion-perfusion mismatch. 7) Perform atlas-assisted analysis (including the infarct-MCA ratio calculation). 8) Generate report.

The infarct and penumbra are segmented by a combined automatic-interactive approach and the diffusion-perfusion mismatch is quantified. Atlas-assisted analysis employs the atlases to quantify the infarct and penumbra. The size of the infarct versus that of MCA territory is calculated automatically by means of the BST atlas. The CAD system provides functions for image viewing; diffusion image processing; perfusion map processing; diffusion-perfusion mismatch quantification; 3D display and manipulation of the infarct and penumbra; atlas to scan mapping; and atlas-assisted analysis.

3.3 Infarct Segmentation

Infarct segmentation from DWI is done in three ways (at three levels): global automatic, local semi-automatic, and local interactive. The automatic segmentation is based on processing of energy images followed by post-processing enhancement [15]. The local semi-automatic segmentation can subsequently be applied to the currently displayed slice or any ROI if the global segmentation is not accurate enough. Finally, the user can interactively fine tune the outline of the infarct by means of the contour editor. A 3D model of the infarct can be generated, displayed, and manipulated. The volume of the infarct is measured on the fly (i.e., also during its interactive editing). The 3D display of the infarct, showing the spatial relationship among the contours on consecutive sections, may eventually lead to an improvement of infarct's delineation and quantification.

As early ischemic signs in CT scans are subtle, infarct identification consists in comparison of the corresponding ROIs in both hemispheres. The system first calculates the midsagittal plane (MSP) and when the user draws an ROI in the studied area, the symmetric ROI is drawn in the opposite hemisphere and statistics calculated in both ROIs. Several ROI templates are provided with editable location, size, and shape.

3.4 Penumbra Segmentation

The penumbra is segmented from PI at two levels: global automatic and local interactive. The global automatic segmentation method thresholds (typically MTT) images. The thresholded images can further be edited by using the contour editor. Penumbra segmentation is facilitated by displaying the outline of the infarct and other perfusion maps (CBF, CBV, and TTP).

A 3D model of the penumbra can be reconstructed from the 2D contours, and displayed and manipulated in 3D to better understand 3D relationships and to enhance, if needed, penumbra's segmentation. The penumbra's volume is also measured. To better assess the mismatch, the 3D infarct and penumbra can be displayed together with a user-controlled degree of blending.

3.5 Atlas to Scan Mapping

Numerous methods have been developed for brain warping. A choice of a warping technique for atlas to scan mapping is application dependent. For acute ischemic stroke, when "time is brain", we apply very fast dedicated techniques.

We have earlier developed the Fast Talairach Transformation (FTT) which maps automatically the atlas onto a scan in about 5s [16]. The FTT is a rapid version of the Talairach transformation [6] with the modified Talairach landmarks [17] validated for T1-weighted scans. When an anatomical T1-weighted scan is not available, the atlas is fit directly to DWI and PI images by calculating the MSP [18] and employing a statistical approach which correlates the shape of the cortex with cortical and subcortical landmarks [19]. The same approach is used for CT scans.

3.6 Atlas-Assisted Analysis

After atlas to scan mapping, both atlases are superimposed (in image or contour representation) with a user-controlled blending onto the studied scans or maps and can be used to get the underlying anatomy and BSTs. The user can point to any location in the displayed image and get the anatomy and BST labels as well as inspect which anatomical structures and BSTs are within the infarct and penumbra.

The concept of atlas-assisted analysis of acute ischemic stroke images has been introduced earlier [10] to speed up the process of analysis. The system automatically analyzes entire regions occupied by the infarct and penumbra and calculates: 1) names of all anatomical structures and blood supply territories within the infarct and penumbra, 2) volume of occupancy for each structure and territory, and 3) percentage of occupancy for each structure and territory. In addition, the system calculates the infarct-MCA and penumbra-MCA territory ratios.

4 Hemorrhagic Stroke

Our hemorrhagic stroke CAD system supports the evacuation of hemorrhage by thrombolytic treatment. The procedure requires a catheter to be inserted into the ventricular system, t-PA administered through it, and a series of CT scans acquired to monitor the outcome of clot lysis. The CAD system aims at progression and quantification of blood clot removal. The clot is automatically segmented on each scan and it can be further edited by means of the contour editor, Figure 2. It can be displayed and manipulated in 3D, and its volume measured. In addition, the system provides tools for stabilization assessment, progression assessment by analyzing time series, and visualization of the catheter along with the clot.

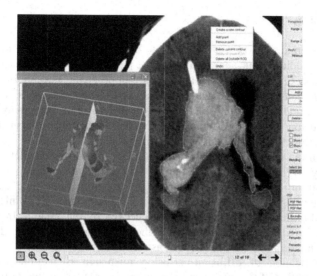

Fig. 2. Blood clot segmentation and its 3D display. A CT slice with the catheter and the segmented clot along with a pop-up contour editing window (right). The 3D clot along with the MSP and brain's bounding box (left).

5 Stroke CAD in Emergency Room

A stroke CAD system in the emergency room (ER) supports rapid and automatic decision making and localization analysis. It analyzes, statistically, the differences between the left and right hemispheres in multiple ROIs delineated by the previously outlined atlases showing anatomical structures, blood supply territories, and arteries. This CAD system facilitates interpretation of stroke images by non-neuroradiologists in ER and increases the confidence of their interpretation by applying complementary, mutually co-registered brain atlases.

6 Results

The acute ischemic stroke CAD system was designed and developed in C++, and its successive versions have been demonstrated as an infoRAD exhibit at the Radiological Society of North America annual meeting RSNA 2005 [20] (awarded), informatics exhibit at RSNA 2006 [19] (awarded), stand alone computer exhibit at the American Society of Neuroradiology annual meeting ASNR 2006 [21], and as a novel solution at the IMAGINE exhibition, European Congress of Radiology ECR 2007 [23]. This CAD system has already been installed or is in the process of installation in a number of hospitals in North America, Europe, Asia, and Australia for testing.

The hemorrhagic stroke CAD is still in the research phase and algorithm development. It is planned to be applied in a large scale clinical trial in 2008. A prototype of the stroke CAD in ER is developed and will be presented at RSNA 2007 [22].

7 Discussion

The acute ischemic stroke CAD system is, to our best knowledge, the first developed for stroke. In addition, our approach shifts the paradigm in stroke image processing. This CAD system has several advantages. It supports the thrombolysis algorithm; provides rapid, automatic and quantitative assessment; and increases both accuracy of results and confidence in them. The first two conditions of the thrombolysis algorithm (i.e., the diffusion-perfusion mismatch and the size of the infarct versus that of MCA territory) are calculated rapidly and quantitatively.

The ratio of the volume of infarct to that of MCA territory is calculated quickly and automatically by means of the BST atlas. This gives more flexibility in decision making regarding prediction of hemorrhagic transformation. For example, [14] predicts hemorrhagic transformation for the ratio greater than 1/2, while [24] greater than 1/3, and either situation can easily be checked by our system. In addition, our method calculates this condition with a higher BST parcellation, i.e., for the MCA penetrating and terminal branches as well as the other territories.

The quantification of diffusion-perfusion mismatch is facilitated by a semi-automatic extraction of the infarct and penumbra; interactive editing of the infarct and penumbra contours; 3D display of the infarct and penumbra along with the midsagittal plane and brain's bounding box; measurement of volume of the infarct, penumbra, their ratio and difference; and a simultaneous display of multiple modalities as mutually blended images. Decision making is further facilitated by listing and quantifying all anatomical structures and BSTs within the infarct and penumbra; this additionally may lead to formulation of more advanced conditions uncovering the relationships among the infarct, penumbra, anatomy, and BST.

The vessel occlusion condition is checked visually in 3D. Initially (the RSNA 2005 version [20]), we extracted a 3D vascular model from the MRA. However our algorithm [24] may take several minutes (depending on data size and accuracy) so this solution is not acceptable. The recent version (RSNA 2006 [19]) provides volume rendering of MRA with a user defined volume of interest.

3D display and manipulation of the infarct and penumbra with user-controlled transparency increases their segmentation accuracy. In addition, displaying the 3D models in relation to the MSP and brain's bounding box with its orientation facilitates spatial correlation of the infarct and penumbra, which increases confidence.

Processing of MR images is very fast, as almost all operations are near real-time (excluding interactive editing of infarct's and penumbra's contours). The most time consuming is the FTT taking approximately 5s.

Having the first stroke CAD system developed and deployed facilitates our work on subsequent solutions. The work on the hemorrhagic stroke system is already advanced. In 2008, this CAD system is planned to be used for clinical trials. The stroke CAD in ER will be presented at RSNA 2007, and if the clinicians express interest in it, we will begin deployment.

In summary, our CAD systems facilitate and speed up image data analysis and support decision making. They increase image processing accuracy and interpreter's confidence. These systems are potentially useful in diagnosis and research, particularly, for clinical trials.

Future work includes enhancements of the atlases and employment of more accurate yet fast warping methods, construction of new brain atlases, validation of the methods on a larger number of cases, and deployment of our solutions.

References

1. Jiang, Y.: Computer-aided diagnosis of breast cancer in mammography: evidence and potential. Technol Cancer Res Treat 1(3), 211–216 (2002)
2. Mani, A., Napel, S., Paik, D.S., et al.: Computed Tomography Colonography: Feasibility of Computer-Aided Polyp Detection in a "First Reader" Paradigm. Abdominal Imaging. J Comput Assist Tomogr. 28(3), 318–326 (2004)
3. Van Ginneken, B., Ter Haar Romeny, B.M., Viegever, M.A.: Computer-aided diagnosis in chest radiography: A survey. IEEE Trans Med Imag. 20(12), 1228–1241 (2001)
4. Ilkko, E., Suomi, K., Karttunen, A., et al.: Computer-assisted diagnosis by temporal subtraction in postoperative brain tumor patients - A feasibility study. Acad Radiol. 11(8), 887–893 (2004)
5. Nowinski, W.L., Thirunavuukarasuu, A.: The Cerefy Clinical Brain Atlas on CD-ROM, Thieme, New York (2004)
6. Talairach, J., Tournoux, P.: Coplanar Stereotactic Atlas of the Human Brain, Thieme, Stuttgart-New York (1988)
7. Nowinski, W.L., Fang, A., Nguyen, B.T., et al.: Multiple brain atlas database and atlas-based neuroimaging system. Comput. Aided Surg. 2(1), 42–66 (1997)
8. Nowinski, W.L.: Electronic brain atlases: features and applications. In: Caramella, D., Bartolozzi, C. (eds.) 3D Image Processing: Techniques and Clinical Applications. Medical Radiology series, pp. 79–93. Springer, Heidelberg (2002)
9. Nowinski, W.L.: The Cerefy brain atlases: continuous enhancement of the electronic Talairach-Tournoux brain atlas. Neuroinformatics 3(4), 293–300 (2005)
10. Nowinski, W.L., Qian, G., Bhanu Prakash, K.N., et al.: Analysis of ischemic stroke MR images by means of brain atlases of anatomy and blood supply territories. Acad. Radiol. 13(8), 1025–1034 (2006)
11. Nowinski, W.L., Thirunavuukarasuu, A., Volkau, I., et al.: Three-dimensional atlas of the brain anatomy and vasculature. Radiographics 25(1), 263–271 (2005)
12. Nowinski, W.L., Thirunavuukarasuu, A., Volkau, I., et al.: Interactive atlas of cerebral vasculature. In: 92 Radiological Society of North America Scientific Assembly and Annual Meeting Program 2006, Chicago, USA, November 25 – December 1, p. 884 (2006)
13. Lorensen, W.E., Cline, H.E.: Marching Cubes: A high resolution 3D surface construction algorithm. Comput. Graph. 21(4), 163–169 (1987)
14. Parsons, M.W., Davis, S.M.: Therapeutic impact of MRI in acute stroke. In: von Kummer, R., Back, T. (eds.) Magnetic Resonance Imaging in Ischemic Stroke, pp. 23–40. Springer, Berlin (2006)
15. Gupta, V., Bhanu Prakash, K.N., Nowinski, W.L.: Automatic and rapid identification of infarct slices and hemisphere in DWI scan. Academic Radiology (in press 2007)
16. Nowinski, W.L., Qian, G., Bhanu Prakash, K.N., et al.: Fast Talairach Transformation for magnetic resonance neuroimages. J. Comp. Assisted Tomogr. 30(4), 629–641 (2006)
17. Nowinski, W.L.: Modified Talairach landmarks. Acta Neurochir. 143(10), 1045–1057 (2001)

18. Nowinski, W.L., Bhanu Prakash, K.N., Volkau, I., et al.: Rapid and automatic calculation of the midsagittal plane in magnetic resonance diffusion and perfusion images. Acad. Radiol. 13(5), 652–663 (2006)

19. Nowinski, W.L., Qian, G., Bhanu Prakash, K.N., Volkau, I., Bilello, M., Beauchamp, N.J.: A CAD system for stroke MR and CT. In: 92 Radiological Society of North America Scientific Assembly and Annual Meeting Program 2006, Chicago, USA, November 25 – December 1, p. 789 (2006)

20. Nowinski, W.L., Qian, G.Y., Bhanu Prakash, K.N., et al.: Atlas-assisted MR stroke image interpretation by using anatomical and blood supply territories atlases. In: Program 91st Radiological Society of North America Scientific Assembly and Annual Meeting RSNA 2005, Chicago, Illinois, USA, November 27– December 2, p. 857 (2005)

21. Nowinski, W.L., Qian, G., Bhanu Prakash, K.N., et al.: A CAD system for stroke MR. In: Proc. American Society of Neuroradiology 44th Annual Meeting ASNR 2006, San Diego, CA, USA, May 1– 5, pp. 425–426 (2006)

22. Nowinski, W.L., Qian, G., Leong, W.K., Liu, J., Kazmierski, R., Urbanik, A.: A Stroke CAD in the ER. 93 Radiological Society of North America Scientific Assembly and Annual Meeting Program 2007, Chicago, USA, November 25–30, 2007 (2007)

23. Nowinski, W.L.: ECR - Efficient Cerebral Routines. From bench to bedside in neuroradiology. In: ECR Today, 10 March 2007, European Congress of Radiology ECR 2007, Vienna, Austria, March 9-13, p. 28 (2007)

24. Hacke, W., Donnan, G., Fieschi, C., et al.: Association of outcome with early stroke treatment: pooled analysis of ATLANTIS, ECASS and NINDS rt-PA stroke trials. Lancet. 363, 768–774 (2004)

25. Qiao, Y., Hu, Q., Qian, G., Nowinski, W.L.: Thresholding based on variance and intensity contrast. Pattern Recognit 40(2), 596–608 (2006)

Author Index

Lecture Notes in Computer Science

Sublibrary 6: Image Processing, Computer Vision, Pattern Recognition, and Graphics

For information about Vols. 1–3951
please contact your bookseller or Springer

Vol. 4538: F. Escolano, M. Vento (Eds.), Graph-Based Representations in Pattern Recognition. XII, 416 pages. 2007.

Vol. 4522: B.K. Ersbøll, K.S. Pedersen (Eds.), Image Analysis. XVIII, 989 pages. 2007.

Vol. 4485: F. Sgallari, A. Murli, N. Paragios (Eds.), Scale Space and Variational Methods in Computer Vision. XV, 931 pages. 2007.

Vol. 4478: J. Martí, J.M. Benedí, A.M. Mendonça, J. Serrat (Eds.), Pattern Recognition and Image Analysis, Part II. XXVII, 657 pages. 2007.

Vol. 4477: J. Martí, J.M. Benedí, A.M. Mendonça, J. Serrat (Eds.), Pattern Recognition and Image Analysis, Part I. XXVII, 625 pages. 2007.

Vol. 4472: M. Haindl, J. Kittler, F. Roli (Eds.), Multiple Classifier Systems. XI, 524 pages. 2007.

Vol. 4466: F.B. Sachse, G. Seemann (Eds.), Functional Imaging and Modeling of the Heart. XV, 486 pages. 2007.

Vol. 4418: A. Gagalowicz, W. Philips (Eds.), Computer Vision/Computer Graphics Collaboration Techniques. XV, 620 pages. 2007.

Vol. 4417: A. Kerren, A. Ebert, J. Meyer (Eds.), Human-Centered Visualization Environments. XIX, 403 pages. 2007.

Vol. 4391: Y. Stylianou, M. Faundez-Zanuy, A. Esposito (Eds.), Progress in Nonlinear Speech Processing. XII, 269 pages. 2007.

Vol. 4370: P.P. Lévy, B. Le Grand, F. Poulet, M. Soto, L. Darago, L. Toubiana, J.-F. Vibert (Eds.), Pixelization Paradigm. XV, 279 pages. 2007.

Vol. 4358: R. Vidal, A. Heyden, Y. Ma (Eds.), Dynamical Vision. IX, 329 pages. 2007.

Vol. 4338: P.K. Kalra, S. Peleg (Eds.), Computer Vision, Graphics and Image Processing. XV, 965 pages. 2006.

Vol. 4319: L.-W. Chang, W.-N. Lie (Eds.), Advances in Image and Video Technology. XXVI, 1347 pages. 2006.

Vol. 4292: G. Bebis, R. Boyle, B. Parvin, D. Koracin, P. Remagnino, A. Nefian, G. Meenakshisundaram, V. Pascucci, J. Zara, J. Molineros, H. Theisel, T. Malzbender (Eds.), Advances in Visual Computing, Part II. XXXII, 906 pages. 2006.

Vol. 4291: G. Bebis, R. Boyle, B. Parvin, D. Koracin, P. Remagnino, A. Nefian, G. Meenakshisundaram, V. Pascucci, J. Zara, J. Molineros, H. Theisel, T. Malzbender (Eds.), Advances in Visual Computing, Part I. XXXI, 916 pages. 2006.

Vol. 4245: A. Kuba, L.G. Nyúl, K. Palágyi (Eds.), Discrete Geometry for Computer Imagery. XIII, 688 pages. 2006.

Vol. 4241: R.R. Beichel, M. Sonka (Eds.), Computer Vision Approaches to Medical Image Analysis. XI, 262 pages. 2006.

Vol. 4225: J.F. Martínez-Trinidad, J.A. Carrasco Ochoa, J. Kittler (Eds.), Progress in Pattern Recognition, Image Analysis and Applications. XIX, 995 pages. 2006.

Vol. 4191: R. Larsen, M. Nielsen, J. Sporring (Eds.), Medical Image Computing and Computer-Assisted Intervention – MICCAI 2006, Part II. XXXVIII, 981 pages. 2006.

Vol. 4190: R. Larsen, M. Nielsen, J. Sporring (Eds.), Medical Image Computing and Computer-Assisted Intervention – MICCAI 2006, Part I. XXXVVIII, 949 pages. 2006.

Vol. 4179: J. Blanc-Talon, W. Philips, D. Popescu, P. Scheunders (Eds.), Advanced Concepts for Intelligent Vision Systems. XXIV, 1224 pages. 2006.

Vol. 4174: K. Franke, K.-R. Müller, B. Nickolay, R. Schäfer (Eds.), Pattern Recognition. XX, 773 pages. 2006.

Vol. 4170: J. Ponce, M. Hebert, C. Schmid, A. Zisserman (Eds.), Toward Category-Level Object Recognition. XI, 618 pages. 2006.

Vol. 4153: N. Zheng, X. Jiang, X. Lan (Eds.), Advances in Machine Vision, Image Processing, and Pattern Analysis. XIII, 506 pages. 2006.

Vol. 4142: A. Campilho, M. Kamel (Eds.), Image Analysis and Recognition, Part II. XXVII, 923 pages. 2006.

Vol. 4141: A. Campilho, M. Kamel (Eds.), Image Analysis and Recognition, Part I. XXVIII, 939 pages. 2006.

Vol. 4122: R. Stiefelhagen, J.S. Garofolo (Eds.), Multimodal Technologies for Perception of Humans. XII, 360 pages. 2007.

Vol. 4109: D.-Y. Yeung, J.T. Kwok, A. Fred, F. Roli, D. de Ridder (Eds.), Structural, Syntactic, and Statistical Pattern Recognition. XXI, 939 pages. 2006.

Vol. 4091: G.-Z. Yang, T. Jiang, D. Shen, L. Gu, J. Yang (Eds.), Medical Imaging and Augmented Reality. XIII, 399 pages. 2006.

Vol. 4073: A. Butz, B. Fisher, A. Krüger, P. Olivier (Eds.), Smart Graphics. XI, 263 pages. 2006.

Vol. 4069: F.J. Perales, R.B. Fisher (Eds.), Articulated Motion and Deformable Objects. XV, 526 pages. 2006.

Vol. 4057: J.P.W. Pluim, B. Likar, F.A. Gerritsen (Eds.), Biomedical Image Registration. XII, 324 pages. 2006.

Vol. 4046: S.M. Astley, M. Brady, C. Rose, R. Zwiggelaar (Eds.), Digital Mammography. XVI, 654 pages. 2006.

Vol. 4040: R. Reulke, U. Eckardt, B. Flach, U. Knauer, K. Polthier (Eds.), Combinatorial Image Analysis. XII, 482 pages. 2006.

Vol. 4035: T. Nishita, Q. Peng, H.-P. Seidel (Eds.), Advances in Computer Graphics. XX, 771 pages. 2006.

Vol. 3979: T.S. Huang, N. Sebe, M. Lew, V. Pavlović, M. Kölsch, A. Galata, B. Kisačanin (Eds.), Computer Vision in Human-Computer Interaction. XII, 121 pages. 2006.

Vol. 3954: A. Leonardis, H. Bischof, A. Pinz (Eds.), Computer Vision – ECCV 2006, Part IV. XVII, 613 pages. 2006.

Vol. 3953: A. Leonardis, H. Bischof, A. Pinz (Eds.), Computer Vision – ECCV 2006, Part III. XVII, 649 pages. 2006.

Vol. 3952: A. Leonardis, H. Bischof, A. Pinz (Eds.), Computer Vision – ECCV 2006, Part II. XVII, 661 pages. 2006.